the
woman's
heart
book

FREDRIC J. PASHKOW, M.D., AND CHARLOTTE LIBOV

the woman's heart book the complete guide to keeping your heart healthy and what to do if things go wrong

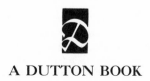

A DUTTON BOOK

NOTE TO THE READER
The ideas, procedures, and suggestions contained in this book are not intended as a substitute for consulting with your physician. All matters regarding health require medical supervision.

DUTTON

Published by the Penguin Group
Penguin Books USA Inc., 375 Hudson Street, New York, New York 10014, U.S.A.
Penguin Books Ltd, 27 Wrights Lane, London W8 5TZ, England
Penguin Books Australia Ltd, Ringwood, Victoria, Australia
Penguin Books Canada Ltd, 10 Alcorn Avenue, Toronto, Ontario, Canada M4V 3B2
Penguin Books (N.Z.) Ltd, 182–190 Wairau Road, Auckland 10, New Zealand

Penguin Books Ltd, Registered Offices:
Harmondsworth, Middlesex, England

First published by Dutton, an imprint of New American Library, a division of Penguin Books USA Inc. Distributed in Canada by McClelland & Stewart Inc.

First Printing, June 1993
1   3   5   7   9   10   8   6   4   2

 REGISTERED TRADEMARK—MARCA REGISTRADA

LIBRARY OF CONGRESS CATALOGING-IN-PUBLICATION DATA:
Pashkow, Fredric J.
    The woman's heart book : the complete guide to keeping your heart healthy and what to do if things go wrong / Fredric J. Pashkow and Charlotte Libov.
        p. cm.
    Includes bibliographical references and index.
    ISBN 0-525-93611-4
    1. Heart—Diseases.   2. Women—Diseases.   3. Heart—Diseases—Sex factors.   4. Heart—Diseases—Prevention.   I. Libov, Charlotte.   II. Title.
RC682.P353 1993
616.1'2'0082—dc20   92-42988
                                                                                CIP

Printed in the United States of America
Set in Caslon No. 3 and Palacio

Designed by Steven N. Stathakis

*This book is dedicated
in loving memory of
Laura and Ben
Sister and Brother*

A Note to Readers

The Woman's Heart Book is the result of a unique collaboration between Dr. Fredric J. Pashkow, medical director of cardiac rehabilitation at the Cleveland Clinic Foundation, and Charlotte Libov, a journalist who underwent open-heart surgery. To best convey her own story, Charlotte Libov speaks directly to readers in italics throughout this book.

Contents

Foreword

The most astonishing thing about the human heart is not that it fails but that it works as long, as hard, and as efficiently as it does. The heart is the most effective pump imaginable: it keeps about five quarts of blood circulating through a pathway of arteries, veins, and blood vessels that would measure approximately 75,000 miles if laid end to end—and it does so twenty-four hours a day, every day, for a lifetime. Not bad for a mere muscle that weighs about a pound.

Mentioning these impressive facts about the heart seems an appropriate way to introduce a book that contains a wealth of important facts about the human heart. But this book differs from other works about the cardiovascular system in speaking both from hard medical information as well as from the heart to address the concerns of, not Everyman, but rather Everywoman: how a woman can keep her heart healthy and what she should do when she suspects that something has gone wrong with her heart.

One of the great myths of modern medicine has been the notion that most women are not at risk for heart disease. In fact, one in nine women between that ages of 45 and 64 has some cardiovascular disease, and the number increases to one woman in three after the age of 65. Stroke today accounts for a higher percentage of deaths among women than men at all stages of life. Not only has heart disease often gone undiagnosed in women, but even when a woman suffers a heart attack, which should certainly serve as convincing proof that she has cardiovascular disease, she is less likely to receive the same level of care as a man. A study of mortality presented by the American Heart Association shows, for example, that about 44 percent of women die within one year of suffering a heart attack, compared with only 26 percent of men. Physicians, however, are not entirely to blame.

Part of the problem is that medical researchers, until very recently, have taken the Renaissance idea of "man as the measure of all things" too literally. As a result, most clinical studies of heart disease have used men as the normative standard. For example, as late as the 1980s, a major study on the preventive effects of aspirin in treating coronary disease involved some 22,000 men, but not a single woman, while another study focused on the role of estrogen in preventing heart disease, but only in men. We still do not know when, and if, estrogen replacement therapy is indicated in treating post-menopausal women and precisely what effect it has on a woman's cardiovascular system.

To answer such questions and to increase the medical community's understanding of women's health in general, the National Institutes of Health has launched a $625 million study of women's health. The Women's Health Initiative is the largest clinical study ever undertaken in the United States. Over the course of fourteen years, the study will involve some 16,000 women nationwide. By focusing on the major diseases that imperil the lives of women—heart disease, cancer, osteoporosis, and depression—within the context of a woman's total health and well-being, the initiative will answer questions about how these diseases and conditions interact. Like the lifesaving and mindsaving tips that are found in this book, the Women's Health Initiative will also yield practical guidelines: tips about diet, exercise, vitamin supplements, and hormone therapy.

Implicit in the approach of this book and the Women's Health Initiative are two closely related principles. First, the principle that health is a positive state, not merely the absence of disease. Health is, in short, a state of physical, mental, and emotional well-being too precious to be described by what it is not—and too precious to entrust entirely to other people. Doctors are merely our partners in preserving health. The corollary principle is that each of us has primary responsibility for maintaining this most precious asset. Being well informed about our bodies is the key to staying healthy. *The Woman's Heart Book* offers the reader an important opportunity to learn about how to care for the remarkable pump that is, literally, at the heart of preserving health.

Bernadine Healy, M.D.,
Director,
National Institutes of Health

Preface
by Fredric J. Pashkow, M.D.

For me it was a typical Saturday on call. I had just walked into the kitchen from the garage after making rounds at the hospital almost all day, and the phone was already ringing. "Yes?" I said, knowing it would be the answering service. "Dr. Pashkow, the ER called; they need you back right away. They have a lady with a heart attack and the ER doctor thinks she's unstable."

I didn't even bother yelling "Hello . . . Goodbye!" to my unseen family. I just got back into the car and sped back to the hospital. I found the woman on a mobile cart in the cardiac room of the ER. Nurses were hovering, their hands busy. An EKG technician was running a second tracing. The patient was in obvious pain. The ER doctor looked relieved to see me. He handed me the first tracing: The heart attack was a big one. I started to gently question the patient about her history and any recent symptoms. I noticed that she was lying stiffly with her fists clenched and her lips tightly pursed. I thought at first it was the discomfort. Wrong—she was grievously irate.

"This really stinks," she finally blurted out. "He's the one who should be here." By "he" I knew instantly she meant her husband. "He smokes like a factory, and I quit ten years ago. He eats everything and anything he wants, usually garbage, and all I eat is "grass" (diet food). I'm always on a diet." She continued her angry soliloquy. "He works day and night in that crummy car dealership of his and he never exercises. Bending over to tie his shoelace for him is a big-time workout, while I slave away at Gloria Stevens three days a week." By this point she was seething. I was preoccupied with the details of getting her medically stabilized, and I nodded absently while a nurse tried to placate her. "You're absolutely right, it should be your husband here instead of you," the nurse said. "Well, if that's the case," the patient shot back, getting my full attention, "why isn't he?"

But her husband Ralph wasn't on the table; he was in the adjacent waiting area, an anxious spouse. Josephine had had the heart attack. But women don't have heart attacks, she was sure (the prevailing medical misbelief of that time)—only if they're "old," and she wasn't old, she was in the prime of her life. What had happened?

What had happened was that the odds had caught up with Josephine. Her individualized risk of a heart attack was about half that of her cigarette-smoking, coffee-swilling couch potato of a husband. But since *his* risk of a coronary was about one in six, *her* risk was about one chance in twelve. That may not sound like heavy odds—but if you play the lottery, where the chance of winning is one in 4 or 5 million, one chance in twelve seems almost a sure thing. The point is, heart attacks can happen to women as well as men, only a little less frequently and usually at a slightly different point in the life cycle. Ironically, despite the hundreds of women with heart disease I'd treated up to that point in my career, particularly women with the coronary variety, I found each and every case of a young woman (under forty-five) so afflicted "unusual."

It took about ten years for me to fully awaken to my bias. Once that happened, however, I became increasingly sensitive to the similarities and differences in the comprehensive manifestations of my female patients' heart disease. When a woman has heart disease, for example, her ancillary problems are often different from a male's. She doesn't get "disability" or much time off from her responsibilities to family and home. Care of a recovering spouse for many men means ordering out for a pizza.

What this book means to do is to provide women with the

knowledge they need to obtain the best of care for their hearts. This book doesn't pretend to offer all the answers. But when a woman is told, "Forget about it," and she can't, or "We'll take care of it, you don't need to worry about a thing," and she wants to know more, she'll have this book to help her. I owe it to Josephine and all her sisters.

Preface
by Charlotte Libov

Since it was November, it was already growing dark outside, though it was still afternoon. I watched the deepening dusk from the window behind the cardiologist's desk. Before this afternoon, I'd never been to a cardiologist. In fact, I'd never anticipated having to see one, not for thirty or forty more years, anyway. Only old people get heart problems, right?

Wrong, I was to learn. Even a baby boomer of forty can have something go wrong with her heart. What was wrong with mine had happened before I was born, I heard the cardiologist saying. The problem was an "atrial septal defect," a hole in the wall separating the chambers of my heart. It had to be fixed. I would have to undergo open-heart surgery.

I only half-listened. I was wondering how I'd manage the drive home without steering my car into a tree.

The news that there was something wrong with my heart came as a complete shock. I'd always considered myself robustly healthy. Over the years, whenever I had a routine physical, the doctor performing it would usually mention that I had a heart murmur, then hasten to assure me that the murmur was "innocent," that there was nothing whatsoever wrong with my heart.

That is, until I arrived at the Waterbury, Connecticut, office of Dr. Jeffrey Stern for a routine exam. Unlike all the doctors I'd ever seen, Dr. Stern (a superb diagnostician who never assumes anything) paused when he came across that murmur. "You do have a heart murmur, but I don't know whether or not it's harmless," he said.

He sent me for an echocardiogram, which clearly identified the problem. Six weeks later, I underwent open-heart surgery. Physically, I was fine. Psychologically, I was shaken. I was nagged by the thought that if I had not stumbled upon a truly astute doctor, my heart problem might never have been identified in time. For although this type of heart defect can be corrected relatively easily, if it goes untreated too long, it can irrevocably damage the heart. This was too close a call.

So I set out to find out more about women and their hearts. At first, seeking answers to my questions was a means of dealing with my own anxiety. Before my surgery, I searched for every bit of information I could find. I arrived at the Cleveland Clinic lugging a satchel filled not with toiletries, but with medical books. You'd have thought I was going to perform the surgery rather than undergo it.

After my surgery, I fully expected my interest to wane as I went back to my life as a free-lance writer, which includes writing about everything from the economy to the environment to circus sideshows. Instead, my interest in women's hearts continued to grow. The more I learned, the more there was to learn. Before long, I had teamed up with Dr. Fredric Pashkow to write this book.

I was to spend some two years learning the answers to all my questions about women's hearts. My research took me to women's bedsides, to heart support groups, to cardiology conferences. Before the book was done, I'd even had the opportunity to observe open-heart surgery. I am truly grateful for this unique "insider's" view of women's hearts, from both sides of the bed.

My hope is that this book will convey information. That may not sound dramatic, but information can be powerful, as was illustrated for me a few months ago. I received a telephone call from a woman named Marie. We've never met, but I was instantly drawn to her, as we had been born with the same type of congenital heart defect. Marie was sixty-two, and her heart defect had just been diagnosed. Her doctor had declared she was not a candidate for surgery (she wasn't certain why, but she thought her age might be a factor). Her situation was hopeless, she'd concluded. She'd been sent home to eventually die.

From my research, I knew that surgery to correct this heart defect had been performed on women older than Marie. That was all Marie needed to hear. She sent her test results to a major heart center for a second opinion. This past summer, she underwent surgery. The operation went fine. Marie comes from a line of indomitable Minnesota farmers. Her mother is in her nineties, and Marie is now looking forward to reaching that age herself. All she'd needed was accurate information—information that was available in medical textbooks and journals but had never filtered down to her.

Although I didn't realize it at the time, this book began that November afternoon I spent in my cardiologist's office. That day, which at the time seemed the gloomiest of my life, turned out to be unimaginably bright. That was the day I began seeking information about my own heart—and about every woman's heart.

Acknowledgments

A book is far more than the work of its authors. Many people gave generously of their time and expertise to assist us in the preparation of this book.

Special thanks go to the Cleveland Clinic Foundation and the following members of its staff: Andrea Baldyga, M.D.; Delbert L. Booher, M.D.; Paul N. Casale, M.D.; Betty Ching, R.N.; Michael Cressman, D.O.; Sue Dehner, R.N.; Fetnat M. Fouad-Tarazi, M.D.; Maria Geraci; Sharon Harvey; Loretta Isada, M.D.; Sally Koulousek; Bruce W. Lytle, M.D.; Pam Marinelli, R.N.; Daniel J. Murphy, M.D.; Steven E. Nissen, M.D.; Russell E. Raymond, D.O.; Eliot R. Rosenkranz, M.D.; John Royer, R.N.; Elena Sgarbossa, M.D.; Betsy Stovsky, R.N.; Michelle Tobin, R.N.; Eric J. Topol, M.D.; Cheryl E. Weinstein, M.D.; Deborah Williams, M.D.; and Randall Yetman, M.D.

Many experts at other institutions gave of their time and knowledge as well. They included Janice Anderson, R.N., M.S.N., Norwalk Hospital; Anita Arnold, D.O., Olympia Fields Osteopathic Hospital and Medical Center; Susan J. Blumenthal, M.D., Alcohol, Drug Abuse and Mental Health Administration; Trudy L.

Bush, Ph.D., Johns Hopkins University; Bernard R. Chaitman, M.D., St. Louis University Medical Center; Margaret A. Chesney, Ph.D., University of California at San Francisco; Richard P. Devereux, M.D., Cornell University Medical College; Erica Frank, M.D., Stanford University School of Medicine; Ellen Hall, Ph.D., Johns Hopkins University; Florence P. Haseltine, Ph.D., M.D., National Institutes of Health; Anne S. Kasper, Ph.D., Older Women's League; Shiriki Kumanyika, Ph.D., Penn State College of Medicine; Charles Maynard, Ph.D., University of Washington School of Medicine; Irma L. Mebane, Ph.D., National Institutes of Health; Catherine A. Neill, M.D., Johns Hopkins Hospital; Judith K. Ockene, Ph.D., University of Massachusetts Medical School; Valerie M. Parisi, M.D., University of Texas Medical School; Lynda Powell, Ph.D., Yale School of Medicine; Lynda E. Rosenfeld, M.D., Yale School of Medicine; Carol Shively, Ph.D., Bowman Gray School of Medicine; Jeffrey T. Stern, M.D.; Judith S. Stern, Sc.D., University of California at Davis; and Nanette K. Wenger, M.D., Emory University School of Medicine.

While most of the research for this book was done at the Cleveland Clinic Foundation, thanks also go to Yale–New Haven Hospital, and in particular to John A. Elefteriades, M.D., and Sheila Hogan.

Special thanks also to the staff at the American Heart Association for promptly answering so many inquiries during the past two years.

We are exceedingly grateful for the enthusiasm and support of our agent, Carole Abel. To Alexia Dorszynski, senior editor at NAL/Dutton, special thanks for accepting our proposal and getting us under way. Thanks also go to our editor, Deborah Brody, for shepherding this manuscript to its completion.

A very extra-special thank-you to Joanne Kraynak for helping in so many ways. Thanks also to Frances Chamberlain for her research help. Special thanks also to Jeffrey Loerch, manager of the medical illustrations department of the Cleveland Clinic Education Foundation, for his cooperation, and to Nancy Hein, senior medical illustrator, for the drawings which enhance this book. We want to also acknowledge the Cleveland Clinic Office of Health Affairs, especially Cheryl Jensen and Phyllis Marino.

Dr. Pashkow offers very special thanks to Peg, the woman who shares his life. It was her willingness to share what little time was left over that allowed this book to be written. It was also through her experience with her "cardiacs" that he realized the potential of exercise, education, and psychological support.

Charlotte Libov would like to thank Gerry Shanahan, Dick Madden, and all the editors that she's learned so much from over the years, with particular gratitude to George Ralston for first hiring her as a reporter and Larry Williams for teaching her how to do her best. She gives very special thanks to the most important person in her life, Terry Montlick, for his invaluable support throughout all the writing of this book.

Most of all, the authors owe a great debt to the women who helped us by sharing their stories. These included those interviewed at the Cleveland Clinic, and, in Connecticut, the Norwalk Hospital's Cardiac Rehab Second Chance Association and the Greater Waterbury Heart Club. A heart-felt thank-you to all of you for sharing your stories.

1
Female Hearts
at Risk

Lois zealously eliminates every gram of cholesterol from her husband, Dan's, favorite dishes, convinced him to give up smoking, and surprised him with membership in a health club for their anniversary. So the fifty-two-year-old homemaker is stunned when her doctor tells her that she, not Dan, will soon face coronary bypass surgery.

Allison, a thirty-nine-year-old financial analyst, lies on the table in a New York hospital emergency room as waves of unbearable chest pain sweep over her. Tucked into her green leather shoulder bag among her keys, lipstick, and appointment book are packets of birth-control pills and cigarettes. With her unusually strong family history of heart disease, this combination is potentially deadly. But no one ever warned Allison.

Formerly a strong swimmer, Joan, age sixty-three, must now be content to paddle slowly up and down the pool. Her enlarged heart has grown so weak that it can't keep up with the demands of much exertion. Early medical treatment could have allowed her to remain active longer, but her family doctor scoffed at her complaints of chest pain for years, telling her, "It's all in your head."

Like most American women, including me, Lois, Allison, and Joan lived their lives without much thought to their hearts. I had barely turned forty when my congenital heart defect was discovered. Had it not been found out, it could have shortened my life. I'd had no reason not to assume my heart was fine.

For years women, and too often their doctors as well, have shared these assumptions. Health-care books, articles in women's magazines, even television commercials convey the impression that heart disease strikes men, not women. "I worried about my husband's cholesterol, but now it's down to one sixty-eight," exults a woman in a TV commercial about the joys of switching to vegetable shortening. "My husband eats right, works out, and he's feeling great," says another beaming TV commercial wife, shown picking up her husband at the gym.

It's now becoming clear that these assumptions fly in the face of reality. Although the rate of heart disease in the United States has declined in recent years, it is still the number one killer of American women, far outranking stroke, lung cancer, and even the disease most dreaded by women, breast cancer. But women remain largely unaware of their risk. Repeatedly, they voice their fears about breast cancer, never dreaming of a threat that looms much larger.

Since this threat to their lives has been so widely overlooked for so long, even now many women remain unaware of how vulnerable their hearts are. Sometimes this can be tragic, as many of these risks can be avoided or their impact lessened. What's more, although the past few decades have been marked by dramatic progress against heart disease, these innovations have been denied to many women. Such potentially lifesaving procedures as coronary bypass surgery, in which a new blood supply to the heart is created; balloon angioplasty, in which narrowed coronary arteries are dilated to allow the flow of more blood; and thrombolytic therapy, the administration of "clot busters" to minimize damage after a heart attack, are all performed far less frequently on women than on men. While experts argue among themselves whether this is scientifically justified, the fact remains that as a woman, it's less likely these procedures will be offered to you.

Even though there is now a new awareness of heart disease

in women, other problems which affect women's hearts remain too often overlooked: irregular heart rhythms (known also as arrhythmias), mitral valve prolapse, and congenital heart defects, all of which more often affect, or manifest symptoms in, women than men.

CORONARY HEART DISEASE: THE "MALE" DISEASE?

Each year 240,000 women in the U.S. die from heart disease. Heart disease is the second leading killer of U.S. women over the age of forty, second only to cancer; by age fifty-five heart disease assumes the lead. By comparison, 90,000 women die annually from stroke, 41,600 from lung cancer, and 40,500 from breast cancer. These other devastating diseases must not be overlooked, but the numbers make it clear that, for women, preventing heart disease is of utmost importance. Still, polls repeatedly show that when women are asked to rank their biggest health worry, cancer comes out on top, with heart disease listed far below.

Faced with this threat, the best way for a woman to safeguard her heart is through knowledge. You must learn about the changing risks which may damage your heart over the course of your life.

As you age, your risk of heart disease increases. Typically, women develop heart disease fifteen to twenty years later than men, although once they reach menopause, their rate of heart disease begins to climb. Once past the age of sixty-five, every woman is a candidate for heart disease, no matter what her state of health. She may be a nonsmoker, exercise, and qualify as a health-food "nut." At this stage of life, her heart becomes as vulnerable to heart disease as her male counterpart's.

YOUNG WOMEN—"IMMUNE" FROM HEART DISEASE?

The fact that older women have a higher risk of suffering a heart attack than younger women contributes to another dangerous belief: that only they are in jeopardy. While it's true that heart attacks usually kill elderly women, young women are not necessarily immune. An estimated 6,000 U.S. women under age sixty-five die each year of heart attacks, and nearly one-third of them are under age forty-five.

In fact, heart disease in middle-aged women is far from uncommon. Such women are seen daily in cardiology clinics across the country. There are many reasons that a middle-aged woman is at risk for developing heart disease. She may be diabetic, a factor more strongly related to heart disease in women than in men. She may have gone through menopause early, resulting in a loss of estrogen—which may turn out to be the most important contributor to the development of heart disease in women. Or she may have inherited abnormal blood cholesterol levels.

Some women can appear deceptively robust, like Linda, a nonsmoking gym teacher who suffered a heart attack in her early fifties. In her gym shorts, with her whistle hanging around her neck, she once seemed the very picture of good health. But her body harbored two hidden time bombs. The first was hyperlipidemia, a metabolic disorder which results in abnormal levels of blood cholesterol. The second was that her ovaries had been removed years earlier, propelling her body into premature menopause.

Although it's unusual for a woman under the age of forty-five to suffer a heart attack or develop heart disease, it happens more often than most doctors suspect. Sometimes the risk factors go unrecognized until it's almost too late. That was the case with Randi, a thirty-five-year-old mother of two who was unaware she had hyperlipidemia. When she complained to her doctor of chest pain, he brushed her worries aside. He did reluctantly order a treadmill exercise test, a measure commonly used to help diagnose heart disease. But because he ordered a type which is less accurate when used on women than on men, Randi's results were interpreted as normal. Randi's doctor told her she was "too nervous" and that if she worried less her symptoms would disappear. Fortunately, she saw another doctor who used a more sensitive version of the test. The results clearly showed that two of her coronary arteries were seriously blocked. If her condition had remained undiscovered, she most likely would have suffered a major heart attack.

Because heart disease is so rarely suspected in young women, if you're a young woman suffering cardiac symptoms for which there is no other explanation, it's up to you to make certain your doctor investigates the possibility of heart problems. It may save your life.

SOCIETY'S RISKS TO WOMEN'S HEARTS

Over the years, women's place in society has changed, in many ways for the better. However, there has been one dangerous change: In recent years, more and more women have taken up smoking, a deadly habit for a woman's heart.

Stress also poses a risk for women and their hearts. Although the link between stress and heart disease is not as clear as the connection between smoking or diabetes and heart disease, some studies show that stress can present risks to your general health and to your heart. Some say that women's new roles in the workplace may lead to heart attacks, but this is not necessarily so. As we discover more about stress, it appears that it's not the typical hard-driving "Type A" personality which contributes to heart problems, but anger, frustration, and powerlessness which may be unhealthy. Women trapped in dead-end jobs or workplace discrimination may be the ones who find their emotions tied up in knots, under just the type of stress that may contribute to damaging their hearts.

HEART ATTACK: HIGH RISK FOR WOMEN

Some studies have found that when women suffer heart attacks, they fare even worse than men. Research has shown that a woman's first heart attack is more likely to kill her, or to be followed by a second attack. A major study at the University of Massachusetts Medical Center in Worcester found that more than double the number of women suffering a heart attack died within six weeks. Studies have also shown that women are less likely than men to survive over the long term.

The picture is not completely bleak. Most of the time, women do survive heart attacks. But even if they recover, they tend to suffer more than men from such symptoms as disabling chest pain. This makes them less likely to be able to return to work or enjoy their lives fully. Mary, a supervisor for a high-tech computer company, had a heart attack when she was fifty-seven years old. Afterward, she still suffered chest pains, which forced her to quit her job. Her pains persisted, even after coronary bypass surgery and despite her use of a variety of cardiovascular medications. Although her case was extreme, it's not uncommon for women to be plagued with chest pain and other symptoms even after the physical causes of their heart problems appear to have been resolved.

The feminist revolution not withstanding, women in our society are still burdened with running the household and taking care of the children. These responsibilities don't disappear if a woman has a heart attack or undergoes heart surgery. Many women feel compelled to be up and about managing the household when they should rest. Or they may try to return to their jobs outside the home too early because they can't afford not to or feel anxious about losing their hard-won place on the corporate fast track.

CONGENITAL DEFECTS: HIDDEN DANGERS

Congenital heart defects are a hidden danger which women face more often than men. Although such heart defects are usually diagnosed in childhood, a significant number remain hidden until adulthood. Unless treated, some may cause irreversible damage to the heart.

HEART SURGERY FOR WOMEN: RISKY BUSINESS

Coronary bypass surgery is now one of the most common operations in the United States, and the risk for the procedure has decreased sharply over the years. Still, despite some three decades of experience, studies nationwide persist in showing that coronary surgery remains riskier for women than men. This is also true of balloon angioplasty and similar interventional procedures used to treat coronary artery disease (also known as coronary heart disease). While experts debate the reasons, these dangerous discrepancies for women persist.

A "GENDER BIAS" IN HEART DISEASE?

"Can't I count on my doctor to recognize a heart problem?" you might very well ask. The unfortunate answer to this is "Sometimes, but not always." The truth is that while women have mistakenly believed they're not vulnerable to heart problems, this belief is often shared by their doctors.

Although women visit doctors more often than men, their problems are often given short shrift, especially when it comes to their hearts. Not so long ago, doctors were taught to respond differently to women. If a medical student approached an instructor to discuss the case of a woman with chest pain, he or she would almost always be told to dismiss it. "She must be psychosomatic. It's all in her head" was the standard line. Studies have shown that when doctors are asked to diagnose women with chest pain, the problem is more likely to be attributed to "psychiatric" causes.

A major reason that doctors may tend to ignore women's cardiac problems is that consciously or subconsciously, women are viewed as less important than men in the economic marketplace. Also, because women develop heart disease later in life than men, a doctor may erroneously assume that the snowy-haired woman seated before him cannot withstand the rigors of surgery. It's true that coronary bypass surgery is riskier for women than men, but by not being objectively evaluated a woman may be denied a potentially lifesaving treatment.

That women's hearts are treated differently than men's can be seen in the rate and type of diagnostic tests performed on women. In 1991, major studies at the Oregon Heart Institute in Portland and the Brigham and Women's Hospital in Boston revealed convincing evidence that doctors treat women with heart disease less aggressively than they do men. These studies, involving tens of thousands of women, showed that they were at most half as likely as men to undergo cardiac catheterization, a common diagnostic procedure required before such treatments as balloon angioplasty and coronary bypass surgery.

Not all studies support the contention of gender bias. A 1992 study which compared the treatment after heart attacks of 2,473 patients in Boston found that women were as likely to receive balloon angioplasty as men. This study also found that although men were more likely to be referred for coronary bypass, the difference was very slight.

Over the years, some studies have intimated that coronary bypass surgery and other "aggressive" treatments may be overused. If these procedures are indeed being performed too often on men, women certainly don't want to fall into the same trap. Still, the sharp difference between the way men and women are treated has generated an important discussion.

OUR UNDERSTANDING OF HEART DISEASE

Such treatment differences may not be surprising when you consider that coronary heart disease has been viewed as a man's disease, from the early days of modern cardiology. Our modern understanding of coronary disease was shaped, in part, in the 1950s, when pathologists examining the corpses of young Korean War soldiers discovered to their amazement the fatty streaking that is the first step on the path to clogged arteries. Since then, coronary heart disease has been perceived as a male problem. In the ensuing years, this emphasis on men has not only persisted, but has helped to shape our national health policy.

A major example is the Framingham Heart Study, the nation's largest continuing study of coronary artery disease, which began in 1948. While women were included in this major study, the early results concluded that chest pain in women was not a serious problem. Even though this was later found to be wrong, the damage had been done. "The myth that 'women don't get heart disease' had taken root," says Dr. Nanette K. Wenger, a cardiologist and professor of medicine at Emory University School of Medicine in Atlanta. But, she notes, times are changing. "Years ago, older women were less visible. There were fewer of them, they had retired from the work force, and they had fulfilled their family duties. Heart disease in women was not perceived as a major problem. But now that the life span of women has increased, and they live on average six to seven years longer than men, we are seeing a tremendous change."

The emphasis on men and heart disease has also meant that far less clinical research has focused on women; some believe that potential treatments may have been overlooked. "If we had a disease like breast cancer and most of the research had been done on men, we would not use the male model and say, 'Oh, let's see how we can adapt it to women.' We would want to take a fresh approach," says Dr. Erica Frank of the Stanford Center for Research and Disease Prevention at the Stanford University School of Medicine.

This male perspective has also shaped the methods by which drugs are tested in this country. Cardiovascular drugs, the medications which control blood pressure, reduce cholesterol, and ease the symptoms of heart disease, are of particular concern because they're prescribed for women as often as for men, yet have been tested almost exclusively on men. Traditionally women have been excluded from medical research because of the concern that if they're young, they might become pregnant, or if they're older, they most likely have developed other diseases which will complicate the results.

"The argument is spurious. It says we cannot study women because they are so different, but yet they should take medicines developed on the basis of work done on men," says Dr. Florence Haseltine, a founder of the Society for the Advancement of Women's Health Research in Washington, D.C. "You can't have it both ways."

In recent years, however, some promising developments have emerged. At the National Institutes of Health, which directs America's taxpayer-supported scientific and medical research, the Women's Health Initiative, a $625-million, ten-year research project on the health problems of older women, is under way. As the first female director of the NIH, Dr. Bernadine Healy, a cardiologist, has pledged to include women in the NIH's medical trials.

"There has been a general awakening to the fact that all too many articles published in the medical research literature and publicized by the mass media have been based on studies of men," notes Dr. Healy. "This is unfortunate as coronary heart disease is the major killer of both men and women."

The NIH has also pledged to include members of minority groups in such clinical studies. The vast majority of medical research in heart disease has targeted not just men, but white men. If information on how heart disease affects women is slim, information on how heart disease affects women of different racial groups, such as blacks and Hispanics, is far scantier.

Because of this past lack of emphasis on heart disease in women, women are only now discovering the importance of caring for their hearts. The urgency extends not only to older women, who make up the majority of heart disease patients, but to younger women as well. The most "heartening" news of all is that women of all ages can benefit from taking care of their hearts.

2

How Your Heart Works

My heart stopped at precisely 4:55 P.M. on Monday, November 12, 1990. Or at least that's how it felt. I remember the moment vividly. I was seated across from my cardiologist, who was telling me I would need heart surgery. And that's when I could have sworn I felt my heart momentarily stop beating. Actually, my heart was performing its assigned duty, beating as it had for the forty years of my life. But because I was so stunned, for a moment it seemed to me that it had literally stopped.

This dual role played by our hearts—the beating that keeps us alive, and the way they seem to reflect our emotions—is the reason our hearts so fascinate us. The heart is a biological organ. Unless something goes wrong, we're usually unaware of its tireless pumping. But in times of high emotion, of deep sadness, fear, or joy, our hearts seem to take on a life of their own. They jump, skitter, ache, pound, and sometimes even seem to soar! Today's scientists know such heartfelt reactions are the result of hormones which act on our hearts in times of crisis. For centuries, though, this response has led us to see our hearts not only as biological organs, but as strong symbols, too.

Since prehistory, people have puzzled over the mysterious workings of the human body. A prehistoric drawing of a mammoth is believed to represent the earliest anatomical rendering of a heart. Drawn on a cave wall some 25,000 years ago, the animal has a mass of paint below its back, roughly heart-shaped. In different cultures throughout history, the greatest thinkers subscribed to the belief that the heart was the powerful source of life. Ancient Babylonians believed a sharp pain in the chest signified the presence of demons. The ancient Egyptians ascribed to the heart many purposes; they believed it was not only the seat of intelligence and the central force of life, but also the source of love. Aristotle thought along similar lines, concluding that the heart was the body's vital source as well as the seat of the soul.

Around the first century A.D. medical knowledge of the heart began to develop, in a gradual process that took centuries. Great anatomists such as Galen, a Greek renowned as the greatest physician of his day, and Leonardo da Vinci, who dissected human bodies to learn how to illustrate them more accurately, gradually began to surmise how the heart worked. In the seventeenth century, the brilliant English doctor William Harvey put it all together.

Since then, modern science has unlocked many mysteries about the heart. We recognize now that it's not in the heart but in the brain where what we consider our soul resides. Still, though, we exchange cards on Valentine's Day, festooned with images of hearts not unlike those found on that cave wall. We can all understand the yearnings of the Tin Man in *The Wizard of Oz*, who wanted a heart so that he could feel love. We shed tears over sonnets that talk of our hearts' losses, and we write songs that sing of our hearts' joy. Medical evidence to the contrary, this is still how we feel in the bottom of our hearts.

A FIRST LOOK AT YOUR HEART

The heart is one of the main organs which make up your circulatory system, the network of vessels whose job it is to deliver oxygen and nutrients to your body's organs and remove the carbon dioxide which is generated during the process known as metabolism. Your circulatory system includes your heart, lungs, arteries, and capillaries (extremely small blood vessels), as well as your veins, through which blood flows on its return to the heart.

Anatomically speaking, a woman's heart is virtually the same as a man's, except for its size. An adult male's heart weighs about ten ounces, a woman's heart about two ounces less. The size of the heart varies with the size of the individual. If you want a rough idea of the size of your heart, make a fist. Your heart is about that size, or a little larger if you have unusually small hands.

A cone-shaped organ, your heart is situated centrally in your chest. It fits snugly in an area known as the mediastinum of the thoracic cavity, just behind your breastbone and between your lungs. To get an idea of how the major part of your heart's left ventricle (or chamber) is shaped, hold a Styrofoam cup with its bottom tilted toward the left. This may not seem very scientific, but it's a reasonable approximation of how your heart is shaped and positioned. Although your heart is located centrally, between your lungs, the bottom corner juts forward a bit from beneath the breastbone, coming closest to the surface of the chest. This position accentuates the sounds your heart makes as it beats and makes it appear that your heart is located on the left side of your body.

Your heart is a strong muscular organ composed of a special type of tissue known as cardiac muscle. A translucent sac called the **pericardium** envelops both the heart and the roots of the major blood vessels which emerge from it, the **vena cava** and the **ascending aorta**. The walls of your heart are made from specialized muscle, called the **myocardium,** which differs from other types of muscle in your body in that it can contract rhythmically when stimulated by the currents of your heart's electrical system. This rhythmic contraction is the origin of your heartbeat.

YOUR HEART'S JOB

Even if it's been ages since you studied biology, you probably recall learning that your heart is a pump, and this is true. A pump is defined as a machine for the raising, driving, or compressing of fluids. Your heart is such a pump—such an efficient one, in fact, that engineers have borrowed from its design.

Your heart is quite specialized in its purpose. Some of your other organs perform a variety of functions. Your kidneys, for example, have a multitude of jobs. They filter your blood, excrete waste products, control your blood's acid-base balance, and excrete or conserve fluid. Scientists are still learning new things about the heart, but, when it comes down to the heart's main function, it's to perform one crucial task: pumping blood.

Actually, to be more accurate, your heart is two pumps which act separately but in concert. The left side of your heart acts as a high-pressure pump which forces oxygen-rich blood out into all the parts of your body. The right side of your heart receives the oxygen-depleted blood and passes it into the lungs, where it is replenished with oxygen. The blood then flows into the left side of the heart, to begin its journey again. Every organ in your body needs blood to live. This is why if your heart is not working properly the resulting lack of oxygenated blood can damage your brain, kidneys, and all other organs which depend on it.

As the blood makes its journey through the heart, it's very important that it flow only in one direction. Four heart valves ensure this proper flow and see to it that blood does not flow backward through the pump.

YOUR HEART'S STRUCTURE

The heart has two halves. Each of two halves, left and right, is also divided into lower and upper chambers. This is what's meant when the heart is referred to as a four-chambered pump. The left side of the heart is divided into the **left atrium** (the upper chamber on the left side) and the **left ventricle** (the lower chamber on the left side), and the right side of the heart is divided into the **right atrium** (the upper chamber on the right side) and the **right ventricle** (the lower chamber on the right side). These four chambers have similar jobs: they all pump blood.

The atrium and the ventricle on each side of the heart act as a duet. The atrium feeds blood to the ventricle, which then pumps the blood out. The atrium's job is very important, however, because it is this chamber of the heart which supplies a consistent blood flow to the ventricle. In this way, the atrium forms a buffer for the ventricle and makes sure that the pump never runs dry. This flow of blood acts to prime the pump, and explains why, even if you radically change position, your heart's ventricles are always assured a constant supply of blood to pump. This is one reason that your heart can perform its job so steadily, without your being aware of it. It's one of the many brilliantly evolved features of the heart.

To enable the two sides of your heart to perform their separate but critically important functions, your heart is divided vertically into right and left sides by the **septum,** a thick central muscular wall. Large blood vessels also emerge from the top and sides of your heart. These vessels deliver blood to and from the heart. The right side of your heart receives deoxygenated blood. The left side of your heart sends blood out to the rest of your body.

YOUR CARDIAC VALVES

The proper functioning of your heart depends on the four valves, which in essence control traffic through the individual chambers of your heart, making certain your blood flows in the right direction. These heart valves are fascinating structures in themselves.

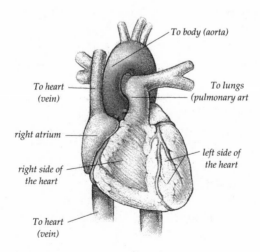

The Heart. The heart pumps blood to all the organs of the body through arteries. The sequence starts when the right side of the heart pumps blood to the lungs through the pulmonary artery. The oxygen-rich blood returns to the left side of the heart and is then pumped through the aorta out to the body. Oxygen-depleted blood returns to the heart's right atrium through the veins, completing the sequence.

The four valves of your heart are the **tricuspid valve,** between the right atrium and the right ventricle; the **pulmonary valve,** between the right ventricle and the pulmonary artery; the **mitral valve,** between the left atrium and the left ventricle; and the **aortic valve,** between the left ventricle and the aorta. The mitral valve was so named, by the way, because its shape reminded anatomists of a bishop's miter.

Although the word "valve" may conjure up an image of a mechanical device with gears designed to control the flow of liquid, that image does not truly capture what these structures look like. Your heart valves more closely resemble the structure of a flower, moving and flowing in a sort of ballet choreographed to the changes of pressure in the heart. Each valve is outfitted with a set of "petals" (also called leaflets or cusps). The mitral valve normally has two leaflets; the others have three. Motion pictures taken within the heart reveal the motion of these leaflets. They billow open gently, like sails on a sailboat, and allow the blood to pass. After the blood flows out, the leaflets close or fold down against themselves, effectively sealing the passageway. Valves normally leak a tiny bit, and this can show up on an echocardiogram, but they should not leak significantly. Blood flow occurs only when there's a difference in pressure across the valves, causing them to open and close.

Considering the delicacy of these leaflets, it's easy to understand why if, for example, a leaflet becomes stiff because of valvular heart disease, it becomes harder for the heart valve to perform its vital function. Although valve disease usually progresses gradually, there are exceptions. The aortic valve can fail suddenly if the aorta tears (this is called aortic dissection) or balloons out and bursts (an aortic aneurysm). If either occurs, death can come quickly because the heart is overwhelmed by the blood cascading back into it.

The tricuspid and the mitral valve are the largest of the heart's four valves. They're also more delicate in structure, and their leaflets are larger and need to be mechanically supported. Just as a parachute or tent is supported by cords, so are these valves in the heart. Delicate cordlike structures known as the **chordae tendinae** are attached to the papillary muscles, fingerlike projections that hold the leaflets to the walls of the ventricle. Sometimes in the mitral valves these leaflets can be oversized and can billow too much, like drapes made with too much material.

In this case, the leaflets can't snap shut properly. When this occurs, as it sometimes does in women, it results in a condition known as mitral valve prolapse (see Chapter 7).

HOW YOUR HEART PUMPS BLOOD

Blood is pumped to the lungs and all of the tissues of the body in a highly organized sequence which involves all four of the heart's chambers. Your heartbeat has two phases, **diastole** and **systole**. They make up your blood pressure measurement. Diastole is the period when the heart is said to be relaxed; systole is the phase when the ventricles contract and blood is ejected. Together, these two movements, squeezing and relaxing, make up your heartbeat. A heart normally goes through this cycle an average of 60 to 100 times a minute, with adults averaging 70 beats a minute. That's 100,000 times a day!

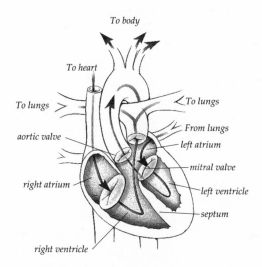

Blood Flow through the Heart. The heart with its front walls removed revealing its four-chambered structure: the right and left atria and the right and left ventricles. Valves control the flow of blood from the atria to the ventricles and out of the heart. A tissue-like divider, the septum, separates the heart's two halves.

The purpose of the cardiac cycle is to guide your blood through its journey from your heart into your lungs, where it receives oxygen, and then eventually through your arteries to every cell in your body. Your blood then returns into your heart, where the cycle is repeated over and over for as long as you live.

Your heart never stops its cyclical pumping—but to visualize how the process works, let's interrupt one cycle. We'll interrupt it just as the right atrium is receiving blood returning from the body via the veins. This is venous blood, oxygen-depleted and loaded with carbon dioxide, and darker than bright-red arterial blood, the oxygenated blood which flows through your arteries. At this point, your heart is relaxed. The deoxygenated blood flows through your open tricuspid valve and starts to fill your right ventricle. This causes your right atrium to contract, completing the priming of the ventricle. The right ventricle squeezes, the tricuspid valve closes, and the deoxygenated blood is pumped past the pulmonary valve into the pulmonary artery and on into the lungs.

Once in the lungs, an important exchange takes place. The blood spreads through a vast and numerous network of alveoli, the tiny grapelike air sacs within the lungs. Here the carbon dioxide in the deoxygenated blood is exchanged for a fresh supply of oxygen, which comes from the air you breathe. The addition of fresh oxygen turns the blood bright red. This oxygenated blood is now ready for its trip to nourish the rest of your body. It returns to the left side of the heart. The left atrium contracts, sending blood past the mitral valve into the left ventricle. Once filled, the left ventricle contracts, pumping the blood through the aortic valve. The blood immediately enters the aorta, your body's largest artery. From the aorta, the blood flows through a branching system of arteries throughout your body.

As your blood travels through your body via your circulatory system, it flows through vessels which become progressively smaller until it reaches the tiniest vessels of all, the capillaries. These are thin-walled blood vessels located in organs and tissues which play an important role in your body's functioning. They're so tiny that the oxygen-carrying red cells move through them in single file. In the capillaries another important exchange takes place. This process is basically the opposite of what occurred in the lungs: At this point the red cells of the blood give up some of their oxygen in exchange for carbon dioxide.

This is only part of the story, however. Now transformed into venous blood, the blood must return to the heart for a fresh supply of oxygen. This deoxygenated blood travels back to the heart through a network of veins which grow progressively larger until the swelling stream of blood empties into the vena cava, the two major veins that are interconnected to the right atrium leading back into the heart. Then the journey begins again. It's estimated that your blood makes this trip a mind-boggling 2.5 *billion* times over a life span of seventy years.

YOUR CORONARY ARTERIES

It's very important for the functioning of your body that blood reach every organ, including the heart itself. Your heart, after all, is living tissue that requires oxygenated blood to survive. Since your heart is so busy pumping, you might wonder how it gets enough blood for itself. Some oxygen and carbon dioxide are exchanged to the superficial cells adjacent to the inner lining of the heart, but this is not nearly enough to supply your heart with the amount of oxygen it requires. The answer to this riddle shows how cleverly the heart has evolved. To provide for itself, your heart is equipped with its own specialized vascular system, the coronary arteries.

In appearance, these arteries encircle the heart like the winding tubes of a coronet, which gives the coronary arteries their name. Although they're actually two arteries, the left one quickly divides into two, which is why they're usually referred to as *three* coronary arteries.

The coronary arteries lie on the surface of your heart muscle. They branch from the aorta, right above the leaflets of the aortic valve. Once your blood is pumped by the left ventricle through the aorta, a portion of it flows back directly to the heart via the coronary arteries. This occurs during the diastolic part of the heart's cycle, while the heart is momentarily relaxing. This incredibly well-designed system has evolved over millions of years. Your coronary arteries are only the width of a strand of spaghetti, which is why any narrowing which occurs, as it does during atherosclerosis (coronary artery disease), can be devastating.

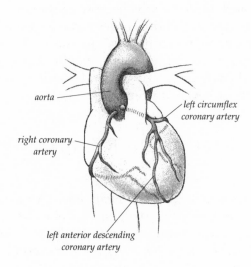

aorta

left circumflex
coronary artery

right coronary
artery

left anterior descending
coronary artery

Coronary Arteries. The heart has two main coronary arteries, the left and the right. The left coronary artery branches off into the left circumflex and the left anterior descending arteries. Collectively, they are referred to as the heart's "three" coronary arteries.

YOUR HEART'S ELECTRICAL SYSTEM

Your heart's cardiac cycle is coordinated by an intrinsic electrical system which began operating in your heart before you were born. This system has its own "timers" and "wiring" that stimulate it to contract on average 100,000 times per day. Each heartbeat originates in a specific area of the right atrium called the sinoatrial node. This is often referred to as your heart's intrinsic pacemaker. If anything goes wrong with this electrical system, the result can be disruption of the heart's rhythm, also known as an arrhythmia.

YOUR BLOOD PRESSURE

Just as the chambers of your heart respond to the electrical signals generated by the heart's electrical system, your heart also responds to changes in the pressures within it. Since your heart is not actually one pump but two, two systems of blood pressure are involved. The left side of your heart, which is responsible for pushing the blood out through your entire body, functions as a high-pressure system. The right part of your heart, which is responsible for spreading your blood out into your lungs so that the exchange of carbon dioxide and oxygen can occur, functions as a low-pressure system. If your blood pressure is elevated, it indicates that your heart is working harder than normal, putting both your heart and arteries under greater strain.

YOUR HEART AND YOUR NERVOUS SYSTEM

You may wonder why when you're startled or surprised—say you suddenly realize your purse is missing—your heart may pound or even seem to stop beating momentarily, or why it may feel as if your heart is bursting when you receive joyous news, such as that you have a new grandchild or you've received an award. These responses have to do with the workings of your nervous system.

The function of your nervous system, which is located mostly in your brain and spinal cord, is to act as your body's overall information-gathering system. Based on the information your brain collects, it sends out messages to all the parts of your body. Some of these messages can be voluntary, such as the message to rise when your alarm clock goes off. Other messages can be involuntary, such as when your body jerks as a car backfires or a firecracker explodes. The latter is an example of a spinal cord reflex.

Messages between the nervous system and the cardiovascular system are relayed by chemicals called neurotransmitters. These chemicals travel between cells and can provoke a response in the target organ. There are different types of neurotransmitters. Norepinephrine, an adrenaline-type substance, can increase your heart rate and the force of your heart's contractions in response to a threat, causing more blood to be pumped out to your muscles so that you can fight or run (hence the name the "fight or flight" hormone). This response is believed to stem from our primitive beginnings, when "fight or flight" was an everyday dilemma.

Thus the link between heart and brain was not totally a figment of the imagination of early scientists. Your heart is more than a nonresponsive pump; it does beat in step with your emotions. Since those early days, though, scientists have learned a great deal about how you can keep your heart functioning well.

3

What's Your Risk of Heart Disease?

After spending fifteen years in the secretarial pool, Helen was finally promoted to supervisor last year. At first she was delighted, but lately she's been having second thoughts. She's caught in the middle. Her boss is pressuring her to pile the work onto her staff, but these are the same women who used to be her coworkers and friends. Now she sees them glaring at her as if she's the enemy. Helen doesn't know what to do. She's smoking more now, she finds herself grabbing for doughnuts, and her blood pressure is skyrocketing.

Helen is a heart attack just waiting to happen. But you don't have to be exactly like Helen to be at risk for coronary artery disease or a heart attack. Take Melanie, a thirty-six-year-old lawyer. She exercises regularly, enjoys meditation, and is the envy of her friends, who think she's got it all under control. Yet she's at high risk for a heart attack because she's unaware that she has inherited hyperlipidemia, which causes abnormally high blood cholesterol levels. Carolyn, thirty-one, whose mother died young from a heart attack, unwittingly risks the same fate by smoking cigarettes and taking birth-control pills.

Only by learning about risk factors can you realistically determine your individual risk profile. Then you can decide which changes will bring you closest to your goal of preventing heart disease.

IMPORTANT RISKS

A risk factor is an element which has been proved to contribute independently to the development of heart problems. Smoking and diabetes together, for example, increase your chance of developing coronary artery disease, but studies have shown that women who smoke but are not diabetic and those who are diabetic but don't smoke also have an increased risk of developing disease.

Traditionally, risk factors have been divided into two groups: those which are considered changeable and those which are not. This is misleading; even though you may think a risk is nonchangeable, such as your age, race, and family history of early coronary artery disease, that's not really the case, as you'll see.

Here are the risk factors for coronary artery disease and heart attacks:

- Your age
- Your family's medical history
- Your race
- Smoking
- Oral contraceptives (if you're a smoker)
- Overweight
- Abnormal cholesterol pattern
- High blood pressure
- Diabetes
- Sedentary lifestyle
- Stress

In evaluating your personal risk factors for heart disease, it's useful to bear in mind that risks indicate that you have an increased probability of developing heart disease, but are not necessarily definite predictors.

My father died at the age of fifty-nine of a heart attack. For me to throw up my hands and say, "That's it—there's nothing I can do about it; I'll probably die young of heart disease," is neither correct nor useful. Although my father did have coronary artery disease, his having diabetes contributed to its development. Since I may have inherited a tendency toward diabetes as well, this motivates me to control my weight and exercise, which lessens the probability that I will become diabetic. This in turn reduces my chances of developing coronary disease.

You can evaluate your risk factors in much the same way. If you're a black woman, knowing you have a greater risk of developing high blood pressure can motivate you to watch your blood pressure carefully. If you have several risk factors for heart disease and you're approaching menopause, knowing your risks will help you evaluate whether to begin hormone replacement therapy, which some studies have shown can help guard against coronary disease.

Consider the case of Rhonda. Her mother, Alice, was overweight and had not been to a doctor in twenty years, so she didn't realize she was diabetic and had high blood pressure when she suffered a heart attack at the age of fifty-seven. Shaken by her mother's experience, Rhonda quit smoking, lost weight, and began exercising. In fact, she and her mother now walk two miles a day together.

♥ **Lifesaving Tip: Risk factors have been found to increase in combination. So having two risks factors more than doubles your total risk for developing coronary artery disease.**

YOUR AGE

As you grow older, your risk of developing coronary artery disease increases. This is true of both men and women. By virtue of simply being a woman, though, you have about a fifteen-year "grace period" over men—for most of their lives, women develop coronary artery disease about fifteen years later than men, according to findings of the Framingham Heart Study. After menopause, though, your natural protection against heart disease begins to disappear. If you're fifty-five, your risk of dying from heart disease is about equal to that of a man about ten years your senior. By the time you reach seventy, this drops to only five years. By age seventy-five, you have an equal chance of dying from heart disease as a man your age.

IS FAMILY HISTORY DESTINY?

If you have a parent, grandparent, brother, or sister who suffered a heart attack or developed coronary artery disease at an early age, your chance of developing it increases. But exactly how much the probability rises remains a question.

Any discussion of family medical history revolves around genetics, the study of how traits are passed down from one generation to another through the genes, the units of inherited material contained in the body's cells. While coronary artery disease is not considered an inherited trait, it does appear to run in families.

A Harvard 1991 study of 45,317 male health professionals showed, for example, that those with parents who developed heart disease early were more likely to develop it themselves. This study also found that the younger the parent at the time of the heart attack, the greater the odds against the son. While few such studies have focused on females, a 1986 study of seventy-three Utah women who died before the age of fifty-five of coronary artery disease discovered that 62 percent of them had a family history of early coronary disease, as compared with 12 percent who died from non-cardiac-related causes. According to most research, it doesn't matter whether the affected family members are male or female; in the Utah study, however, the risk was higher for women whose female relatives had the disease.

YOUR RACE

The frustrating lack of research about women and heart disease is even greater and more frustrating when it comes to race. Still, there is enough known to draw some conclusions. Statistics show that if you are a black woman and you develop coronary artery disease, you're more likely to die from it than your white female counterpart.

Although black Americans generally have more risk factors than whites—they are more likely to be overweight and to have diabetes and high blood cholesterol—they tend to develop coronary artery disease less frequently but have a less favorable outcome. Although the reason for this contradiction is not known, researchers are looking into the possibility that blacks may have more of a certain type of potentially deadlier cholesterol in their blood, which makes their blood more likely to clot and, even in the absence of coronary artery disease, result in a heart attack and stroke. But this is an area which needs more study.

♥ Lifesaving Tip: If your age, race, or family's medical history seems to put you at a disadvantage, make this knowledge work for you. Use it to motivate you to make the changes that can lower your risk. In the long run, you can become healthier than women who don't have these particular risks but don't live as healthy a lifestyle.

SMOKING: THE BIGGEST RISK YOU CAN CHANGE

Estelle, who was diagnosed as having angina pectoris (chest pain caused by coronary artery disease), didn't realize she might have had a heart problem for months. Although she was experiencing shortness of breath and chest pain, she was unaware that her two-pack-a-day habit was ruining her heart. "I just assumed the shortness of breath was from my lungs," she said. "I always figured lung cancer would kill me."

Estelle is not alone: Polls show that women believe cancer is their number-one health risk. Women surveyed usually believe that it's not even lung cancer, but breast cancer that will kill them. As we said earlier, they're wrong: Heart disease is the biggest killer of women. But because women don't recognize this, they continue to smoke, says Dr. Margaret Chesney, a professor of epidemiology and biostatistics at the University of California at San Francisco.

"Women know that cigarette smoking is unhealthy," says Dr. Chesney. "They have a general idea that it is unhealthy, but they do not realize the very powerful link between smoking and their leading cause of death, heart disease. That is because they think their leading cause of death is breast cancer. So, although they know that smoking is unhealthy, that doesn't give them a compelling reason to quit."

In men, smoking has long been recognized as an important risk factor for heart disease, and research has shown that this is true for women as well. A 1989 Milwaukee study conducted by researchers at The Medical College of Wisconsin, St. Luke's Hospital, and the Milwaukee V.A. Medical Center found that heavy female smokers were twice as likely to suffer a heart attack as their nonsmoking counterparts. Not only that; these women were 60 percent more likely to suffer from advanced coronary artery disease. The younger the woman, the worse the odds. Nothing erases your natural gender protection against developing heart disease early in life more thoroughly than smoking.

You also may not realize that you don't have to be a heavy smoker to damage your heart. Although heavy smoking will cause more damage, a 1987 nationwide study of nearly 120,000 nurses showed that smoking as few as one to four cigarettes a day increased their risk of a heart attack two to three times. This study also found that smoking was an independent risk factor that accounted for 40 percent of the heart attacks, and this figure climbed to an incredible 90 percent for women who smoked more than forty-five cigarettes a day.

HOW CIGARETTE SMOKE DAMAGES YOUR HEART   Each time you inhale cigarette smoke, you're drawing into your body a mixture of 4,000 chemical substances, many of which are poisonous. Cigarette smoke contains carbon monoxide, one of the deadliest of substances. When you inhale cigarette smoke, sulfuric acid not only eats away at the tissue of your lungs, but damages the blood vessels of your heart as well. And the toxic list goes on.

Researchers believe that cigarette smoke damages your heart in two ways. First, the toxic materials injure the walls of your coronary arteries, and in attempting to repair them your body inadvertently creates conditions which make it easier for atherosclerotic plaque—the fatty deposits that cause coronary artery disease—to develop. It's also believed that tobacco smoke works independently to activate your body's blood-clotting system, promoting clots which can block your arteries and cause a heart attack. Substances in some birth-control pills can do the same thing; this is why taking the pills and smoking can be particularly dangerous.

Besides promoting conditions which can lead to coronary disease, smoking has been linked in women to coronary spasms, a potentially dangerous constriction of the heart's blood vessels. In some cases, even women with apparently healthy hearts can experience chest pain leading to heart attack and death. Cocaine is known to cause coronary spasms, but recently a small 1992 study linked cigarette smoking to this problem as well.

Smoking can also lead to the development of high blood

pressure, another major risk factor for coronary artery disease. You know nicotine as the substance which causes addiction to cigarettes. What you may not know is that nicotine stimulates the release of the hormone epinephrine into your bloodstream, which can raise your blood pressure.

As if this were not enough, smoking is also one of the biggest risk factors for peripheral vascular disease, a narrowing of the blood vessels that carry blood to the legs, kidneys, and brain, which is often found in people with heart disease. In fact, peripheral vascular disease occurs almost exclusively in smokers.

These dangers to your health exist even if you chose "low-tar" and "low-nicotine" cigarettes. Choosing such cigarettes may lead to your smoking more under the misguided notion that they're safe.

> ♥ **Lifesaving Tip:** If you smoke, and do nothing more upon reading this book than quit, you'll sharply decrease your chance of developing coronary artery disease. Giving up smoking is the healthiest thing you can do for your heart.

HOW MANY WOMEN SMOKE?   Take a look around at the shopping mall, the office, and your neighborhood restaurants: Women are lighting up. When they first began smoking decades ago, women started later, smoked fewer cigarettes, and did not inhale as deeply as men. As time went on, women began smoking more like men—earlier, more heavily, inhaling deeply—and their health risks climbed.

Learning about the harmful effects of cigarette smoking has had some effect. Since 1964, when the landmark warning on the hazards of cigarette smoking was issued, the proportion of U.S. smokers dropped from 40 percent to about 25 percent, according to the federal Centers for Disease Control in Atlanta. But women make up a large portion of America's smokers. In fact, between 1930 and 1967, the proportion of adult women who smoked rose from 10 to 35 percent. Since then the percentage of women smokers has declined, but a quarter of the female population still smokes. Young women are starting to smoke earlier and are less likely to quit than men. Some young people are still taking up the habit in junior high or even elementary school. If you don't consider the risk to your own health sufficient motivation to quit, consider the model you're providing for your children.

WHY WOMEN SMOKE Given the tremendously detrimental effect that smoking has on their health, why do women smoke? They may not realize just how hazardous it is. And, not surprisingly, the tobacco industry won't tell them. On the contrary, tobacco companies have worked hard for years to convince women that smoking is glamorous and slenderizing.

Consider Nina, who underwent a balloon angioplasty because of heart disease at the Cleveland Clinic. "When I was growing up, smoking was oh so glamorous. All the Hollywood stars smoked," Nina says as she pantomimes smoking a cigarette in a long holder.

To appeal to women, the tobacco companies have even co-opted the flag of feminism. The Virginia Slims tag line, "You've Come a Long Way, Baby," may seem to promise female equality, but delivers disease and death. Tobacco companies are big supporters not only of athletic and sports activities, but of women's causes as well. According to an article in *Mirabella* magazine, thirteen women's organizations reported receiving contributions from the tobacco industry.

If smoking is so dangerous to a woman's health, you might wonder why you don't read more about it in women's magazines. An answer to that question comes from Dr. Kenneth Warner of the University of Michigan School of Public Health. He conducted studies which showed that magazines that accept cigarette advertising are less likely to run articles publicizing the health risks of smoking. He found this "censorship phenomenon" prevalent in women's magazines.

If you smoke, you may also believe it's not that dangerous because your doctor has not advised you to quit. But Dr. Erica Frank of the Stanford Center for Research in Disease Prevention conducted a study, published in 1991, which found that only about half of the smokers surveyed had ever been told by their doctors to quit. This is not because doctors believe smoking is healthy, but more likely because they don't remember to inquire about smoking, are not reimbursed for smoking cessation counseling, or view advising their patients to quit as interfering with their private lives. Dr. Frank says, "I believe it is a physician's obligation to advise patients to quit, because quitting smoking is the most important thing people can do to improve their health."

SMOKING AND PREGNANCY Smoking is one of the most harmful things you can do to your unborn child. According to the U.S. Surgeon General, smokers give birth to babies who are, on average, half an inch shorter and seven ounces lighter than babies of nonsmokers. Babies born to smokers are more likely to have birth defects, chronic breathing problems, and learning disabilities.

> ♥ Lifesaving Tip: If you quit smoking before you become pregnant, or even during your first trimester, you reduce your risk of a low-birth-weight baby to that of a woman who has never smoked.

SMOKING AND WEIGHT CONTROL (AND WRINKLES) Most health professionals hate to admit it, but cigarette smoking does keep your weight down. You may naturally assume that this is because when you smoke you're less likely to snack. While this is true, research also shows that nicotine affects your metabolism and appetite, keeping your weight low. But if you're so concerned about your appearance that you smoke to keep slim, think of what you may be doing to your face. Most doctors say they can pick out the longtime female smokers in their practice by the crow's-feet and age lines above their upper lips.

> ♥ Lifesaving Tip: Remember, quitting smoking pays off big. According to a recent report from the Surgeon General, after one year you'll decrease by 50 percent the risk to your heart that smoking had produced. After fifteen years, your risk will be the same as that of a woman who never smoked.

NONSMOKERS TAKE NOTE! Even if you don't smoke, your health is at risk from the deadly fumes which curl from the cigarette dangled by your spouse, your best friend, your coworker, or even a stranger seated at a nearby restaurant table. Researchers are finding that passive smoke, also known as environmental or secondary smoke, is a culprit in the development of heart disease and heart attacks.

Sitting in a smoky room raises your heart rate and blood

pressure. Ingesting passive smoke also increases your demand for oxygen during exercise, which can be harmful if you have heart disease. So even if you don't smoke, smoking is not necessarily one less risk to worry about.

ORAL CONTRACEPTIVES

Since their introduction, oral contraceptives, known to a generation as The Pill, have become a very popular means of birth control. For most women, they're perfectly safe. But if you smoke, they may pose a threat to your heart.

Birth-control pills are generally made up of two hormones, progesterone and estrogen. Taken orally, they prevent pregnancy. When they were first developed, it was discovered that women taking them faced a higher risk of cardiovascular problems, including heart attack, stroke, and blood clots in the lungs (pulmonary embolism).

The question of oral contraceptives and cardiovascular disease was reviewed at a 1992 meeting of leading cardiologists, gynecologists, and obstetricians. The participants found that because of the scare in the 1970s, mentioned above, oral contraceptives tend to be underprescribed. Since most birth-control pills have been reformulated, the risk has been greatly reduced, the experts agreed. However, they noted that some higher-dosage pills remain on the market. Also, since the question of the potential for cardiovascular disease, stroke, and high blood pressure was raised in the past, you should keep this in mind if you're at risk for any of these problems. In any case, the decision to take oral contraceptives should be made by you and your doctor after a review of your medical history.

> ♥ Lifesaving Tip: If you smoke cigarettes, you should definitely not use oral contraceptives. Studies show that taking birth-control pills and smoking, in combination, can increase your risk of suffering a heart attack up to thirty-nine times. This is because both smoking and oral contraceptives increase your blood's tendency to clot, which can lead to heart attack or stroke.

ABNORMAL CHOLESTEROL PATTERN

"What's your cholesterol number?" In the 1980s, this question echoed through doctors' offices, shopping malls, and fitness centers. Cholesterol-watching became a fad. As so often happens, confusion reigned. What was the best way to bring down cholesterol? Oatmeal? Rice cakes? Critics also emerged, charging that Americans were being unduly frightened about cholesterol.

So what's the truth? The first important thing to know about cholesterol-watching is that it's not a fad. Studies have shown that high blood cholesterol levels are associated with coronary artery disease. But whether you should be concerned about cholesterol or not depends on your risk history.

A pearly, fatlike substance, cholesterol is an essential component of your body. It's found in the membranes of cells, is used in the formation of the bile acids which help digest food, and it even contributes to sex hormones.

The important news about cholesterol for women is that recent research shows that if you have other risks for coronary heart disease, just knowing your total cholesterol level is not enough. You need to know what types of cholesterol comprise your total level. This is your blood cholesterol or lipid pattern. An abnormal lipid pattern is a risk factor for coronary artery disease. There are different ways in which these patterns can be abnormal. For example, one inherited lipid disorder (hyperlipidemia) results in a blood cholesterol pattern of too much low-density lipoprotein, or LDL cholesterol, when compared to high-density lipoprotein, or HDL cholesterol. Women may also develop an abnormal cholesterol pattern after menopause.

If you are concerned about your cholesterol, you need to know about the following levels, as opposed to just your total cholesterol number:

- Low-density lipoprotein, or LDL cholesterol
- Triglycerides
- High-density lipoprotein, or HDL cholesterol

Low-density lipoprotein (LDL) is the so-called "bad" cholesterol. This substance contributes to the development of heart disease by depositing cholesterol in the arterial wall, which can form the fatty accumulations that result in the narrowing of arteries.

High levels of LDL increase your chances of developing heart disease.

Triglycerides are fatty compounds found in combination with LDL and low HDL cholesterol, and are increasingly being implicated as important in causing coronary artery disease in women.

High-density lipoprotein cholesterol, or HDL, reverses the accumulation of LDL cholesterol by transferring it away from the artery. In a sense, it does for your arteries what Drano does for your plumbing.

A simple finger-prick blood test will give you your total cholesterol level, which may be enough if you have *no* other risk factors for coronary heart disease. For more information on whether you should have your cholesterol level checked, see Chapter 6.

If your blood cholesterol level is undesirable, your doctor will most likely suggest you try lowering it through diet and exercise. If it's severely high and can't be controlled through diet and exercise, your doctor will probably recommend you take one of the cholesterol-lowering drugs on the market, especially if you have coronary artery disease.

DIABETES

For a woman, having diabetes, like smoking, effectively erases the "grace period" for heart disease afforded by gender. Studies show that if you develop diabetes before menopause, your risk of getting coronary artery disease rises to a level equal to that of a man your age. Studies also show that diabetes can contribute to other risk factors associated with heart disease, like high blood cholesterol and high blood pressure. But even in the absence of any risk factors at all, a large-scale medical study of residents living in the California community of Rancho Bernardo in 1991 showed that diabetic women run a higher risk of developing heart disease than do even diabetic men. Also, if you're diabetic and you suffer a heart attack, your chance of survival drops. A major Israeli study of the survival of 5,839 heart attack victims found that diabetic women had twice the risk of dying during their hospitalization than did diabetic men. These women were also more likely to die during the following year.

What is diabetes? If you don't produce enough insulin, the hormone which metabolizes sugar into energy, or if your body doesn't react correctly to the insulin you have, the resulting condition is called diabetes. Diabetics are grouped into two major categories. Type 1, formerly known as juvenile-onset diabetes, is an inherited disorder which usually appears before the age of forty. Type 2, formerly called adult-onset diabetes, is the type which develops after that age. A third type, gestational diabetes, may occur while you're pregnant and disappear afterward. It's an important warning sign, however—if you have gestational diabetes, your chances of developing diabetes later increase.

The exact reason that diabetes is so damaging to women's hearts is not known, but it may be that diabetic women have less HDL cholesterol in their blood. This makes them less resistant to atherosclerotic plaque and blood clots. Diabetes is also serious because it can cause changes in your nerve cells which result in your body's misinterpreting pain signals, such as chest pain. You might even suffer a "silent" heart attack, one you don't realize you're having.

Although Type 2 diabetes is not inherited, your likelihood of developing it increases if you're overweight. Being overweight makes it more difficult for your body to properly metabolize sugar and fat. Keeping your weight under control and exercising help prevent diabetes.

OVERWEIGHT

Many women believe they weigh too much. In discussing overweight as a risk factor for coronary heart disease, though, we are talking about obesity. Obesity is defined as weighing 20 percent or more over your ideal weight. Results of the Nurses' Health Study, which followed 121,700 registered nurses over eight years, found that 70 percent of coronary disease occurred in women who were obese. The study by Harvard Medical School and Brigham and Women's Hospital, published in 1990, also attributed 40 percent of this heart disease primarily to overweight. Obesity, the study concluded, is a major cause of coronary heart disease among women in the United States.

Earlier, in 1983, the Framingham Study, in its follow-up of 2,828 women over twenty-six years, found that the risk of cardiovascular disease rose as overweight increased. For women under fifty, the heaviest were nearly two and a half times more likely to develop coronary heart disease. Also, the study found that very overweight women under the age of seventy had more than four times the rate of stroke.

Researchers are only now beginning to appreciate the complexities of obesity, such as the roles played by genetics, metabolism, and body weight distribution. For example, research has shown that if your fat is concentrated in your stomach, making you "apple"-shaped, you're worse off, in terms of health, than your pear-shaped friends. The fat around your middle makes you more vulnerable to such ailments as hypertension, diabetes, and coronary artery disease.

Eventually, the scale in the doctor's office may become a thing of the past as more doctors pull out a tape measure instead. To learn whether you're apple-shaped (technically, android) or pear-shaped (gynoid), you simply need to look in the mirror. But deciding you're a pear should not automatically put your mind at rest; you may be a pear, but still unhealthily overweight. Here's how to determine whether you have a healthy waist-to-hip ratio:

Take a tape measure and measure around your waist at the navel (no cheating—don't pull in your stomach). Then measure your hips at their widest. Divide the waist measure by the hip measure. What you're after is a waist-to-hip ratio of 0.80. For example, say your waist is 38 inches and your hips are 43 inches. Divide the 43 into the 38 and you'll get 0.88. That's too high. (If you're curious about your husband or boyfriend, the ideal waist-to-hip ratio for a man is 0.95).

HIGH BLOOD PRESSURE

High blood pressure, or hypertension, is found in 10 percent of the adult population and poses a serious threat to your heart. It's known as the silent killer because undiagnosed hypertension can damage your heart, brain, and kidneys before you notice any symptoms.

Just as gender provides women with protection against coronary artery disease, you're afforded a similar "grace period" in the development of high blood pressure. Women usually don't become hypertensive until after menopause. However, as you age, you become as vulnerable as men to hypertension and its deadly complications: heart attack and stroke.

This premenopausal gender advantage doesn't apply if you're black. As are black men, black women are at higher risk than whites for hypertension. Statistics have shown that twice as many black women over the age of twenty-five have high blood pressure as white women.

No matter what your race, you're much more likely to develop hypertension if you have risk factors. These risks are similar to those of heart disease: a family history of early hypertension, age, smoking, obesity, and diabetes.

HOW HYPERTENSION DAMAGES YOUR HEART   With each contraction, your heart pumps a small amount of blood into your coronary arteries, which in turn distribute the blood to the heart muscle itself. Oxygen-containing blood similarly nourishes all of your body's organs, including your heart, kidneys, and brain.

Hypertension damages your heart in two ways. If undetected, high blood pressure can result in a form of heart disease called hypertensive cardiovascular disease, in which your heart becomes enlarged and eventually weakens. While many people are screened for high blood pressure nowadays, this disease is still quite common. High blood pressure can damage your heart by contributing to atherosclerosis, the buildup of fatty deposits within your arteries, which narrows them and results in coronary artery disease.

Think of your circulatory system as a river. At some places, where the river is narrow, pressure can build up and create turbulence, which can damage the banks of the river. The same thing can occur within your body. If your arteries are too narrow, blood pressure can build. High blood pressure can damage the walls of the arteries, and as your body attempts to repair the damage, atherosclerosis, or coronary artery disease, can result.

In most cases, high blood pressure occurs for no discernible reason. This is called essential hypertension, and accounts for about 90 percent of hypertension cases. Much less often, hypertension can stem from an underlying disorder. Some originates in the kidneys, the adrenal glands, or, in rare cases, a congenital disorder. This type of high blood pressure, called secondary hypertension, occurs far less often than essential hypertension. But if you have secondary hypertension, it's imperative that the underlying cause be diagnosed so that it can be corrected.

♥ Lifesaving Tip: Although uncommon, secondary hypertension occurs more frequently in women. So if you are diagnosed with high blood pressure, be certain your doctor checks for secondary causes.

HYPERTENSION IN PREGNANCY   A third type of hypertension can occur during pregnancy. Such hypertensive disorders, which are among the most serious complications of pregnancy, are discussed in Chapter 9.

WHITE COAT HYPERTENSION   Some people become so anxious when visiting the doctor that their blood pressure may rise, and they may be mistakenly diagnosed as having high blood pressure. This is called white coat hypertension. Stephanie was treated for high blood pressure for two years. When she switched physicians, her new doctor noticed that when she first arrived at the office her blood pressure was elevated. As the visit continued and Stephanie felt more relaxed, her blood pressure returned to normal. After evaluating Stephanie further, her doctor became convinced she did not have high blood pressure after all.

Your doctor should check your blood pressure over several visits before deciding that you have high blood pressure, especially if he or she is considering putting you on medication. If you become anxious in a doctor's office, you can purchase a kit to take your blood pressure at home.

If you have borderline high blood pressure, your doctor may advise you to control it by losing weight, quitting smoking, and cutting down your consumption of salt and caffeine. If you have severe hypertension, these steps, as well as medication, will most likely be prescribed.

SEDENTARY LIFESTYLE

Although many experts have long suspected that a sedentary lifestyle contributes to the development of coronary heart disease, the American Heart Association issued a statement in 1992 which every couch potato feared. "There is a relation between physical inactivity and cardiovascular mortality, and inactivity is a risk factor for the development of coronary heart disease," was the official word. The association also issued a revised statement on exercise, coming out stronger in favor of the benefits of regular exercise. For more about how to transform your lifestyle into a heart-healthy and active one, see Chapter 16.

STRESS

What stress is and whether it affects a woman's heart is a complex subject, so we've devoted Chapter 14 to it.

To summarize, you're at risk of developing heart disease if:

- You're past menopause
- You have a family history of early heart disease
- You smoke
- You smoke and take oral contraceptives
- You have an abnormal blood cholesterol pattern
- You're diabetic
- You're overweight
- You have high blood pressure
- You lead a sedentary lifestyle
- You're under stress

> ♥ Mindsaving Tip: No matter what your risk profile, bear in mind that it's within the power of all of us to modify many of these risks and increase the probability of living a healthier life. In the next chapter, we'll tell you how to do just that.

YOUR HEART AND IRON

Often, medical information is presented with such certainty that you'd think it was carved in stone. This is not the case. Medical knowledge is constantly changing. Findings gleaned from studies today may later be confirmed, but they also may be modified, contradicted, or even refuted.

An example of this is a 1992 study which found that high levels of iron seem to contribute to the development of coronary heart disease. The media wasted no time in trumpeting the study's results in television, radio, and newspaper reports, and even on the cover of the September 21, 1992, issue of *U.S. News & World Report*.

But while that study is very intriguing, it raises many questions which must be answered before any firm conclusions about heart disease and iron are drawn.

The study followed 1,900 men from eastern Finland for five years. It found that men with more ferritin, a protein that binds iron in the blood, were more likely to have heart attacks. Likewise, those with less than normal amounts appeared protected.

This finding provides some possible evidence for a theory involving the narrowing of the coronary arteries. It is known that LDL cholesterol plays a role in this. But what occurs to make LDL cholesterol bind with white cells and other substances to form plaque, the dangerous material that narrows coronary arteries and results in heart disease? Many scientists believe the answer to this question lies in a process called oxidation. Research indicates that cholesterol must be oxidized—combined with oxygen— before it will do its damage. Once the LDLs are oxidized, they attract white cells and other fibrous substances which lead to the dangerous plaque. Proponents of the iron theory contend that it is stored iron in the body which facilitates this oxidation process.

If this is true, the iron theory would help explain why women generally develop heart disease later than men. Iron may also provide another piece to the puzzle. The Finnish study indicates that just as excess iron may contribute to heart disease, a lack of iron may protect against it. Since premenopausal women menstruate, this monthly bleeding helps rid them of excess iron.

Now the question remains, "What do these findings mean to you?" The answer is nothing, yet. Although this finding about iron is intriguing, it doesn't provide evidence that it is excess iron, rather than some other factor, which resulted in the increase in heart disease. After all, this study was done on men living in Finland, and the reasons why Finnish men are different from American women seem obvious—gender, diet, and lifestyle. While results of this study may eventually prove significant, much more research needs to be done to determine whether we should take measures to alter our consumption of iron.

HOW TO EVALUATE MEDICAL NEWS

The intense media interest paid to the iron study brings up a much broader topic, which is how much attention you should pay to medical studies and other health news reported in the media.

Health information disseminated in the media can be very useful, and even lifesaving. But you should exercise some caution, and not necessarily believe everything you read.

Ever since the media recognized that health is an important topic to Americans, there has been a health information explosion. New medical findings are not only reported in medical journals but also make the front pages of newspapers and the nightly news broadcasts.

This raises several concerns. Because journalists are trained to present news stories in a most exciting manner, these findings are usually presented in the strongest way possible. Unless you read very carefully, it's easy to misinterpret a theory or speculation as fact. Also a particular study's findings may be only the latest development in a long-standing debate. For example, some reports have found that caffeine is dangerous for your heart; others that it will not do your heart any harm. Such conflicting information can be very frustrating when you're deciding whether or not to indulge in your morning brew. (By the way, the latest word is that caffeine is not harmful for most people.)

Another problem is that research is often very preliminary, so to draw firm conclusions from it would be dangerous. For example, it would be unwise for people taking iron supplements because they are anemic to forgo them because of the iron study discussed earlier.

Here are some tips on how to separate the facts from the hype:

- **Be a discriminating reader.** News stories written by medical writers for such major publications as the *New York Times* are generally far more informative than those appearing in smaller newspapers or tabloids. However, many newspapers carry wire stories, which they get from news services they subscribe to, such as the Associated Press. Wire stories are specially constructed so that subscribing newspapers can run as much of the story as they like. The original story may be well written and complete, but your newspaper may run a shortened version. So you may never see important information contained in the original story.
- **What kind of study is it?** There are basically three different types of studies: experimental, epidemiologic, and clinical.

Experimental studies are usually animal studies. These are often preliminary studies which need to be verified later using human subjects before determining if the findings are relevant at all.

Epidemiologic studies make observations from a given group of participants over time but do not involve any intervention. For example, some very important findings have come from the Framingham Heart Study over the decades, such as the observation that cigarette smoking is a risk factor for heart disease. Such findings were obtained from studies which observed the health status of people who were smokers and nonsmokers before they participated in the study.

On the other hand, sometimes clinical studies are needed to back up epidemiologic studies before firm conclusions can be made. These are studies in which an intervention is done. For example, the Nurses' Health Study found that estrogen lowered a woman's risk of heart disease. But a lower rate of heart disease may have been influenced by other factors, such as the increased health-care monitoring of women taking estrogen. Clinical trials to further study the effects of estrogen are under way. These studies, the Post-Menopausal Estrogen/Progestin Intervention Trials, are discussed further in Chapter 13.

- **Is this the first time the results have been reported?** If so, it will take awhile for studies to be done to back it up. There is a big difference between the results of a single study or two, such as the iron study, and consensus statements reported by organizations like the American Heart Association. For example, in 1992 the heart association added a sedentary lifestyle to the list of major risk factors for heart disease. The association took this step after reports from numerous studies were published and experts from many fields reached agreement.

- **Do the findings make sense?** If there is sound reasoning behind the findings, the chances are better it will hold up over time. This is one reason why scientists are excited about the iron study; it poses a logical theory consistent with other scientific findings. Another example of this is recent data indicating that the consumption of certain vitamins, particularly vitamin E, but also C and beta carotene—a parent molecule of vitamin A—may protect against heart disease. As with the iron theory, the answer may lie with the oxidation process. Iron fa-

cilitates oxidation, which can lead to damage-causing cholesterol, but these vitamins seem to block the oxidation process,
rendering the LDL cholesterol less harmful. This is logical and
consistent with other findings, as researchers have observed
that people taking these vitamins do appear to have lower rates
of heart disease. In fact, a 1992 study found the 87,245 women
participating in the Nurses' Health Study who had been taking
vitamin E supplements for over two years had about half the
risk of heart disease as women who did not (and this decline
rose to 64 percent for those taking the supplement for eight
years). Men taking supplements for two years had their risk cut
by only 26 percent. But prospective clinical studies (studies
which set out to determine whether something is so, not
studies which simply look back at data and draw conclusions)
are still needed to make certain the benefits are indeed from the
vitamins and not from other factors.

· **Is the treatment worse than the disease?** Excellent examples
of this are the studies showing that drinking a moderate
amount of alcohol is beneficial to a person's cholesterol level.
But drinking leads to a whole host of other medical ailments
and social ills, such as drunk driving. As we note in the next
chapter, it would be exceptionally foolhardy for a nondrinker
to begin imbibing just to ward off heart disease.

4

Beating
the
Odds

"I'm exercising three times a week, but it's trying to stay on a diet that's driving me nuts. Friday night is pizza night at our house and it's hard to eat only one piece," says Lindsay, with a sigh. She was examined at the Cleveland Clinic two months before, after her family doctor had brushed off her worries about chest pain. Because of her family's strong history of early heart disease, she refused to take the doctor's word for it when he told her, "Don't worry. Women your age don't get heart disease." Good thing, too. Lindsay's test results showed that though she is only thirty-six, her coronary arteries are already becoming narrowed by fatty deposits. If untreated, this could someday result in a heart attack.

Lindsay had hoped for some easy answers. She was prescribed medications to relieve her chest pain, but that's only a symptom of her problem. The real job is up to her. To improve the odds that she won't end up having a heart attack, Lindsay learned at the clinic, she should lose about thirty pounds, follow a low-fat diet, and get regular aerobic exercise. In that way, it's hoped, Lindsay can bring her cholesterol level down enough— without cholesterol-lowering drugs—to halt, or at least significantly slow, the progression of coronary disease. So, since then, Lindsay has been faithfully going to an aerobics class. But pizza night is a real struggle.

This chapter is not only for Lindsay—it's for all of us at risk of developing coronary disease. Most of us have at least some risk factors for heart disease. Transforming ourselves from chip-munching couch potatoes to healthy-eating regular exercisers isn't easy. But it can be done.

And it's worthwhile, say Dr. William P. Castelli, director of the Framingham Heart Study. A silver-haired, distinguished-looking man, Dr. Castelli fairly bursts with enthusiasm when he talks about our ability to protect ourselves against heart disease. "Women have to understand that we are saying that half of them in America are going to die of atherosclerosis, and they could prevent it," he says.

A key way to do that is to adopt a diet low in fat. For Dr. Castelli, this presents no problem. "Just give me your ten favorite recipes and I could take you on a shopping trip and show you how you could make them."

But when you go to the supermarket, you don't have Dr. Castelli at your side. You do have a pizzeria on nearly every corner. How can you fight such temptation? Much of the problem is that women tend to sabotage themselves by clinging to long-held beliefs that are, in reality, self-defeating myths. For example:

The Myth: I must attain some "ideal" weight that seems impossible to achieve.

The Truth: The latest research shows that even if you're very significantly overweight, a loss of as little as fifteen pounds can raise your self-esteem, improve your health, and reduce the probability of your developing heart disease.

The Myth: "No pain, no gain" applies to exercise when I'm trying to strengthen my heart and cardiovascular system.

The Truth: Studies have shown that moderation is okay. Doing nothing more strenuous than brisk walking can lower your risk of heart disease.

The Myth: To improve my heart's health, I'm going to have to make dramatic changes in every single part of my lifestyle.

The Truth: Just turn the myth around. It's true that because many heart disease risks are related, you may have to make more than one lifestyle change to significantly reduce your risk of heart disease. But the rewards are interrelated as well. Take exercise: If you undertake a regular exercise program, you'll not only become more fit but will also increase your chances of losing weight or maintaining a weight loss, and you'll reduce your level of stress. That's a lot of benefit from just one change.

♥ **Lifesaving Tip: The more risk factors you have for developing heart disease, the more important it is to reduce them.**

CHANGING RISKY HABITS

As we noted in the preceding chapter, there are several risks for heart disease in women. One is your genetic makeup. Obviously, you can't change your biological parents. Black women are more at risk for heart disease as well. So are women with a close family member who suffered a heart attack under age fifty-five.

But some of the most powerful risk factors are within your power to change. If you're at risk for heart disease, or if you simply want to live a healthier lifestyle, these are the risks you should modify:

- Smoking
- Overweight
- Sedentary lifestyle
- Stress

Because heart risk behaviors are related, it's futile to consider them independently of one another. For example, a woman who is under stress, research shows, is often overweight, is sedentary, smokes, and feels angry most of the time. All of these are risk factors for heart disease. Sometimes just learning about these risk factors is enough to help you reform. But if it's not, berating yourself won't help. "Self-control is not a personality trait. You can have good self-control in some aspects of life and poor self-control in others," says Dr. Michael McKee, director of the Biofeedback Program at the Cleveland Clinic. "The secret is to learn self-control in the important things."

♥ **Mindsaving Tip: Ridding yourself of self-destructive thinking is a good place to start making changes. If you** smoke, weigh too much, or exercise too little, don't hate yourself. You're still a worthwhile person; your value has nothing to do with these habits. These are nothing more than unhealthy behaviors which you can change.

QUITTING SMOKING

If you've tried to quit smoking and failed, staying away from cigarettes may seem impossible. In fact, studies show that women sometimes find it more difficult than men to envision life without cigarettes. But there's plenty of hope. Each year, about 1.3 million Americans quit smoking. All you have to do is become one of them.

If you've suffered a heart attack or have just learned you have a heart problem, you may think it will be easy to quit. This is not necessarily true. A study of 310 smokers in a coronary care unit showed that only 25 percent were able to quit without help.

Here are some tips for quitting smoking, compiled with the invaluable help of Dr. Judith Ockene, director of Preventive and Behavioral Medicine at the University of Massachusetts Medical School and coauthor of the 1992 book *Prevention of Coronary Heart Disease:*

- Whether it's better to quit cold turkey or taper depends on the individual. Contrary to popular belief, tapering can work, but it's important to set goals. For example, you can say, "Next week I'll smoke half of what I'm smoking now, then the next week half of that, and then zero."
- Whether you design your own plan or join an established program, the important thing is to figure out what works for you. Talk to your friends about programs they like. Studies show that women tend to prefer small groups as opposed to larger "lecture-type" settings.
- No matter which method you choose, make sure it includes ways to prevent weight gain and handle stress. Both are key reasons women smokers tend to backslide. Be prepared to gain a couple of pounds as your body adjusts to going without the metabolic changes brought on by nicotine.
- Cigarette smoking is a complex addiction. Some people can smoke rather heavily but not become dependent, while light

smokers can suffer extreme withdrawal symptoms, such as restlessness, irritability, nervousness, anxiety, stomach disorders, and even seizures. If you are addicted, you might want to consider nicotine gum or the more recently marketed patch system. Remember, though, such aids are not an easy answer; you can increase your chances of success by taking a stop-smoking course, such as those offered by the American Cancer Society or your local chapter of the American Heart Association.

Here's our favorite tip for quitting smoking: Set aside the money you've spent on cigarettes each day and, when you've saved enough, indulge in something frivolous. If you backslide, donate the money to your local lung or heart association or favorite charity. This type of incentive system provides the extra oomph you may need to stay with your program. By the way, some people find this system even more effective if they pledge to donate the money to a cause to which they are strongly opposed!

> ♥ Lifesaving Tip: If you've just suffered a heart attack, nicotine in any form can be dangerous, so check with your doctor before using a patch, gum, or other nicotine products. Also, wearing the patch while you smoke may be dangerous, especially for those with heart disease.

A GUIDE TO WEIGHT LOSS AND EXERCISE

"I can lose weight! I've done it a thousand times" goes the old joke. As most unsuccessful dieters will tell you, losing weight is easy; it's keeping it off that's hard. Our country's obsession with weight loss has fueled a multibillion-dollar diet industry.

But you don't have to shell out big bucks to lose weight. Dr. Judith S. Stern, a professor of nutrition and internal medicine at the University of California at Davis, studied women who had successfully lost weight and kept it off. She found, for example, that besides eating less, the women who maintained their weight loss had developed a whole new set of habits, such as exercising regularly and handling stress and problem solving more effectively. The women who lost weight initially but gained it back had tried to change only their eating habits. These "relapsers" exercised little, ate unconsciously in response to their emotions, avoided problems by overeating or sleeping, and took on too many tasks themselves.

Dr. Stern's study also found that the women who were most likely to succeed had designed a weight-loss program to suit themselves. This doesn't mean that a formal weight-loss program might not help you. It does indicate that you can lose weight by yourself. If you decide to join a program, you should choose one well suited to your needs. "Most diets work initially, but you have to think about long-term success," says Dr. Stern.

For our tips on losing weight, see "Every Woman's Eating Plan for Life" in Chapter 16.

DON'T FORGET EXERCISE!

If you could buy a pill which could help you not only lose weight, but also keep it off, stay off cigarettes, cope with stress, avoid osteoporosis and diabetes, and even sleep better, wouldn't you buy it? Unfortunately, there is no magic pill that can do this for you. But exercise can. To learn how you can build exercise into your daily schedule, see "Every Woman's Exercise Plan for Life" in Chapter 16.

BEATING STRESS

Currently among cardiologists, debate rages on whether stress is a major cause of heart disease and heart attacks. But most researchers agree that it's at least a contributing factor. For this reason, we've devoted an entire chapter—Chapter 14—to the types of stress that can affect a woman's heart and what you can do about it.

AGE

Growing older is a major risk factor for women. In the past, the process of aging was viewed as a fact of life we couldn't do much about. But with estrogen replacement therapy, studies have shown, women can actually delay some of the adverse effects of aging on their hearts. Whether or not to opt for such therapy is a dilemma more and more women are facing. This topic is discussed in depth in Chapter 13.

WHAT ABOUT WINE?

If you want to see a roomful of health professionals squirm, bring up the studies which show that drinking one or two glasses of wine a day can decrease your risk of heart disease. The experts who have no problem telling us to give up cigarettes, fats, and sweets become very uneasy when faced with research which shows that alcohol may actually be good for our hearts.

In 1991, researchers at Harvard's School of Public Health looked at 44,000 men and discovered that those who drank a small to moderate amount of alcohol had a 25 to 40 percent lower chance of developing heart disease. While one small study indicated that the subjects had to drink red wine to reap the benefit, the Harvard study showed that it didn't matter whether alcohol was in the form of beer, wine (red or white), or hard liquor.

But before you decide to drink a toast to benefit your heart, consider these sobering statistics. Although the study showed that moderate drinking (defined as one or two drinks a day, a standard drink being twelve ounces of beer, four ounces of wine, or one and a half ounces of eighty-proof spirits) will not harm your heart, alcohol is a potent and potentially addictive substance which should be approached with caution. Studies show that the number of female problem drinkers is growing, and that women alcoholics are more likely to commit suicide than men. Overconsumption of alcohol has been shown to cause not only heart disease, but stroke, liver disease, fetal damage in pregnant women, some forms of cancer, and the dangers of drinking and driving. So while an occasional drink may not harm your heart, quitting smoking, adopting a low-fat eating plan, and exercising are far healthier ways to reduce your risk of heart disease.

♥ Lifesaving Tip: In addition to these cautions, if you are pregnant, have diabetes, elevated triglycerides, or heart failure from any cause, you should only consume alcohol with the specific permission of your doctor.

BLACK WOMEN AND HEART DISEASE

It's generally acknowledged that black women face a higher risk of cardiovascular disease than do white women, probably because of their tendency to have high blood pressure.

Dr. Shiriki K. Kumanyika, an associate professor and associate director for epidemiology at Penn State College of Medicine, Hershey Medical Center, Hershey, Pennsylvania, has published several papers on black women and overweight.

According to Dr. Kumanyika, black women are more likely to be overweight than white women, a fact which has serious ramifications when you consider that excess weight can increase the probability of high blood pressure, diabetes, and such disabling problems as osteoarthritis in the knees.

In one 1991 study, Dr. Kumanyika and her colleagues examined the results of two weight-loss trials and found that black women lost an average of four and a half pounds less than their white counterparts. In trying to understand why this might be so, Dr. Kumanyika noted that studies have revealed a more tolerant attitude toward overweight in the black community. Also, she noted, cultural food preferences may play a role: In general, blacks consume more meat, especially pork, and fried foods than do white persons, and certain beloved traditional southern and black-American foods are very high in fat. Dr. Kumanyika remarked too that black women may be less successful than whites in losing weight and keeping it off because they tend to exercise less. But here, she cautioned, the research is scanty.

One problem facing black women who want to lose weight is the same as that facing white women: Conventional weight-loss programs are not highly effective. One way, Dr. Kumanyika has found, that black women may increase their chances of losing weight and keeping it off is by joining a church-based or community-based weight-loss program. She studied a church-affiliated program in Baltimore called "Lose Weight and Win," a behaviorally oriented eight-week course of diet, counseling, and exercise designed for moderately overweight adults. A specific diet is not prescribed; participants eat the food they are accustomed to, but make small incremental changes to reduce their fat and caloric consumption. They also learn strategies to avoid overeating. Participants during the two-month program lost an average of six pounds, and after six months 65 percent of the women who returned for follow-up had maintained their weight loss.

According to Dr. Kumanyika, programs like "Lose Weight and Win" are models which could be initiated by women where they work and live, no matter what their race. The key, she believes, is making such groups a part of the community. To get started, she suggests contacting the local health department to find someone who can lead the group and distribute proper nutritional information. "People see an ad for Weight Watchers or Overeaters Anonymous and they go across town for a while until their interest peters out," Dr. Kumanyika says. "Most people in the black community know how to create programs for other needs. If they were more aware of this need, they could probably create these programs for themselves."

To sum up: If you don't have heart disease and are trying to avoid developing it, you're working on primary "prevention." If you have heart disease and want to slow or halt its progression, your efforts are known as "secondary prevention." Either way, working to beat the risks of heart disease is a very worthwhile goal.

5

When to See
a Doctor

A sturdy-looking woman of thirty-eight, Maggie was determined not to let this bout of indigestion interfere with the church supper she had promised to oversee. True, her vague intestinal discomfort had intensified lately; handfuls of antacids didn't help anymore. But no one was going to call Maggie a weakling. After all, her mother had never shirked her responsibilities because of her health problems; the family still talked about the time Bridgette had refused to go to the hospital and had delivered Maggie and her twin brother, Patrick, at home. Maggie did indeed finish working at the church supper, but when she got home, she collapsed on the bed. When she could scarcely struggle out of bed the next day, she finally agreed to let her husband, Michael, take her to the doctor. He'd been begging her to go for months.

Maggie was lucky. Tests showed she had a heart problem; in fact, she'd come within a hairsbreadth of suffering a heart attack.

There are many women like Maggie. In a way, I was like her myself. In the spring of 1990, my physician first recommended I undergo a cardiac test at a local hospital; I managed to put it off until the fall. Things just came up; the car broke down, I had a magazine article to finish, we were going on vacation. I was so certain that my heart was fine, I actually feel sheepish when I finally did go to the hospital for the test. An old pal of mine from college was too terrified to tell anyone about her chest pain for over a year, so convinced was she that she had coronary artery disease. She finally spilled out the story to me in tears after learning about my surgery.

You should see a doctor if you have any of the following signs or symptoms:

- Chest pain
- Palpitations (a pounding heart)
- Fainting
- Shortness of breath
- Fatigue
- Bodily swelling
- Heart murmur

♥ **Lifesaving Tip: If you're experiencing what may be a heart attack, seek immediate medical help. The symptoms of a heart attack are dealt with in detail in Chapter 10. If you have other symptoms, make an appointment with your doctor. The information in this chapter is not offered so that you can diagnose yourself, but so that you can help your doctor arrive at a correct diagnosis.**

CHOOSING A DOCTOR

If you experience chest pain or the other symptoms described in this chapter, start off with a visit to your family doctor. This can be an internist, a family practitioner, or a general practitioner, also known as a primary care physician, the doctor to whom you turn for the majority of your health-care needs.

Every woman should have a primary doctor who specializes in the health problems of adults. Too often women rely on their gynecologist for all their medical advice. Remember, your total well-being involves more than your reproductive system. Querying your husband's or mother's doctor or your child's pediatrician is not good enough. Certainly you and your family can share the same doctor, but the physician should be familiar with your medical history and physical health as well.

PRIMARY DOCTOR OR CARDIOLOGIST?

The reason for beginning with a visit to your primary physician rather than a cardiologist is that, especially in women, symptoms such as chest pain usually turn out to be unrelated to the heart. If necessary, your primary physician can refer you to a cardiologist, or, if you don't receive what you consider adequate diagnosis and treatment, you can always decide to see a cardiologist on your own.

But we can't stress this too strongly: *Never* overlook the importance of choosing an astute primary doctor. Some people carefully select a specialist but when it comes to their primary doctor they aren't so choosy. They figure that if they have a serious problem, their physician will refer them to a specialist. The fallacy in this thinking is this: If your primary doctor overlooks a problem, you may not be referred to the appropriate specialist until the problem has become severe.

The process of choosing a good doctor is far from foolproof. Jeffrey Stern, a physician in Waterbury, Connecticut, enjoys asking his new patients this riddle: "What do you call the person who graduates last in his medical-school class?" The answer, of course, is "Doctor." The meaning behind the joke is all too serious: When everyone is called "Doctor," how do you know who's good and who's not?

If you don't have a primary doctor, find one now, while you're well. This provides a "baseline" by which to measure what your health normally is like so that your physician can see more easily when something is amiss.

One place to start is by asking friends for a recommendation. If you're older, your friends probably have plenty of knowledge about doctors in your area, but if you're younger, this is usually not the case. If you're new to your area, contact your county medical society or local hospital for names of recommended doctors. Large public libraries and many hospital libraries have directories of doctors and their credentials.

Some doctors are willing to schedule a brief appointment to meet a prospective patient free of charge, but many doctors prefer not to do this or are too busy. Still, you can tell a lot from your first visit.

Here are tips on choosing a doctor. Many of these tips hold true whether you're seeking a primary physician or a specialist.

- **Be a diploma reader.** Make sure the doctor graduated from a reputable medical school and performed his or her residency at a major hospital. If the medical-school degree says "Alpha Omega Alpha," even better; it means your doctor was in the top ten of the class.

- **Is the doctor board-certified?** This is an added assurance of quality; it means the doctor has successfully completed an intensive testing program in one of twenty-three medical specialties, such as internal medicine or family practice. This is obviously important if you're seeking a specialist, but it also ensures minimum competence if you're choosing a primary physician. A doctor might be "board-eligible," which means he or she has had the requisite training but has not passed the necessary examinations. If the doctor is young, this is certainly understandable. In some specialties, certification regulations can change; a good cardiologist, for example, might not necessarily be board-certified, but may have considerable experience and a solid professional reputation.

- **What hospital is the doctor affiliated with?** You're healthy now, but eventually you may need a hospital stay. Doctors receive "privileges" to practice only at certain hospitals. Bear in mind that in choosing your doctor, you may also be choosing a hospital.

- **Does your doctor stay abreast of medical developments?** The way most doctors do this is by reading medical journals, especially those in their specialty. In talking with a prospective doctor, you should be able to get a general feeling of how well he or she keeps up with medical developments.

- **Does the doctor respect your time?** Any doctor may have an occasional emergency that keeps you waiting, but this should not be the norm. Your doctor's time is valuable, but so is yours.

- **When does the doctor return calls?** Being able to reach your doctor by telephone is important; ask when the doctor returns calls. The correct answer should be "as soon as possible" or during a specific time that same day set aside for answering patients' telephone calls. Who wants to find out she needs a prescription change long after the pharmacy has closed?

- **Does your doctor invest in laboratories or services you might**

be referred to? Your doctor should earn a fair fee for treating you; you should not need to wonder whether the tests or treatments being ordered for you are designed to line his or her pockets.

· **Does the doctor communicate well?** Two-way communication is an essential part of keeping you well. You should never be made to feel stupid for asking a question. It's important that you feel comfortable asking for information, and you should receive answers in terms you can understand. As Dr. Valerie Parisi, director of maternal fetal medicine at the University of Texas Medical School at Houston, puts it, "If a woman feels comfortable talking to me, she can say, 'You know, I heard about such-and-such a test. Should I have it?' A lot of times, that test is not appropriate. But it gives us an opportunity to talk which can be very valuable. You should never be talking to a doctor and feel that you can't bring something up to discuss."

> ♥ Lifesaving Tip: Your doctor is most likely a busy person, but you should feel as if your visit, your concerns, and your well-being are the major focus of his or her attention.

CHANGING DOCTORS

Some people are "doctor shoppers" and go from one to the other. Others tend to stick to the same doctor out of loyalty long after their confidence has evaporated. Doctors are not infallible. If you can't talk comfortably to your doctor about your problems, think your doctor doesn't take your problems seriously, or lack faith in your doctor's expertise, by all means consider a change.

> ♥ Mindsaving Tip: Remember that you and your doctor are members of a team whose goal it is to keep you in good health.

THE ALL-IMPORTANT SECOND OPINION

Yvette's face glows as she watches her mother, Esther, run across the road to greet her. "Isn't that wonderful? I never thought I would see that again," Yvette says, beaming. After her mother's heart attack, Yvette was told that her mother would die. She bitterly recalls the day the doctor told her and her sister that "we should take Mom home and make her life pleasant, because there was nothing more that could be done for her."

Fortunately for Esther, her daughters took her to another doctor, who recommended a coronary bypass operation. In Esther's case, getting a second opinion literally saved her life by enabling her to have the surgery she needed. A second opinion can also keep you from undergoing unnecessary surgery.

WHEN TO GET A SECOND OPINION Unfortunately, there's often no clear-cut answer as to whether or not you should seek a second opinion. Certainly do so if there is any doubt in your mind that your doctor's recommended course is the wisest one. You might seek a second opinion if you're troubled about symptoms which seem cardiac-related but your doctor dismisses your concerns; or if you're taking cardiovascular drugs but your symptoms are getting worse and your doctor is not inclined to investigate further; or if you're told you need open-heart surgery but are too old to survive it.

♥ Lifesaving Tip: It sometimes seems that we're more willing to seek a second opinion about a problem with our car than with our heart. You should consider a second opinion if you have *any* doubt about your doctor's recommendation.

HOW TO GET A SECOND OPINION "Sometimes people are very afraid they'll hurt their doctor's feelings," says Dr. Cheryl Weinstein, an internist at the Cleveland Clinic. "But if your doctor is angry about your wanting another opinion, or a consultation, then he or she really should not be your doctor."

If you value your relationship with your doctor, you'll want to maintain it. So be diplomatic about your request for a second opinion.

Consumer advocates disagree on how to find a doctor to give a second opinion. Some contend that doctors tend to stick together, so someone recommended by your doctor is likely to be only a "rubber stamp." Others contend that since your doctor knows your medical problem best, asking him or her for a recommendation is only logical. It's best to obey your instinct. If you're confident your doctor's recommendation will be objective, follow it. If you're uncertain, contact your county medical society for a list of names, or check your library for a multivolume reference set called *The Directory of Medical Specialists.*

AND A THIRD OPINION?   You've gotten your second opinion, and it's the opposite of the first. This can happen, especially in an area such as heart problems, where experts often disagree. You may have to seek a third opinion to be the tiebreaker. Once you have three opinions, it's probably time to make a decision. Some people will keep looking until they find a doctor who agrees with them; eventually they may, but that's no guarantee that they're getting the best medical advice.

If you have any doubt about the wisdom of seeking a second opinion, here's what Esther, Yvette's mother, who is now fully recovered from her surgery, has to say: "I remember asking my doctor if I'd be feeling good in time to put up my winter storm windows. He said, 'Sure.' It turns out he didn't even think I'd live that long! Now, whenever I put those windows up in the fall and take them down in the spring, I think of that."

ALL ABOUT CHEST PAIN

Joanne, forty-three, is a crackerjack realtor who thrives on the pressure of meeting sales deadlines. When not working, she enjoyed going out to dine on her favorite meal, a cocktail followed by a well-marbled steak. Lately, though, she'd been having chest pain, attacks which left this usually fearless woman scared to death. "It was a very sharp pain and seemed to be coming right from the center of my heart," she says. "I was terrified. I was sure I was having a heart attack."

Roberta began feeling lousy when she was vacationing in the Caribbean. After dining, she became conscious of "an odd feeling in my chest." The pain seemed so mild, she thought it was indigestion.

The chest pain Joanne was convinced was heart-related turned out to stem from a problem in her esophagus, while Roberta's mild "indigestion" was her first warning sign of coronary artery disease.

Confused? You're not alone. Especially in women, heart problems can be tricky to diagnose from symptoms such as chest pain. When chest pain occurs in men, the chances are greater that the problem is heart disease. Chest pains in women, particularly younger women, usually indicates a problem unrelated to the heart.

♥ **Mindsaving Tip: Symptoms of heart problems can be very worrisome, but remember that many nonserious conditions can manifest themselves in truly frightening symptoms. Only your doctor can decide whether they're cause for concern.**

CHEST PAIN IN WOMEN

Because men are more likely to develop coronary artery disease, their chest pain often turns out to be from blockage of their coronary arteries. Since women are at least as likely as men to suffer from chest pain, it's less likely that your ache stems from heart disease. But pinpointing the cause of your chest pain may prove either straightforward or infuriatingly difficult.

Historically, women who complained of chest pain were not taken seriously. Such pain in women was initially interpreted as not dangerous, and though this was later proved false, the conclusion stuck, and a doctor might be too quick to assume that the woman seated before him did not have heart disease because "women don't get heart disease." Although much of that thinking has changed, some doctors still seem to follow it.

That cardiac tests cannot always pinpoint the cause of chest pain only adds to the problem. Your doctor may tell you your chest pain is "all in your head." Since chest pain is sometimes caused by anxiety, this can compound the confusion. Further complicating matters is the fact that, of all cardiac symptoms, chest pain is the scariest. Pain in the chest makes the phrase "heart attack" leap to mind the way finding a lump in your breast raises instantaneous fears of breast cancer. But just as most breast lumps are not malignant, chest pain usually doesn't mean you have a heart problem. Read on; you'll discover there are ailments which manifest themselves as chest pain but aren't related to your heart at all.

DIAGNOSING CHEST PAIN

Your own observations can provide your doctor with the most useful clues of all. Doctors often forget this and order uncomfortable, expensive, and sometimes risky tests in lieu of spending the time to listen to you.

To understand chest pain, let's talk about how you perceive pain. You feel pain not directly, but as it is interpreted through your central nervous system. Your central nervous system is made up of your brain, spinal cord, and your peripheral nerves, which contain nerve cells, or neurons, within every part of your body. These neurons can be stimulated by an outside force, as, for example, when you stub your toe. Any stimulation along the pain pathway from your toe to your brain may also be perceived as "stubbed toe."

Another system of your body also comes into play here: your autonomic nervous system. This system regulates the functions of your body without your being aware of it, and can modify your perception of pain as well. The autonomic nervous system does some of its work through hormonelike substances, chemicals which your body secretes and which keep your body functioning smoothly.

Individuals vary in their responses to these substances. Take the hormone adrenaline. Caffeine serves as a stimulus for the production of adrenaline, but some people are more sensitive to the effects of this hormone than others. So while one cup of coffee is enough to give one person the jitters, another may guzzle cup after cup without much effect.

How you perceive cardiac pain depends in part on your sensitivity to adrenaline and another hormone substance, adenosine. Those who are more receptive may be hypersensitive to chest pain and feel rapid or skipped heartbeats more intensely.

Think of pain as a continuum. On one end are people with heart disease so advanced that they should feel excruciating pain, yet they feel nothing, a condition known as silent ischemia. On the other end of the continuum are those who experience severe chest pain for no known clinical cause. Both these groups suffer from malfunctions in their cardiac pain sensitivity. This sensitivity may affect the quality and intensity of pain you feel, whether it's caused by heart problems or by something that has nothing to do with your heart.

CHEST PAIN FROM CORONARY OBSTRUCTION

HEART ATTACK   A heart attack, medically known as a myocardial infarction, occurs when the flow of oxygenated blood to the heart is completely cut off, resulting in the injury of all or part of the heart muscle. Coronary artery disease is the most common cause of heart attack. A rarer cause is a sustained coronary spasm, which pinches off blood flow in arteries that appear otherwise healthy. For a detailed discussion of a heart attack, see Chapter 10.

ANGINA PECTORIS: "CLASSIC" HEART PAIN   Angina pectoris is the classic type of chest pain, which occurs when the heart muscle doesn't receive enough oxygen because of a narrowing in the coronary arteries. It most often occurs during physical exertion or "stress" and is similar to, but less severe than, the chest pain from a heart attack. Since the arteries are narrowed, but not blocked, the pain is relieved when the need for increased blood flow subsides.

Such pain is usually the result of coronary artery disease. If you're a young woman, it's unlikely, but by no means impossible, that you're experiencing it. Such pain can also result from coronary spasm, from malfunctioning heart valves, or from a congenital birth defect, although the mechanism that causes the pain is slightly different.

You may be having angina if:

* You experience pain which is dull, aching, tingling, or burning, or you experience tightness, squeezing, heaviness, constriction, or a sensation of pressure. You may instinctively clench your fist close to your heart when describing the pain.
* The pain sometimes moves around, often radiating from the middle of your chest, to the base of your neck, to your left shoulder, down either your left or right arm, or into your jaw and sometimes your shoulder blade.
* The pain lasts at least a few minutes and is relieved by rest, or by taking a nitroglycerin tablet under your tongue.
* The pain comes on when you're exerting yourself—running for a bus, exercising, carrying heavy bundles, walking in the cold, or climbing stairs. Or you may feel it in times of stress—during arguments or in an atmosphere of tension.
* With the pain, you may also feel anxious or unable to breathe.

> ♥ Lifesaving Tip: Even if you've only begun experienc-
> ing it, the pain from angina can be a signal that you may
> be close to suffering a heart attack. Do not delay; make
> an immediate appointment with your doctor.

VASOSPASTIC ANGINA　　Lately, almost every night at midnight, Irene's heart begins racing and keeps her up most of the night. The dull pain, which radiates to her back and down her arm, scares her because it's "just like the warning sign of a heart attack." When she manages to fall asleep, the chest pain awakens her. Her symptoms never come on when she's active, only when she's resting. Irene is experiencing the symptoms of vasospastic or variant angina, known also as Prinzmetal's angina for the doctor who first described it. This type of angina results from a blockage of blood flow to the heart caused not by permanent narrowing of the coronary arteries, but by a spasm of the coronary artery.

You may have vasospastic angina if:

· The nature and the location of the chest pain are similar to those of angina pectoris, but the pain occurs when you're at rest or in the early hours of the morning, sometimes repeatedly each night.
· The pain lasts longer, sometimes up to a half hour, and intensifies quickly.

Variant angina seems most often (but not always) to affect women who are relatively young and heavy smokers. Sometimes episodes seem to be brought on by stress; in Irene's case, she suspects that the burden of caring for her aging mother has contributed to her condition.

> ♥ Lifesaving Tip: If you're suffering from what appears
> to be angina, no matter what type it seems to be, be seen
> by a physician.

ATYPICAL CHEST PAIN SYNDROMES

Sometimes women experience chest pains which are caused by their heart but don't fall into these two larger categories of angina. These are known as atypical chest pain syndromes, and they can be among the most difficult problems to diagnose. A syndrome, by the way, is a group of symptoms which occur together and constitute a specific condition.

MICROVASCULAR ANGINA This is a type of chest pain which is not caused by disease of the larger coronary arteries or coronary spasm. It affects mostly women; according to one study, 72 percent of 200 patients suffering from this kind of pain were female. They weren't old, either; they ranged in age from twenty-eight to sixty-five, and their average age was forty-nine.

There are no specific tests to pinpoint this problem, and it doesn't turn up on X rays, which is why it can be so difficult to diagnose. The chest pain in this case results from problems in the functioning of your microvascular circulation system. This problem also goes by the somewhat mysterious-sounding name "Syndrome X."

Ever since the mid-1960s, when the problem was first recognized, the existence of Syndrome X has been hotly debated. Some believe this chest pain is psychological, but evidence is mounting that it does come from the heart. Dr. Philip M. Sarrel, a professor of obstetrics/gynecology and psychiatry at the Yale University School of Medicine, believes this type of chest pain may be caused by a decrease in estrogen during menopause and that, in some cases, may be eased by estrogen replacement therapy. In the past, it was also thought that this syndrome rarely developed into a serious heart problem, but this may not be the case.

Your heart receives blood from the large coronary blood vessels which are part of your cardiovascular circulatory system. But you also have a microcirculatory system, a network of tiny blood vessels that branch from the large coronary vessels and which in turn feed oxygen to each of the millions of cells which make up your heart. If these tiny vessels go into spasm and the blood flow is impeded, anginal chest pain results. If you're a person with heightened cardiac sensitivity, the pain will feel even worse.

This chest pain sometimes comes on during or after exertion and is indistinguishable from the pain of angina pectoris. It usually lasts at least thirty minutes. Diagnosing this problem is largely a matter of eliminating the most common cause of such pain, which is coronary artery disease. If you suffer from angina-type pain but have *absolutely* no risk factors for coronary heart disease, your doctor may decide to treat you for microvascular angina without ordering further tests. If there's a reason to suspect you may have coronary artery disease, you'll probably undergo further testing.

Although microvascular angina may not lead to serious heart problems, it can be disabling. Susan, a twenty-nine-year-old secretary, suffered chest pain so severe she often ended up in the emergency room before her problem was diagnosed. Fortunately, the chest pain of microvascular angina can often be relieved by using commonly available cardiovascular medication.

CHEST PAIN FROM MITRAL VALVE PROLAPSE Mitral valve prolapse, a common heart valve anomaly, sometimes results in chest pain, although the reason for this is not clearly understood. For more information, see Chapter 7.

You may have an atypical chest pain syndrome if:

· The pain occurs to the left and usually below the breast.
· The pain is usually achy, sharp, "knifelike," or stabbing. If dull, it may last hours; if sharp, only seconds.
· The first time you feel the pain it starts so suddenly you can remember what you were doing when it began; after that, it comes and goes.
· You may experience additional symptoms such as a pounding heartbeat, dizziness, and fatigue.

OTHER CARDIAC CAUSES OF CHEST PAIN

Chest pain from other causes related to your heart can sometimes occur. Two which are uncommon, but serious, are pericarditis and pulmonary hypertension.

PERICARDITIS "It felt like a knitting needle was sticking in my chest every time I took a breath," says Diane of the chest pain which suddenly appeared soon after she recovered from a bout with the flu. It turned out she had pericarditis, an inflammation of the membranous sac which encloses your heart. Pericarditis is usually caused by a viral infection, but it can also occur after a heart attack or open-heart surgery. On occasion, pericarditis occurs for no specific reason. Pericarditis is treated by bed rest and anti-inflammatory drugs, or, if required, steroids. If untreated, pericarditis can become very serious.

You may have pericarditis if:

- The pain comes on suddenly, sometimes after an upper-respiratory infection.
- The pain worsens if you take a deep breath.
- The pain worsens, or is relieved, if you change your posture.
- The pain is accompanied by fever.

PULMONARY HYPERTENSION This very serious type of high blood pressure develops within the blood vessels of your lungs and, if untreated, can lead to heart failure. It sometimes develops in the presence of lung disease or some types of congenital heart defects. A symptom of heart failure from pulmonary hypertension is a generalized swelling of your body, especially noticeable in your abdomen. Pulmonary hypertension is discussed further in Chapters 8 and 9.

NONCARDIAC CHEST PAIN: A CASE OF MISTAKEN IDENTITY

Remember Joanne, whose story was related early in this chapter? She learned that chest pain can be deceiving. Sometimes, although the pain you feel seems to come directly from your heart, that may not be the case at all.

How can this be? Since you perceive pain only as it is interpreted by your brain, your brain may misinterpret or confuse these signals, according to one theory which seeks to explain how some common noncardiac disorders can result in chest pain. Imagine your central nervous system as a telephone system, with a bundle of nerves encased by the spinal cord as the telephone lines, and your brain acting as the switchboard. Pain messages travel along the telephone lines, sometimes sharing them, as would callers on a party line. With all these messages traveling back and forth, occasionally the lines can get crossed. The result is pain from "signal confusion" or "mistaken identity."

Noncardiac causes of chest pain are:

- Esophageal dysfunction and spasm
- Osteoarthritis of the neck
- Gas in the colon
- Ulcers and gallbladder disease

ESOPHAGEAL DYSFUNCTION   Because your esophagus and your heart are so near one another, the theory of "signal confusion" explains why pain signals from your esophagus may be misinterpreted by your brain as coming from your heart. In fact, the symptoms of esophageal dysfunction often mimic the symptoms of pain from coronary artery disease. Such malfunctions can occur as esophageal spasms, or as reflux esophagitis, an inflammation of the esophagus caused by regurgitation of some of your stomach acid into your esophagus.

Your esophagus is a muscular tube which carries liquid and chewed food from the back of the throat to the stomach. Its function is to propel food downward into the stomach, where it is readied for passage into your small intestine. Your esophagus has muscular valves on each end which relax, allowing the food to pass through.

Normally, when food is not passing through, the lower valve remains closed. But if this lower valve does not shut tightly enough, some of the acidic contents from your stomach may splash back, irritating your esophagus and causing inflammation or sometimes spasm. The result can be chest pain.

Often, but not always, reflux esophagitis is seen in overweight women. Carrying packages against your stomach can cause extra pressure which aggravates this condition. So can smoking, anxiety, alcohol, and heavy meals. Some people with a hiatal hernia have this problem as well.

If your doctor suspects you have reflux esophagitis, you'll probably be referred to a gastroenterologist, a physician trained in the management of digestive system disorders. This specialist can perform a test called an esophagogastroscopy, an examination of the esophagus by means of a long, flexible viewing tube inserted through your mouth, which can determine whether the lining of your esophagus is inflamed. Even specialists have their preferred subspecialties, so ask your doctor to refer you to a gastroenterologist who prefers to concentrate on the esophagus.

Usually, just being reassured that you don't have a heart problem, watching your diet, and using some antacids will ease these symptoms. If not, such antiulcer medications as Zantac or Pepcid may provide relief. In the case of severe esophageal spasm, nitroglycerin may sometimes help, further confusing you and your doctor about the source of the pain. People who have increased pain sensitivity can suffer severely from this problem, while others may not even notice anything amiss.

OSTEOARTHRITIS OF THE NECK   Another kind of chest pain that's tricky to discern may occur if you have osteoarthritis of the neck. There, pain which actually originates in your neck may be interpreted as coming from the chest. In fact, this is one of the most common causes of chest pain in women, and may feel just like angina pectoris, the pain from coronary artery disease.

Known as wear and tear arthritis, osteoarthritis is the degenerative type of arthritis which occurs at various joints in your body. If this inflammation occurs in your neck, your body responds by forming calcium deposits, or "bony spurs," which are situated next to the pain neurons that carry pain messages from your chest. These spurs dig into the nerve, and the result is signal confusion, as your brain misinterprets these pain signals as radiating from your heart.

Although osteoarthritis is thought of as an elderly person's disease, it sometimes occurs in younger people, and tends to be inherited. You may have osteoarthritis of the neck if your chest pain occurs when you're carrying a briefcase or doing activities, such as rearranging furniture, that may strain your neck, or after such activities. Anti-inflammatory drugs, heat, neck traction, or other types of physical therapy may provide relief. A diagnosis of osteoarthritis of the neck can be confirmed by the presence of bony spurs seen on an X ray.

GAS IN THE COLON   An old-fashioned problem like gas can occasionally manifest itself as chest pain. In this case, gas becomes trapped in a loop of colon, or large bowel, located just under the left side of your diaphragm, the muscle which divides your abdominal and chest cavities. Distension of the loop of bowel and spasm probably produce the pain. This pain can be misinterpreted as coming from the heart because of the signal confusion discussed earlier.

If gas is a persistent problem, try to find out the cause. Excessive gas can be caused by irritable bowel syndrome (also called spastic colon), which is accompanied by alternating diarrhea and constipation. Another source of excessive gas is lactose intolerance, in which your body is unable to digest the lactose, or milk sugar, in dairy products. This condition also causes cramp, bloating, and diarrhea. Eating a dairy-free diet is the best way to ease symptoms from lactose intolerance.

ULCERS AND GALLBLADDER DISEASE   Peptic ulcers and gallbladder attacks can sometimes cause pain which mimics that associated with angina or a heart attack. To add to the confusion, heart attacks may often be associated with nausea and even vomiting, symptoms that are also associated with the gastrointestinal illness cited above. It's useful to note that pain from peptic ulcers generally occurs more in the lower central area of the chest than does the pain from coronary artery disease, and gallbladder pain more often occurs on the right side of the upper abdomen.

PAIN FROM YOUR CHEST WALL

SHINGLES   Anna, a sixty-nine-year-old woman, was brought to the doctor's office by her worried daughter, Ellen. Over the past several days, Anna had been suffering from sharp chest pains. Anna's husband of forty-five years had died recently of a heart attack, and Ellen was terrified her mother was going to die soon, too.

The pain Anna was experiencing did indeed resemble pain from coronary artery disease, but the cause was shingles, known medically as herpes zoster. Shingles is caused by the same virus that causes chicken pox. As a child, Anna had had chicken pox, and a few of the viral organisms remained dormant in her nervous system for years. The aging of Anna's body, coupled with the stress of her husband's death, provided the virus with the perfect conditions to become reactivated. The excruciatingly painful disease of shingles was the result.

Shingles manifests itself in a telltale rash, but it may not occur until several weeks after the chest pain has begun. An astute doctor can often diagnose shingles based on details about the pain and when it occurred. For example, the pain of shingles characteristically begins under the left arm and radiates around the back. It may start as vague discomfort; the sufferer may think she's pulled a muscle, but instead of disappearing, the pain gets worse.

Shingles is not easy to treat, can cause unbearable pain, and can recur. An antiviral treatment called acyclovir (Zovirax), if started early enough, can be helpful. Until recently, there was no treatment for the painful rash; however, an ointment called capsaicin, made from a derivative of hot peppers, has been found to help. An antidepressant drug called amitriptyline can also relieve the pain.

MUSCULAR PAIN

Very buxom women may suffer chest pain from the weight of their breasts. Sometimes chest pain arises from problems with the muscular and skeletal structure of the chest.

Your rib cage is interconnected with cartilage, a type of hard, rubbery tissue which enables your ribs to flex against the other bony structures of your rib cage. If these rib joints become inflamed, a painful condition called costochondritis can result. It can cause chest pain and lead you to fear you may have breast cancer. Sometimes costochondritis is caused by a virus which follows a respiratory flulike illness, but it can also occur for no apparent reason. A doctor can often diagnose this problem because of a characteristic tenderness. Costrochondritis is treated similarly to arthritis, with heat, anti-inflammatory drugs such as aspirin, and, in severe cases, steroids. For persistent problems, a long-acting steroid is sometimes injected. Tietze's syndrome, a similar type of pain and swelling of the rib joints, is also treated with heat and anti-inflammatory drugs.

CHEST PAIN FROM ANXIETY

From an era when too many women were told their chest pain was "all in your head" and too many tranquilizers were prescribed, we've moved into an era when the pendulum is in danger of swinging too far over to the other side. The simple fact is that there are many different causes for chest pain, and anxiety remains one of them.

In the same way that anxiety can cause a tension headache, it can also tighten the muscles in your chest wall. Tension can also contribute to spasms of both your large coronary blood vessels and the vessels of your microvascular circulatory system. The result can be chest pain.

If your doctor tells you that your chest pain stems from anxiety, don't immediately dismiss the idea. Think about it. Sometimes we don't recognize anxiety in ourselves. It might be worthwhile to seek an evaluation from an expert, such as a psychologist, a psychiatrist, or a psychiatric social worker. Avoid a self-proclaimed therapist or someone who tends to view all problems through a favorite therapeutic prism, such as believing all symptoms are related to allergies which can be cured by dietary changes. If you're convinced anxiety is not the cause, you can choose to return to your original doctor and request a further evaluation. If you are rebuffed or think your symptoms aren't being taken seriously, go to another doctor.

OTHER SYMPTOMS

While chest pain is the most common, and usually the scariest, of symptoms which may seem to be originating in your heart, other symptoms can accompany heart problems as well. They can be caused by coronary artery disease or occur in the presence of other heart problems, such as valvular disease or congenital defects. Such symptoms can occur alone, or you may suffer from two, three, or even all of them.

PALPITATIONS

Alicia, the twenty-nine-year-old owner of a fashionable women's clothing shop, was in the midst of compiling her monthly inventory report when her heart began to pound. It happened again a few weeks later, while she was reading, then again the following week, while she was window-shopping after work. "I just felt like my heart was beating so hard, it was coming out of my chest," she recalls. Alicia discovered she had an arrhythmia, or a disturbance of her heartbeat's rhythm.

Most of us experience arrhythmias all the time and don't even notice them. When you become aware of them, they're called palpitations. The sensation of palpitations has been described as a heart that seems to bump, pound, jump, flop, flutter, or race.

There are different types of arrhythmias, ranging from harmless ones to some which are very serious and can even result in death. If you have an arrhythmia, your doctor will want to determine what type it is and whether it requires treatment. You may have a serious type of palpitation when:

- The palpitation occurs in association with pain or causes severe shortness of breath.
- The palpitation is associated with fainting or severe lightheadedness.
- The palpitation lasts for many hours.
- There is a history of unexplained sudden death of young people in your family.

Arrhythmias are discussed further in Chapter 10.

FAINTING

Laura, a twenty-two-year-old who was working in her first advertising job after graduating from college, passed out in a Manhattan bar where she'd gone with some friends after work. She regained consciousness within minutes and forgot about it until a few weeks later, when she passed out again at work and was brought to a hospital emergency room. Her parents were beside themselves with worry, as was she. "I know there must be something wrong with me, because I've never had fainting spells before," she said.

Fainting can be one of the most frightening of symptoms. It can also be very dangerous if you fall and hurt yourself or faint while driving. But the reason behind most fainting spells is not serious. Medically known as syncope, fainting is a temporary loss of consciousness due to insufficient oxygen reaching the brain.

VASOVAGAL SYNCOPE Laura's case, frightening as it was, turned out to be caused by the harmless syndrome called vasovagal syncope. Typically, vasovagal syncope is caused by overstimulation of the vagus nerve, a major nerve which runs from the brain to the stomach and helps control breathing and blood circulation.

This type of fainting can be triggered by many conditions. Fear or anxiety bring it about in some people; they faint when they hear bad news, or visit the dentist, or see blood. Such fainting can also be brought on by being in a hot, stuffy room, eating a large meal, taking a hot bath, exercising if you're dehydrated or have been hyperventilating, or even straining to have a bowel movement. Episodes of syncope are usually preceded by a brief feeling of warmth, lightheadedness, nausea, and impending collapse. Such fainting spells are relatively harmless and leave no ill effects.

Sometimes women suffer from fainting if their blood pressure falls when they change position abruptly, such as standing up after sitting or lying down. Such episodes can also be a side effect of some forms of antidepressants or drugs to control high blood pressure, or can be caused by nerve damage from diabetes. This type of syncope is called postural hypotension.

While many women occasionally suffer a fainting spell, others can faint with such frequency that their lives become disrupted. This was the case with Mary Ann, a twenty-three-year-old who adores riding roller coasters but has been known to faint when she's doing nothing more strenuous than fixing her hair.

Because of her fainting spells, Mary Ann is participating in a research project run by Dr. Fetnat M. Fouad-Tarazi, who specializes in cardiovascular disease and hypertension at the Cleveland Clinic. When Mary Ann's feet are tilted downward on a tilt table, she can be diagnosed and the underlying circulatory abnormalities can be identified. By studying patients like Mary Ann, Dr. Fouad-Tarazi is hoping to find information to help patients like her.

FAINTING FROM CARDIAC CAUSES   Some heart problems can manifest themselves as fainting. You may have a serious form of fainting if you pass out suddenly, without the warning period of lightheadedness, dizziness, and nausea—one instant you're fine and the next you're on the floor. This type of fainting can indicate a problem with your heart valve or can be a sign of a dangerous arrhythmia. Such problems can even result in sudden death.

> ♥ Lifesaving Tip: If you're in good health and you faint in a hot, crowded room or if you're anxious or scared, check with your doctor, but don't be unduly alarmed. If, on the other hand, you suffer an unexplained fainting spell, or faint repeatedly, and you have heart or circulatory problems or have risk factors for a heart attack or stroke, contact your doctor immediately.

SHORTNESS OF BREATH

Pearl, a sixty-two-year-old town librarian, enjoyed walks with her friend. Lately, though, she'd had to stop frequently to rest. Her husband noticed her huffing and puffing and insisted she see a doctor. The doctor determined that her shortness of breath stemmed from a failing heart valve, the result of rheumatic fever she'd suffered as a child, and the valve had to be replaced. "My shortness of breath came on so gradually I barely noticed it," Pearl says. "I just assumed it was because I was getting older."

As a sign of cardiac problems, shortness of breath, or, as it is termed medically, "dyspnea," can be difficult to pin down. It can come on suddenly or gradually. It can stem from a problem with the heart or with the lungs.

But shortness of breath doesn't always indicate a health problem. Sometimes it's a problem of perception. For example, if you were a star tennis player in college, when you pick up a racket again five years after you graduate, you may find yourself short of breath. Most likely, this simply means you're out of condition. Or if you're older, your body is unable to transform oxygen into energy as efficiently as it used to, so you probably can't walk to the store as briskly as you once did.

Since everyone can become short of breath under certain circumstances, you need to figure out whether your shortness of breath is normal. One way to do this is to see how you feel when you climb one, two, or three flights of stairs. Virtually everyone, no matter how young or old, should be able to climb one flight of stairs and feel only slightly winded, if at all. If you can't, you should tell your doctor. Another form of shortness of breath which may indicate a heart problem occurs when you're lying down, or can awaken you from sleep. If this occurs, and you do not have allergies or asthma which can make sleeping uncomfortable, see your doctor.

If you're short of breath, ask yourself:

· Could your shortness of breath be due to overweight, poor physical conditioning, asthma, or allergies?
· Under what conditions do you get short of breath? Exercising? Relaxing? Sleeping?
· Try to quantify your shortness of breath. Can you climb one flight of stairs without becoming uncomfortable? Two?

♥ Lifesaving Tip: You should contact your doctor if just walking up one flight of stairs makes you very short of breath, you awaken from sleep short of breath, or you have a heart problem and become very short of breath.

FATIGUE

Ellen, a thirty-four-year-old divorced mother of three, juggles her free-lance writing assignments with teaching and research jobs. She's so tired, she's tempted to fall into bed right after dinner. Her friend Pam, a newly minted accountant, works sixty-hour weeks trying to become a partner in her national firm. Pam's sister, Sally, a medical secretary, works full-time, makes a gourmet dinner for her husband when she comes home, then cleans the house. She's exhausted, too. Such instances are so common it's no wonder "chronic sleep deprivation" is becoming our new national malady.

Given all this, it's important to remember that there are plenty of reasons for being tired besides problems having to do with your heart. But since cardiac problems can manifest themselves as fatigue, it's important to determine whether you're just plain tired or may be sick.

As with shortness of breath, perception can come into play here. If you were once an avid ballroom dancer and start whirling around the floor after an absence of ten years, it's normal to get tired quickly. But if you're accustomed to dancing the night away every Saturday and suddenly find yourself spent after a dance or two, that could signal a problem.

If you're always tired, ask yourself:

- Are you sleepy? If you're working very hard, or juggling many activities, and you're ready for bed at 6:30, you probably are suffering from a shortage of sleep.
- Are you depressed? Depression is a very common cause of fatigue, and may come upon you without your realizing it. Some other signs of serious depression are insomnia, crying spells, and suicidal thoughts. If this is happening to you, or you realize you're seriously depressed, seek help.
- Are you eating right? If you're too busy, it's also very likely you're skipping meals or eating on the run. A faulty diet may be the cause of your fatigue.
- Is your hair coarse and brittle and your skin dry, and has your sex drive gradually disappeared? If so, you may have an underactive thyroid gland.
- Do you have other symptoms, such as fever, unexplained weight loss, and loss of appetite? While you may not have a

heart problem, you may have another serious illness, such as mononucleosis, acute hepatitis, or even cancer. Make an appointment to see your doctor immediately.
- Have you suddenly become exhausted by doing the things you're accustomed to doing? If so, seeing your doctor is in order.

SWELLING

Edema, or swelling, can occur throughout your body. In women, the most common cause is the type of bloating you can experience just before your menstrual period. Peripheral venous disease, in which the veins of the leg become narrowed, can also result in swelling. However, edema can also be a sign of congestive heart failure. In this case, it's usually first noticed in the feet and ankles and progressively worsens. If you have this type of progressive swelling, see your doctor.

A HEART MURMUR

For as long as I could remember, I had a heart murmur, but it was "nothing to worry about." It was not until I was forty that a doctor appreciated the significance of my murmur and referred me for tests which showed I had a congenital heart defect. This heart defect, if it had gone untreated, could have shortened my life.

Technically, a heart murmur is not a symptom which you feel; it's a clinical finding discovered by listening to your heart with a stethoscope. However, we're including heart murmur in this chapter because it can provide an important clue whose significance is sometimes overlooked.

Normally your heartbeat consists of two sounds, made by the opening and closing of your heart valves as blood passes through them. This sounds basically like "lub" followed by "dub," or together, "lub-dub." With a stethoscope these sounds can be heard more clearly, along with any abnormal additional sounds, some of which are called heart murmurs. When they don't represent a significant problem, they are termed "innocent" murmurs. However, other heart murmurs can indicate such problems as a malfunctioning heart valve or a congenital heart defect.

Years ago, doctors were often reluctant to mention to patients that they had heart murmurs because they were concerned that the news would turn otherwise healthy adults into cardiac invalids. Today diagnostic procedures can determine whether or not your heart murmur denotes a serious problem.

To check out your heart murmur further, you may need to undergo an echocardiogram. If your doctor demurs, consider asking for a referral to a cardiologist. Your heart murmur may very well be "innocent," but it's always good practice to know for certain. Dr. Eliot Rosenkranz, a Cleveland Clinic surgeon who specializes in correction of congenital heart defects in adults, notes, "Over the years, we've found that many of these 'innocent' murmurs were in fact not so innocent."

> ♥ Lifesaving Tip: It's common for children and adolescents to have "innocent" heart murmurs; pregnant women have them as well. If, however, you're not among these groups and have been told you have a heart murmur, you should consider having it checked further. If the murmur turns out indeed to be "innocent," so much the better.

To sum up: The symptoms discussed in this chapter are the most common seen with heart problems, but they may not signify a problem with your heart at all. The only person who can determine for certain what's going on is your doctor. Remember, though, that your doctor depends on you for an accurate description of your problem.

If you have a problem which may be serious, don't delay in seeking your doctor's advice because you're scared. Heart problems are scary— believe me, I know. But today, virtually all heart problems can be treated. If you develop a heart problem and, like me, learn about it in time, your heart problem can be treated, and possibly even resolved, before your heart has been irreversibly damaged.

6
Diagnostic Differences

Over the years, diagnostic testing has become highly sophisticated, enabling doctors to peer ever more closely into the workings of the human heart. But the best diagnostic tools in the world can't help you if you're not referred for them. Let us tell you about Hope, an energetic woman with a spunky personality befitting her clouds of red hair. A few years before, she had been treated for cancer, but had recovered. Now, she was in despair. She felt poorly, but her concerns were dismissed repeatedly by her family doctor, who kept telling her, "Don't worry, your test results say you're fine."

About six months before, she'd gone to the doctor complaining of exhaustion, shortness of breath, and an achy feeling in her chest. Her doctor admitted her to the hospital for three days of testing, most of which were aimed at ruling out a recurrence of cancer, although a few heart tests were included. When the results came in, her doctor called her into his office, reeled them off, told Hope she was fine, and sent her on her way. But Hope continued to feel below par. She even considered canceling a trip to New York to visit her daughter, who lives in a fourth-story walk-up—the thought of climbing all those stairs filled Hope with dread. Then one day, by chance, Hope picked up a magazine article on women and heart disease. She was shocked. "It was a revelation," she recalls. "I realized I was reading about myself."

She immediately returned to her doctor, who, still insisting that all her test results were fine, told her he would reluctantly test her heart further, as she says, "if it would make me happy." The results clearly showed that Hope was suffering from advanced coronary artery disease. She was admitted to the hospital immediately, where she underwent balloon angioplasty to widen her dangerously narrowed coronary arteries.

"The first time, I didn't question my doctor; in fact, I didn't even know what tests he did," Hope says. "But I ask a lot of questions now."

VISITING THE CARDIOLOGIST

If you suspect you may have a heart problem, the diagnostic procedure actually starts before you undergo your first test. Today doctors too often substitute uncomfortable, expensive, and sometimes risky tests for an in-depth interview with you about your complaints. A detailed recitation of your symptoms, and your risk factors for heart disease, can go a long way to help an astute doctor arrive at the right diagnosis.

> ♥ **Lifesaving Tip: Be wary if, on your first meeting, your cardiologist sends you off on a round of testing without taking time to talk to you. A good physician, like a good detective, ferrets out clues. Only then does the doctor develop a hypothesis, or a tentative diagnosis, and order tests to confirm it.**

Whatever your problem, important clues to its nature may be hidden in your family's medical history. While it isn't necessary to become a walking encyclopedia of every ailment that ever befell a family member, you should know about major illnesses, and the causes of death, of your grandparents, parents, brothers, and sisters. If you don't, try to do a little familial sleuthing before you visit your doctor.

Consider also your own medical background, taking into account your own risk factors for heart disease, as well as any serious illnesses you had as a child. Childhood ailments that can cause heart problems later in life include rheumatic fever, scarlet fever, streptococcal infections, and Kawasaki disease (an increasingly common disease of unknown origin which occurs mostly in children and can result in heart problems).

Answer questions about your lifestyle honestly: whether you smoke, your diet, how much you exercise, and whether you're under unusual stress. All of us (your doctor included) wish we followed a more exemplary lifestyle, but this is not the time to cover up possibly important clues.

On your first visit to a cardiologist, expect an extensive interview and a physical examination. Like creating a picture with broad, fast strokes, these procedures provide the doctor with a general picture of your cardiac health. Then, if needed, diagnostic tests can be used to fill in important details.

THE PHYSICAL EXAMINATION

When performed by a skilled physician, even such seemingly casual measures as checking the color of your fingernails can yield a wealth of information about the health of your heart. Bluish lips or nails, swollen feet, warm or cold skin, or erratic pulse all provide clues.

About the only diagnostic tool your doctor will employ at this point is the stethoscope, still an unbeatable device for listening to your heart. Abnormal sounds, such as a heart murmur, can focus suspicion on such conditions as mitral valve prolapse or a congenital heart defect. At the end of the exam, you should expect your doctor to give you a tentative diagnosis and explain the course of testing needed to confirm it.

This chapter discusses the most commonly performed cardiac tests, along with a few which are less often done, but which you may encounter. They're grouped according to the conditions they're most commonly used to diagnose. Many cardiac tests, though, are multipurpose. For example, a cardiac catheterization can be used not only to diagnose coronary artery disease, but also to gauge the blood pressure within your heart if you have a congenital heart defect. We've noted whether the tests require preparation, but it's always a good idea to ask your doctor, or the lab where you'll take the test, to find out whether you need to take any preparatory measures, such as fasting.

> ♥ Mindsaving Tip: No matter what test you're taking, you'll probably have to wait, so bring along a book or something else to occupy your time.

> ♥ Mindsaving Tip: If you're seeing a new doctor or visiting a consultant for a second opinion, you may be asked to undergo tests you've already had. Ask whether you may bring the earlier test results with you. There are various reasons that those results may be unsuitable, but if they can be used, you can save yourself time, money, and inconvenience. Hand-carry your tests to their next destination, rather than relying on their being sent, even if you're going for treatment out of town.

A note on test terminology: Two words you'll often hear when cardiac tests, or any medical tests for that matter, are discussed are "noninvasive" and "invasive." Noninvasive tests do not involve penetration into your body. Such tests generally carry very little risk and are pain-free; they account for the majority of cardiac tests. Invasive tests do involve such penetration. They generally carry a small degree of risk, can be uncomfortable, and are more expensive. Sometimes, though, there's no substitute for them; cardiac catheterization, the definitive test for coronary artery disease, is one example. In this chapter, you can assume that the tests discussed are noninvasive unless otherwise noted.

BASIC TESTS

Basic tests such as a blood pressure reading, a cholesterol test, a chest X ray, and an electrocardiogram are commonly done when you visit a cardiologist. You probably are familiar with them from visiting your regular physician.

BLOOD PRESSURE

In the same way that the chambers of your heart respond to the electrical signals generated by your heart's electrical system, your heart also responds to changes in the system of pressures within it. These pressures are recorded when you have your blood pressure taken. Your blood pressure reading consists of a top and a bottom number. The top number is recorded at the time of highest pressure, after the aortic valve opens to allow blood to rush from the heart into the rest of your body; this is the systolic pressure. The bottom number, the diastolic pressure, denotes the point when your aortic valve closes and your heart is starting to fill with blood.

Your doctor measures these readings with a sphygmomanometer (blood pressure cuff) and a stethoscope. If your blood pressure is elevated, it indicates your heart is working harder than normal, putting both your heart and arteries under greater strain.

CHOLESTEROL PROFILE

For years the government has waged a public education campaign to persuade people to know their cholesterol numbers. There are two common types of cholesterol tests: a so-called "finger-prick" test, which is often done at health fairs and shopping malls, and the "lipid profile," a more extensive test taken in your doctor's lab. Lipids, and their significance, are discussed in Chapter 3.

Should your cholesterol pattern be checked? If your physician includes such a test in a routine physical, by all means have it done. If your physician doesn't include it, should you insist on having it performed? That depends. The American Heart Association recommends that everyone have his or her lipoprotein profile (or "lipid" profile for short) done at the age of twenty, and every five years after that until the age of sixty, after which it becomes optional. If you have not yet reached menopause and have *no* other risk factors for coronary disease, knowing your total cholesterol level from a finger-prick test should suffice. Such tests are subject to error; if you have the test at a health fair or in a mall, as opposed to a doctor's office, and your cholesterol total is above 220, have the test repeated. If your level is still over 220, see your doctor for a lipid profile.

If, however, you have significant risk factors for coronary disease, particularly if your family has a history of early heart disease or abnormal cholesterol levels (known also as hyperlipidemia), or if you have other risk factors such as over-weight or diabetes, you should consider having your lipid profile checked. This is a relatively simple blood test, although it requires you to have blood drawn from your arm rather than a finger-prick. You need to fast for about twelve hours beforehand.

> ♥ **Mindsaving Tip: There's a common misconception that you must fast before a finger-prick total cholesterol-level test. You needn't. This test can be performed without any special preparation.**

CHEST X RAY

Among the oldest of cardiac tests, the chest X ray can provide very revealing information. It can show whether your heart is enlarged, and sometimes can indicate a congenital heart condition. Taking the test is easy; you just stand against the film cassette and pictures of your chest are taken from different vantage points. The amount of radiation you receive from a chest X ray is considered minimal and within a safe standard—with one important exception: **if you know you're pregnant or think you may be.** The radiation from a chest X ray may damage your unborn baby. Inform your doctor so that other tests can be substituted.

ELECTROCARDIOGRAM

Picture the busy emergency room portrayed in any television medical drama: Most likely, there's a patient being wheeled in on a stretcher while the doctor barks, "Get me an EKG." He's talking about an electrocardiogram, referred to most commonly as an EKG or ECG.

For this test, a technician dabs a bit of conductive jelly on various points along your bare arms, legs, and chest and painlessly applies several electrodes. Each electrode conveys a signal from your heart, which is displayed on a graph. Together, the signals provide such information as the size of your cardiac chambers, whether you have reasonably normal heart rhythms, and whether your heart may have suffered any muscle damage from a previous heart attack. Often a resting electrocardiogram can indicate that an abnormality exists, but cannot pinpoint the exact cause. An EKG also records symptoms which occur only while you're at rest, not chest pain or the pounding heart that can come on when you're hurrying the kids out the door in the morning or running for a bus.

If you're a relatively young woman experiencing heart problems, they're most likely to involve the structure of your heart itself, or its rhythm. The following are the tests commonly used to diagnose such problems.

DIAGNOSING STRUCTURAL HEART PROBLEMS

The structures that make up your heart are crucial to your well-being. To evaluate these structures, the echocardiogram is an unbeatable diagnostic tool.

ECHOCARDIOGRAM

If you consider that your heart is a pulsing organ submerged in the fluidlike environment of your body, you can understand how useful a device that reads sound waves can be. A procedure called a transthoracic echocardiogram, or "echo" for short, uses the sound waves produced by your heart to create an image of it. If you've had children, you're probably familiar with a sonogram, which is basically the same procedure.

To undergo an echocardiogram, you lie on your side on an examining table while a technician moves a sound probe around your chest to various positions. The probe, called the transducer, transmits and then picks up small pulses of ultrasound which reflect off your heart. These sounds are then amplified and visually displayed on a screen. The echocardiagram shows how efficiently your heart and its valves are working, the direction in which the blood is flowing, and the size of your cardiac chambers. It draws a picture of the overall health of your heart muscle.

Echocardiograms are relatively reliable in women, although if you have large breasts, they may insulate your heart, producing a fuzzy image that is more difficult to interpret. Even if breast size is not a problem, the probe still has to "see" through layers of muscle and fat; newer approaches are being developed to provide more precise pictures of your heart.

TRANSESOPHAGEAL ECHOCARDIOGRAM

This measurement provides a clearer image than the traditional echo because the sound waves are actually transmitted from inside your body. In most cases, a traditional echocardiogram is sufficient, but if, for example, a hard-to-see part of a valve must be examined, the transesophageal echo is used. For this type of echo, you actually swallow a smaller version of the probe used in the traditional echocardiogram. You're given a mild sedative to relax you first, and your throat is anesthetized so that you don't gag. The probe then rests inside the esophagus, where it provides a crystal-clear view of your heart. This procedure carries a slightly increased risk because of the slim possibility that you may react to the sedative, or that some bacteria may be introduced into your body via the probe.

While extremely beneficial in studying your heart's structure, echocardiograms done at rest are not especially useful in the diagnosis of coronary artery blockage. However, doctors are finding that the combination of an echocardiogram with an exercise stress test, commonly called an exercise echocardiogram, is quite accurate in women. This test is discussed later in this chapter, under "Tests to Diagnose Coronary Artery Disease." An echocardiogram may also provide useful information in diagnosing and following the clinical course of a heart attack.

TESTS TO DIAGNOSE DISTURBANCES OF HEART RHYTHM

A broad category of problems which tend to affect women more than men are disturbances in the functioning of the heart's electrical system, which regulates the rhythm of the heartbeat and keeps the heart operating perfectly. Called arrhythmias, these disturbances can produce such frightening symptoms as fainting, palpitations, shortness of breath, and chest pain.

ELECTROCARDIOGRAM

The electrocardiogram, explained earlier in this chapter, is probably the first test you'll have if you experience such symptoms. The problem is that if you don't show the symptoms while you're undergoing the procedure, your heartbeat may look normal. That's what happened to Denise, a school nurse. Every time Denise began rushing around to get her three children ready for school in the morning, she says, "My heart started pounding and I felt faint."

Since Denise never experienced symptoms while she was lying down, her echocardiogram results were normal. So, her doctor suggested she wear a Holter monitor, a device which would record her heartbeat for twenty-four hours while she went about her everyday activities. Sure enough, as Denise was scrambling to get her kids off the next morning, her symptoms returned. The Holter monitor revealed that she suffered from an arrhythmia, one which was not serious and was easily treated.

HOLTER MONITOR

The Holter monitor, a small device like a tape recorder, is worn slung over your shoulder or at your waist. The monitor is attached to your chest by five leads. If you're asked to wear the monitor, you'll also be instructed to keep a diary of your activities, noting when symptoms occur. The diary and Holter measurements are analyzed later by your doctor to determine whether you have an arrhythmia, whether or not it's serious, and what measures, if any, should be taken to treat it.

> ♥ **Mindsaving Tip: If you're concerned about others being aware that you're undergoing a cardiac test, you should be able to conceal the Holter monitor fairly easily beneath your clothing.**

TILT STUDY, OR TILT-TABLE TEST

This test has proved very valuable in determining why some people experience blackouts or dizziness. The test is quite simple. You lie on a special table in a quiet, dark room. Your feet are lowered gradually to sixty degrees and your head is tilted upward to the same angle, movements which simulate the changes in your body that occur when you shift your position. During the test, your blood pressure and pulse are monitored, and special blood tests are sometimes performed.

The results can reveal irregularities in your body's vascular regulating system, and in the way your body automatically adjusts itself to changes in posture, such as standing up after you've been lying down. If your body reacts normally, you can change your position without any thought, but in women with vasoregulatory irregularities, such as those sometimes associated with mitral valve prolapse, such changes in posture can bring on dizziness or fainting.

ELECTROPHYSIOLOGIC STUDY

If your doctor suspects you have a serious arrhythmia, or rhythm disturbance, an electrophysiologic study, known commonly as EPS, may be ordered. This is an invasive test that's done in a manner similar to cardiac catheterization, which is described later in this chapter. In an EPS, however, wires are threaded inside your heart to stimulate it electronically in hopes of making the arrhythmia appear. Since this is an invasive test, and not without risk, it's performed only when there is concern that you might develop a life-threatening arrhythmia, or in some cases when the rhythm problem is very disabling and resistant to treatment. For an EP study, you're conscious, but sedated. The preparations are basically the same as those outlined in the section on cardiac catheterization.

TESTS TO DIAGNOSE CORONARY ARTERY DISEASE

Diagnosing coronary artery disease (known also as coronary heart disease or simply coronary disease) has proved more difficult in women than in men. One reason for this is that the exercise stress test, commonly used to diagnose coronary artery disease, appears less accurate when performed on women than on men. Since the stress test is a major method of diagnosing coronary artery disease, you should be aware of different types of stress tests and their pros and cons when used on women.

EXERCISE STRESS TEST

The purpose of the exercise stress test, commonly referred to simply as a stress test, is to evaluate the way your heart responds to the physical stress of exercise—walking and jogging on a tread-mill or pedaling a stationary bicycle. Before the test begins, leads are attached to your chest, as in an EKG, so that changes in your heartbeat can be monitored. Your blood pressure is also mea-sured. You begin exercising at a slow pace and gradually speed up. If you're unfamiliar with a treadmill, don't worry—you'll soon get used to it. If you have severe arthritis or some other con-dition which makes it impossible to exercise with your legs, a drug can be used to alternatively increase the stress on your heart.

> ♥ **Mindsaving Tip:** If you've suffered a heart attack, have recently undergone cardiac surgery, or are experi-encing chest pain or other symptoms, you may be wor-ried that such exercise could be too much of a strain. Relax: During the test, you're carefully monitored, and the test is halted immediately if you're in any danger.

Research has shown that, in women, the exercise stress test alone is too inaccurate to be used as the sole determinant of coronary artery disease. Even when stringent measures are taken, this test has proved inaccurate in women about one-third of the time. There are better tests to determine whether you have coronary ar-tery disease which are discussed later in this chapter.

The problem with the exercise stress test for women is that it too often mistakenly diagnoses coronary disease. This can occur for two reasons: first because although most women and men ex-perience chest pain, in women—particularly in relatively young women—it's less likely that the pain is caused by coronary dis-ease; and second because during exercise, a healthy woman's heartbeat may display changes characteristic of a woman with coronary disease. Precisely why this happens is not known, but it may relate to the fact that women respond differently to exercise than do men. Some researchers believe a woman's fluctuating es-trogen levels may contribute to the response. Dr. Bernard R. Chaitman, chief of cardiology at St. Louis University Medical Center, says, "Some studies have shown that, if you study women through their menstrual cycle, at some points in the month, the exercise electrocardiogram tends to be abnormal."

In interpreting a test that indicates coronary disease, then, a cardiologist takes into consideration the woman's risk factors for coronary disease, as well as how markedly abnormal the test result is. "If a woman is a heavy smoker, is diabetic, is fifty-two years old, and has chest pain, and the test is markedly abnormal, you'd pay attention to a test like that," Dr. Chaitman says. "But if it is a thirty-five-year-old woman who does not have risk factors and the test is only mildly abnormal, you wouldn't be as concerned about it."

This doesn't mean you should refuse to take an exercise stress test; rather, you should discuss with your doctor the purpose for which it's being performed. Although a stress test alone is not accurate enough to pinpoint the existence of coronary artery disease, it's more precise in determining that no such problem is present. So if you have chest pain, a negative test result can be reassuring. The test can also demonstrate that you have a normal capacity and physical response to exercise, or that such activity brings about such symptoms as chest discomfort, shortness of breath, or an irregular heartbeat.

> ♥ **Mindsaving Tip:** If you're asked to take a stress test in a health or fitness club, for a purpose other than testing your exercise capability, you should decline. When used as a broad screening tool for heart disease, these tests are notoriously inaccurate and can cause you unnecessary alarm.

To prepare for your exercise stress test:

- Fast for about four hours before the test. You can drink water.
- For accurate results, your doctor may want you to discontinue certain medications temporarily. Otherwise, continue to take your medications as prescribed.
- Wear loose, comfortable pants or shorts and rubber-soled shoes. A hospital gown will be supplied to cover you on top.
- If you're expecting your period and prefer not to strenuously exercise while you're having it, postpone the test. If exercise doesn't bother you, however, go ahead with the test. (This holds true for all forms of exercise testing.)
- Be prepared for a wait. The test itself usually takes about ninety minutes.

EXERCISE ECHOCARDIOGRAM

The echocardiogram is a particularly fine device for examining the structure of the heart. But when it's done while you're at rest, as it traditionally has been, it can't determine to what degree your coronary arteries may be blocked. However, some exciting research studies have shown that when an echocardiogram is performed in combination with a stress test, the result is a sensitive and reliable procedure for diagnosing coronary artery disease in women. The exercise echocardiogram becomes a most cost-effective and convenient way of providing a comprehensive evaluation of your heart. Most importantly, recent studies show that it's equally reliable when used on women and men, regardless of age or body weight.

The test begins with a technician performing a brief version of an echocardiogram, to obtain images of your heart at rest. Then you undergo an exercise stress test, exerting yourself on a stationary bike or treadmill until your heart reaches its peak rate. At that point, you get off the exercise machine and return to the examination table nearby, where a second echocardiogram is performed.

By comparing the images of your heart at rest with those after exercise, your doctor can evaluate any changes that may indicate coronary artery disease. This test does not furnish images of your actual coronary arteries, however, so if you do indeed have blocked or narrowed arteries, cardiac catheterization, an invasive test discussed later, is still needed to assess the extent of the disease and the methods of treatment.

Exercise echocardiography is proving more accurate and less expensive than thallium stress testing (discussed below). However, since the thallium test has traditionally been more widely used, it may take some time before the exercise echo catches on. Whichever your doctor's choice, the important thing to remember is that both provide noninvasive, risk-free, and relatively effective means of diagnosing coronary artery disease in women.

To prepare for your exercise echocardiogram, follow the steps outlined for the stress test related to fasting, medication, and clothing. This test usually takes about two and a half to three hours.

THALLIUM STRESS TESTING

This test, which combines an exercise stress test with a nuclear scanning procedure, is a better way of diagnosing coronary artery disease in women than an exercise stress test alone; instead of relying solely on a graphic depiction of your heartbeat, the test also produces images of your heart. Before the test, an intravenous drip (IV) will be attached to your hand.

This test begins just like an ordinary exercise test: You exercise on a treadmill or stationary bike until your heart reaches its maximum rate. Then, thallium, a safe radioactive tracer, is injected via the IV and you're taken over to an imaging table. You lie perfectly still on the table, your arms stretched above your head, while the camera circles you, taking pictures. After the picture-taking, you'll still be required to fast, but you'll be allowed to get up and possibly even leave and go about your business. Four hours later, you'll return for a second set of picture-taking, similar to the first.

Here's what happens during the procedure: On entering your bloodstream, the thallium heads for your heart. If there is no blockage or narrowing, it flows freely and highlights all of your heart muscle, which shows up on the special X-ray image. If part of your heart appears to be missing in the first set of images, it indicates that the thallium did not reach all of your heart because one or more arteries are narrowed or blocked. By the time the second set of images is taken, the usual flow of blood should have resumed, and the images of your heart should look normal.

Though a thallium stress test is much more accurate than an exercise stress test alone, it's still not perfect. If you have large breasts, your breast tissue may diffuse the radioactive energy of the thallium and make it appear that the thallium is not being fully absorbed, leading to the mistaken impression that you have coronary artery disease. But this happens far less often than in exercise testing without thallium.

To prepare for your thallium test, follow the preparatory steps for the regular exercise stress test, and add these measures:

· Fast overnight, or several hours before the test if it's scheduled for later in the day. And no coffee!
· Plan nonstrenuous activity between the two sessions of picture-taking. Some hospitals will let you leave to run errands, or

bring something to read. Remember, though, you must continue to fast between the two sessions of picture-taking.

This test takes about six hours.

CARDIAC CATHETERIZATION: THE "GOLD STANDARD" OF TESTING

Think of the morning traffic reports you see on your local television station. Some use graphics which display the roadways with traffic flowing smoothly or, in the case of an accident or other obstruction, with lines of cars backed up. Wouldn't it be useful if your doctor could peer inside your coronary arteries to see whether there are any blockages caused by coronary artery disease?

Your doctor can. An "aerial" picture of your coronary arteries can be obtained through the use of cardiac catheterization, also called coronary angiography. Not only does a cardiac catheterization show whether and where such blockages or obstructions exist, but it also provides your doctor with a road map to be used in deciding the best way to lessen or bypass any obstructions.

Since this is such an important test in cardiology, it's no wonder that when major research studies were released in 1991 which showed that men were twice as likely as women to be referred for it, a furor erupted. To some, this indicated that coronary artery disease was not being addressed as seriously in women. Since coronary artery disease in women tends to be more advanced when it's finally diagnosed, any indication that women are being shortchanged when it comes to diagnosis is cause for concern. Also, cardiac catheterization is not only a diagnostic tool; it's also imperative if you're being considered for such potentially lifesaving treatments as balloon angioplasty or coronary bypass surgery. So, since women are referred less frequently for catheterizations, it's not surprising that they're also underrepresented in undergoing such aggressive procedures as angioplasty and coronary bypass surgery. On the other hand, a study published in a November 1992 issue of the *Journal of the American Medical Association* estimated half of the catherizations in the U.S. are unnecessary or at least could safely be postponed, although some critics of this study disagree. The concern with women tends to run in the opposite direction, so this is a tricky topic. If you suspect you may need a cardiac catherization and your doctor demurs, or if you suspect the catherization may be unnecessary, you might consider seeking a second opinion.

All the tests we've discussed until now are noninvasive. The invasive cardiac catheterization involves some discomfort, is expensive, and entails a small degree of risk. In some places, it also entails an overnight hospital stay. But if you may be a candidate for angioplasty or bypass surgery, there's no substitute.

Cardiac catheterization is also sometimes used to determine, once and for all, whether coronary artery disease exists. Sometimes the test provides the needed proof that it does not, as in the case of Diana, a thirty-seven-year-old guidance counselor who for years had experienced the type of chest pain characteristic of coronary artery disease. Since Diana's mother had died suddenly at the age of thirty-eight from a heart attack, Diana's doctor was concerned. Diana's thallium stress test was abnormal, and the doctor feared she might have one or more blocked coronary arteries. But much to Diana's surprise, when she underwent the catheterization her coronary arteries appeared normal. It was found that her chest pain did not stem from coronary disease. Without the catheterization, she and her doctor would not have been certain.

Cardiac catheterizations are performed:

- To determine whether coronary artery disease is present.
- To determine the extent of coronary artery disease and the best way to treat it.
- If you suffer severe chest pain which seems to have a cardiac cause.
- If your chest pain persists after a heart attack.

These days, most cardiac catheterizations are done on an outpatient basis, but some hospitals still require an overnight stay. Beforehand, you'll undergo some routine tests, like a blood count, a chest X ray, and a resting EKG. You'll fast overnight, or be allowed to eat only very lightly if your test is scheduled late in the day.

For your catheterization, you're awake but sedated. A fine tubing, called a catheter, is introduced into your heart via a blood vessel, and sends a special X-ray dye into your coronary arteries. A 35-millimeter motion picture camera produces images which clearly show any blockages.

In a woman, the catheter is usually inserted by way of the

femoral artery, a large artery accessible in the groin. An artery in the arm is also sometimes used. No matter which site the doctor chooses, the preparation is pretty much the same, except that if your femoral artery is used, your pubic hair is shaved. A local anesthetic is administered, which causes a quick stinging sensation before the area becomes numb.

Once the catheter is in place, the physician guides it to the section of the aorta just before the heart where the coronary arteries originate. Then the dye is injected and traces the route of the blood flow, pinpointing any obstructions. The doctor—and you, if you wish—can watch as the dye travels through your arteries on a video monitor suspended above you. As the contrast dye is flowing, X-ray motion pictures are taken.

When the dye infuses your heart, you may feel an intense, sometimes uncomfortable warmth. If you have coronary artery disease, the process of injecting the dye may cause chest pain. Doctors will be on hand to monitor your condition and provide relief. If you feel pain, let them know, but don't be unduly alarmed. Every cardiac catheterization team has emergency equipment, but it rarely is needed.

Will you find this procedure painful? The injection of local anesthetic usually burns a bit. Most people find this procedure uncomfortable, rather than painful.

After the procedure is over, you'll most likely spend the next several hours resting. If your arm was used to insert the catheter, you'll be free to go as soon as you feel up to it. If, as is most likely, your femoral artery was used, heavy pressure will be applied for about twenty minutes to close the artery. For some, this is the most uncomfortable part of the procedure. You'll also have to lie perfectly still for several hours. It's not painful, but since most of us are not accustomed to lying motionless, it can be very uncomfortable. You'll need to have someone drive you home, since you should bend your leg only sparingly after the procedure.

♥ Mindsaving Tip: The sedative, in combination with the local anesthetic, really works. Reading about cardiac catheterization is more painful than the procedure. No one pretends that a cardiac catheterization is pleasant. But it can reveal an enormous amount of potentially life-saving information about your heart.

"What people tell me they are most afraid of is that we'll find something horrible and they'll have to go straight into emergency surgery. Everyone's afraid of that," says Dr. Anita Arnold, who performs catheterizations at Olympia Fields Osteopathic Hospital and Medical Center in Olympia Fields, Illinois. "But that's so rare. I tell people not to worry, that if they do need surgery, everyone, including the patient and the family, will have plenty of time to prepare for it."

Some patients, particularly those who have already undergone angioplasty or bypass surgery or who have severe underlying disease, are afraid that the catheterization will show that their condition is hopeless. But, says Dr. Arnold, "I tell patients that every month, it seems, there are new drugs and new procedures. Just because they've had a previous procedure doesn't mean we don't have another option that may help them."

A WORD ABOUT RISK   The vast majority of cardiac catheterizations, about 98 percent, go perfectly. But if you are elderly, frail, or have severe heart disease, there is an up to 2 percent risk that moving the catheter around in your blood vessels could result in infection, heart attack, or stroke. On the other hand, successful catheterizations are now being routinely performed on patients in their nineties. If you're in a high-risk category, having the catheterization may be far less dangerous than doing nothing about your heart problem.

> ♥ Lifesaving Tip: If you're a high-risk patient, you should choose the hospital where you undergo the catheterization carefully. Although it's extremely unlikely, if you suffer a heart attack or need to undergo emergency open-heart surgery at the time of the catheterization, there won't be time to transfer you to another hospital.

To prepare for your cardiac catheterization:

· Find out how long you should fast ahead of time, and whether there are any other preparatory steps you should take.
· Arrange for any lab or other medical tests you need beforehand.
· Arrange for transportation home so that you don't have to drive.

• Try to relax; this is one of those procedures that usually sounds worse than it is.

INTRAVASCULAR ULTRASOUND: COMBINING ECHO AND CATH   Dr. Steven Nissen, director of clinical cardiology at the Cleveland Clinic, becomes very animated when he describes Adele, a forty-four-year-old woman with chest pains that sounded like angina. She was hospitalized several times, but her test results showed nothing wrong. In fact, routine coronary angiograms revealed no major blockages of her coronary arteries. A new procedure that uses a miniature sound probe on the tip of a coronary catheter that is threaded through the coronary arteries during catheterization was tried. Images that accurately reflect the status of the blood vessels can thus be seen. "Sure enough," said Dr. Nissen, "we put the probe in her coronary circulation and found cholesterol-laden plaque all up and down her coronary arteries," indicating that serious blockage was really present. "We now have another powerful means of discriminating a normal from a diseased artery," Dr. Nissen said. In Adele's case the information was used to initiate a program of agressive drug and dietary treatment. Since women experience more "negative" catheterizations, this technique may turn out to be especially valuable in the future for the diagnosis of chest pain.

OTHER DIAGNOSTIC TESTS

The tests described thus far are the ones commonly used to diagnose structural problems of the heart, heart rhythm disturbances, and coronary artery disease. The following tests can also provide very useful information, although they're not as commonly performed.

MUGA

The MUGA, or multiple-gated acquisition test, evaluates the strength of your heart. It's particularly useful in assessing whether your heart has been weakened by a virus or damaged by a heart attack, and in measuring your heart's recovery after surgery.

The MUGA uses a special radioisotope which is injected into

your arm as you lie on an examining table. On entering your bloodstream, this "tracer" radioisotope mixes with your blood and races through the chambers of your heart, highlighting them. A special camera takes pictures of your heart.

The results of this very useful test are used to determine the efficiency of your heart as a pump, by measuring the amount of energy present in the course of each heartbeat and doing some arithmetic. The value derived is called the ejection fraction, which is one of the most important indicators of the health of your heart.

PET: ONE OF THE BEST, AND LEAST USED, TESTS

There is a very accurate, noninvasive way of detecting coronary artery disease in women, but you probably won't have the opportunity to avail yourself of it. The test is called positron emission tomography, or PET. Relatively few medical centers are equipped for PET, and their number is unlikely to grow. In case you are referred for PET testing, here's how it works.

The PET scanner looks like a huge doughnut. You lie on your back on a table inserted in the doughnut's hole. A small amount of a radioactive isotope is injected into your body. As the isotope decays, or loses energy, it emits small particles called positrons, which can be detected as they leave the body. PET produces sharp three-dimensional images of your heart. You don't need to exercise, because a drug is used to increase your heart's metabolic workload.

Because of the clarity of the image, a PET scan is the most reliable noninvasive means of identifying coronary artery disease in women, as well as of demonstrating its absence. A PET scan can also provide very valuable information after a heart attack. During a heart attack, the heart muscle is damaged, but some of the muscle which appears dead may actually be viable if the blood flow to that area is increased. A PET scan can determine whether portions of the heart muscle indeed are salvageable.

So why are so few centers equipped for PET? A PET scan is expensive, usually costing several hundred dollars more than a thallium test. The federal government considers PET a "redundant" test, and has discouraged insurers from paying for it. So if you want such a test, you may have to pay for it out of your own pocket.

MRI

Magnetic resonance imaging, commonly referred to as MRI, uses superconductive magnets and radio waves to obtain high-quality, detailed images of your body's internal organs. MRI is not used as commonly as other cardiac tests, such as an echocardiogram, but may be employed in cases where an echo is not considered sufficient. Cardiovascular problems which can be diagnosed with MRI include tumors, valvular disease, and complex congenital defects.

MRI is noninvasive. No radiation is produced, and no special preparations on your part are required. For the procedure, you lie on a scanner bed which is drawn slowly inside a huge doughnut-shaped machine. This machine is basically a large, hollow magnet. You lie motionless during several imaging periods, which last from one to fifteen minutes. You can talk to the technician outside via intercom. If you're prone to claustrophobia, ask for a mild sedative beforehand. While you're inside the machine, you often hear loud clanging noises, so ask for earplugs. An average examination takes about one hour, but this can vary from forty-five minutes to an hour and fifteen minutes.

♥ **Mindsaving Tip: Since the MRI machine is basically a magnet, some people worry that if they have a pacemaker or a mechanical heart valve, or if they have undergone heart surgery and have sternal wires, they could be in danger. This is usually not the case, but ask. Your doctor and the MRI operator will probably have discussed ahead of time whether any such items will pose a problem. It's also a good idea to leave your jewelry at home.**

A final word on testing: Over the years, doctors have amassed an arsenal of sophisticated diagnostic tools, and more are on the horizon. It's easy for both you and your doctor to be seduced by this wealth of fancy instrumentation. Valuable as these tests are, they're no substitute for the kind of valuable information your doctor can glean by taking the time to talk with you. That type of interview, enhanced by the careful, correct use of modern testing, can solve the most puzzling of cardiac problems.

7
Mitral Valve Prolapse

Nancy, a young attorney, was well on her way to a promising legal career until she began developing excruciating chest pains every time she headed into court. Two cardiologists found nothing wrong and attributed her chest pains to job stress. One even put her on Valium, but she feared that the tranquilizer would interfere with her ability to perform at her best. Desperate that she might have to give up the job she loved, she visited a third cardiologist. Additional cardiac testing revealed that she had mitral valve prolapse.

Although Nancy required medication, many women with mitral valve prolapse require no treatment at all. Mitral valve prolapse affects a large number of young women—it's their most common heart complaint. While rarely life-threatening, their symptoms can be truly frightening:

· Chest pain
· Palpitations
· Dizziness
· Fainting

WHAT IS MITRAL VALVE PROLAPSE?

Mitral valve prolapse was first described in medical journals in the 1960s. Doctors differ in their view of it. Some term it a syndrome, a collection of symptoms and signs (medical findings) which occur together. Some call it a disorder, referring to it as a physical irregularity, while others consider it nothing more than a harmless curiosity.

We prefer to describe mitral valve prolapse as an anomaly involving the heart valves. It's more a condition, like being nearsighted, than a disease like cancer. It's important to remember that women with mitral valve prolapse, even those with severe symptoms, almost always live out their normal lives without developing serious heart problems.

UNDERSTANDING MITRAL VALVE PROLAPSE

Your heart is a pump with four chambers. The upper two chambers, the atria, feed blood to the lower two chambers, the ventricles. The ventricles then pump the blood throughout the body. There are four valves which open and close to keep the blood flowing in the proper direction.

Oxygenated blood returns to the heart from the lungs through the left atrium. Once filled, the left atrium squeezes, and the blood goes from the left atrium through the mitral valve into the left ventricle. From there, blood is pumped past the aortic valve and through the circulatory system. The mitral valve serves as the gate into the left ventricle, the main pump of the heart.

If you have mitral valve prolapse, it means that one or both of the leaflets of your mitral valve are larger than they need to be, and that this prevents the valve from snapping tightly shut. Sometimes a small amount of blood regurgitates, or leaks back into the left atrium. Usually the amount of blood is not significant. If it is significant, it results in a problem called mitral regurgitation.

MITRAL REGURGITATION

In an estimated 5 percent of cases, women with mitral valve prolapse develop a serious leakage problem. This is known as mitral valve regurgitation, in which the leaflets which help close the mitral valves become even less effective, resulting in a greater flow of blood back into the atrium. This backward flow of blood can eventually lead to pulmonary congestion and enlargement and weakening of the left side of the heart, and to progressive heart failure. Before that point, however, the problem can be diagnosed, and the mitral valve is usually surgically repaired or replaced.

It's interesting to note that although more women than men are bothered by the symptoms of mitral valve prolapse, studies have shown that men more frequently develop complications such as serious mitral regurgitation.

Symptoms of mitral regurgitation are:

· Weakness
· Difficulty breathing while lying down
· Shortness of breath during mild exercise

> ♥ Lifesaving Tip: Complications such as mitral regurgitation occur very rarely in those with mitral valve prolapse. That said, if you're diagnosed with mitral valve prolapse and notice progressive shortness of breath, fainting, or other unusual symptoms, be sure to check with your doctor.

IS THERE A "MITRAL VALVE PROLAPSE SYNDROME"?

It's generally acknowledged that mitral valve prolapse is a biological entity involving a malformation of the mitral valve's leaflets. However, whether or not this condition accounts for the symptoms suffered by many of those with mitral valve prolapse is a matter of debate.

Initially, mitral valve prolapse was considered to affect only the functioning of a heart valve, but some believe it's a more generalized disorder which may affect other parts of the body's functioning as well. A 1990 study at the Washington University School of Medicine in St. Louis of 100 female and male patients diagnosed as suffering from "panic disorder" showed that a significant number had mitral valve prolapse as well.

Mitral valve prolapse also is often associated with the loss of the body's ability to respond properly to adrenaline. This may account for the panic syndrome, palpitations, dizziness, and chest pains commonly experienced by those with mitral valve prolapse.

Another factor which may play a role in the intensity of mitral valve prolapse in some individuals is their cardiac sensitivity. Cardiac sensitivity, or nociception, is discussed in more detail in Chapter 5. Cardiac sensitivity refers to the way your central nervous system perceives and processes pain messages, and it may be the reason that some people with mild mitral valve prolapse suffer from severe symptoms, while others with severe prolapse are scarcely, if at all, aware of the condition.

Some studies have found that women with mitral valve prolapse seem to experience such symptoms as chest pain, palpitations, fainting, and dizziness more than do others. These studies bear out what doctors see in their patients. They find that, not uncommonly, women experiencing these symptoms, particularly those in the twenty-to-forty age group, are found to have mitral valve prolapse.

But some experts question whether these symptoms are really a result of the mitral valve prolapse. They point out that younger women often suffer such symptoms as chest pain and palpitations, and often no cause, cardiac or otherwise, can be found. This is the crux of the controversy: Does mitral valve prolapse *cause* these symptoms, or is it merely a coincidence that the symptoms appear in combination with mitral valve prolapse?

Adding to this dilemma is the fact that, in the past several years, mitral valve prolapse has received increasing attention in the media, and has become the chic diagnosis of the 1990s. Since the symptoms ascribed to mitral valve prolapse can sometimes be baffling and mimic symptoms of other disorders, some now claim that mitral valve prolapse is associated with a laundry list of symptoms, including vague body aches, difficulty in urinating, insomnia, diarrhea, poor memory, allergies, and excessive gas. It's rare that a person doesn't suffer from one or another of these vague symptoms.

Among those who doubt whether a "mitral valve prolapse

syndrome" actually exists is Dr. Richard P. Devereux, an associate professor of medicine at Cornell University Medical College. He interviewed and performed diagnostic tests on thousands of men and women and failed to find a significant association between most of their symptoms and mitral valve prolapse. These included chest pain, palpitations, anxiety, and symptoms associated with a surplus of adrenaline. However, Dr. Devereux did find that women with mitral valve prolapse more often tended to have low blood pressure, which could account for dizziness and fainting. "There seems to be a real connection there," he says.

If you have mitral valve prolapse or experience the symptoms described in this chapter, you may find it frustrating to learn that a debate exists as to the significance of mitral valve prolapse. It's worthwhile to remember that, in medicine, there are sometimes not as many hard-and-fast answers as you think. Medicine is an ever-changing field and today's medical "truth" may, with research, be proved false tomorrow. However, the information contained in this chapter has been found to be extremely valuable to a large number of women whose symptoms may (or may not) turn out to be linked to mitral valve prolapse.

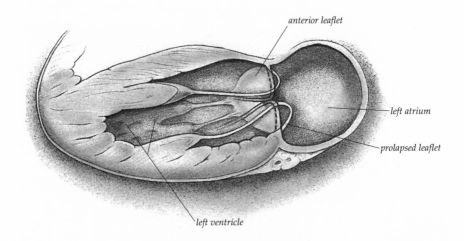

Mitral Valve Prolapse. Dotted lines show where the leaflets are in a normal valve; the solid lines show the leaflets in mitral valve prolapse. The configuration of the leaflets prevents the valve from closing as it normally should.

♥ Mindsaving Tip: Some of the vague complaints which have been lumped in with mitral valve prolapse may have other causes. For example, lactose intolerance, the inability to digest dairy products, can cause such unpleasant symptoms as bloating, excessive gas, diarrhea, and fatigue.

IF YOU HAVE SYMPTOMS ASSOCIATED WITH MITRAL VALVE PROLAPSE ...

Doctors (cardiologists especially) are accustomed to being able to "fix" heart problems, and too often don't have the patience to deal sympathetically with women who are troubled by vague complaints, especially if they don't respond to immediate treatment. Too often, physicians privately label such patients complainers. Women, particularly those who show symptoms associated with mitral valve prolapse, tend to fall into this category, which can diminish their chance of getting effective treatment.

That's what happened to Jean, a forty-five-year-old woman whose lightheadedness had been dismissed by doctors for years. She was sometimes so dizzy that she could barely walk. She was evaluated by doctors for vertigo, with negative findings, so she was told the problem was "all in your head." But virtually every time she got up to walk on some days, she nearly fell down. She even saw one cardiologist who told her to "hang on every time you stand up." It turned out Jean had mitral valve prolapse. Her symptoms responded to a cardiovascular medication, and she was able to resume her normal life.

If you have mitral valve prolapse, you don't necessarily need to be treated by a cardiologist. You should be seen by a cardiologist if you experience cardiac disorders such as mitral regurgitation or serious cardiac arrhythmia. If you don't, you may find treatment by your regular doctor perfectly satisfactory, provided that other heart-related causes of your symptoms have been eliminated and your doctor is willing to treat symptoms which cause you discomfort.

COMMON QUESTIONS ABOUT MVP

How did I "get" mitral valve prolapse?

Mitral valve prolapse is genetically transmitted. This can be seen unusually clearly in the case of the eleven-year-old Colorado girl who suffered from chest pains when she competed in school sports. It was revealed that her mother, who experienced feelings of extreme lightheadedness and abnormal heart rhythms, had mitral valve prolapse as well. So, doctors learned, did her maternal grandmother, who suffered from fainting spells, and her great-grandmother, who had a history of chest pains. Although this example shows mitral valve prolapse being passed down only to females, either parent can pass it down to offspring of either gender.

Do people with mitral valve prolapse always have the same symptoms?

Not at all. People may experience no symptoms, only one symptom, or many symptoms. The symptoms can change over the course of time or occur intermittently. This is most likely connected with normal changes in blood volume related to the endocrine system, which secretes hormones in the body. A woman's hormonal system is more active and changeable than a man's; this is one reason that women may be aware of the symptoms of mitral valve prolapse more frequently and acutely than men.

> ♥ **Mindsaving Tip: If you have what you believe are severe symptoms caused by mitral valve prolapse, bear in mind that usually there is no correlation between the severity of the symptoms and the severity of the prolapse.**

How is mitral valve prolapse diagnosed?

A tentative diagnosis of mitral valve prolapse can sometimes be made by a cardiologist with nothing more than a stethoscope. But mitral valve prolapse can be extremely difficult to pin down because its symptoms can be identical to those caused by other ailments. Sometimes a tentative diagnosis can be made by taking the following factors into consideration:

- **Age.** Although the malformation of the mitral valve occurs during gestation, it usually remains unnoticed until young adulthood. Women usually become aware of symptoms suddenly—they can often pinpoint the day and even the hour when they first occurred. For example, Nancy recalls a sunny day in June when she was outside bathing her dog. Suddenly she felt pain in her chest, which she experienced every few weeks from that point on.

- **Body type.** Body type is often a clue in diagnosing mitral valve prolapse. The condition is most often seen in women with a thin build, possibly because they lack the extra fat that acts as a blood volume buffer. Every pound of fat you carry contains some three thousand miles of tiny blood vessels. Blood can move from the tiny blood vessels to the large blood vessels and smooth the alteration of blood pressure that accompanies changes in body posture and may account for such symptoms as dizziness. Of course, there are exceptions, and women of all shapes and sizes can suffer real discomfort from mitral valve prolapse.

  It's not uncommon for women with mitral valve prolapse to become dancers, gymnasts, and other athletes of slender build. Sometimes the symptoms appear during the spurt of adrenaline which accompanies a performance—as in the case of a forty-five-year-old exotic dancer who used to faint while removing her G-string.

- **The "classical click."** In most cases, heart sounds come into play when making a diagnosis of mitral valve prolapse. By carefully listening with a stethoscope, a doctor may discern, in addition to normal heart sounds, a characteristic high-pitched snapping sound produced near the middle of the heart's ventricular contraction. This is the so-called "classical click." This click is often followed by a characteristic murmur heard in the heartbeat cycle, caused by the leakage of blood back through the mitral valve into the left atrium.

  This click has the tendency to change when you switch positions, so the cardiologist may listen to your heart as you stand, lie down, squat, or sit. But remember that, although the click and murmur are characteristic of most prolapse patients, they're not present in every one. The click can also come and go, depending on other factors. It's also not uncommon for the heart of a woman with mitral valve prolapse to sound perfectly normal.

· **Chest pain.** The type of chest pain associated with mitral valve prolapse is termed by cardiologists "atypical," to differentiate it from "typical" chest pain, the type associated with coronary artery disease. Typically, with heart disease, the chest pain is felt underneath the breastbone, and is a squeezing or pressure-like sensation. The pain usually, but not always, occurs after exercise. If not exercise-related, it may come during other activities which increase the workload of the heart, such as eating a heavy meal. In contrast, the chest pain associated with mitral valve prolapse is usually felt to the left of the breastbone, is sharp, and lasts only several seconds. It's an intermittent pain; it can, for example, be experienced frequently for a few weeks, disappear completely, and then return.

But such "atypical" chest pain as is found in mitral valve prolapse can also occur with other diseases commonly seen in young women. One example is reflux esophagitis, a common inflammation of the esophagus. Or the problem may be due to neuromuscular chest pain, pinching of the nerves of the neck caused by osteoarthritis which is misinterpreted as chest pain. Symptoms of gall bladder disease and stomach ulcers can also manifest themselves as chest pain.

As noted earlier, it's a matter of controversy whether something inherent in mitral valve prolapse "causes" chest pain, whether those with mitral valve prolapse have a heightened sensitivity to such pain, or whether mitral valve prolapse is associated with such chest pain at all.

· **Palpitations.** Women with mitral valve prolapse often suffer from palpitations, or a pounding of the heart, which can be truly frightening. It's believed that women with mitral valve prolapse may be overly sensitive to the secretion of adrenaline, one of the several hormones released by the adrenal glands, which are situated on top of the kidneys. Adrenaline, among other things, increases the heart rate. This hypersensitivity to adrenaline may ultimately result in lightheadedness, dizziness, and fatigue. It may be aggravated by drinking coffee or other beverages that contain caffeine.

Some arrhythmias, however, are serious and, in extreme and very rare cases, can lead to sudden death. An example of this is ventricular tachycardia, which results in an abnormally fast heart rate. If you have potentially serious ventricular tachycardia, your doctor will most likely prescribe a cardiovascular medication.

What diagnostic tests can confirm whether or not I have mitral valve prolapse?

A doctor usually can make a tentative diagnosis of mitral valve prolapse by taking your medical history and listening to your heart. But additional tests may be recommended to confirm the diagnosis or evaluate whether it's likely to cause you any serious problems later on. These tests are also used to rule out any other cardiac-related cause for your symptoms.

The following diagnostic tests can be used to diagnose mitral valve prolapse:

· **Physical examination.** By performing a physical examination, a cardiologist can determine whether you have a heart murmur or whether your heart makes the characteristic click associated with mitral valve prolapse.
· **Electrocardiogram and/or Holter monitor.** An electrocardiogram can show whether your heart is producing the proper electrical impulses to keep it functioning regularly or whether you have any arrhythmias. An electrocardiogram is used to study your heartbeat at rest, while a Holter monitor records your heartbeat as you go about your daily activities.
· **Exercise stress test.** If you have chest pain, an exercise stress test or exercise echocardiogram may determine whether you have coronary artery disease. An exercise stress test is also useful to objectively evaluate your exercise capability.
· **Echocardiogram.** An echocardiogram is often extremely useful in the diagnosis of mitral valve prolapse, because with this image of your heart, your doctor can actually see whether any of your valve leaflets are malformed. Useful as this is, though, mitral valve prolapse is only visible on an echocardiogram image about 50 percent of the time.
· **Tilt study.** If you're suffering from dizziness or fainting, a tilt study may be very useful.

All of these cardiac tests are virtually risk-free and pain-free and are done on an outpatient basis, as we explained in Chapter 6.

Does mitral valve prolapse cause problems during pregnancy?

In and of itself, mitral valve prolapse does not cause problems in pregnancy. For more information, see Chapter 9.

OTHER CONSIDERATIONS FOR WOMEN WITH MITRAL VALVE PROLAPSE

Some doctors believe that women with mitral valve prolapse may be at increased risk of developing bacterial endocarditis, a dangerous inflammation of the heart valves caused by bacteria entering the bloodstream. In its most recent recommendations, updated in 1990, the American Heart Association said preventive antibiotics were unnecessary for people with mitral valve prolapse unless they have a "leaky" mitral valve. For more information, see Chapter 10. Also, over the years, some studies have found that strokes may occur in a tiny percentage of people with mitral valve prolapse, although conclusive evidence of this has not been gathered.

LIVING WITH MITRAL VALVE PROLAPSE

In most cases, simply being reassured that you don't have a serious heart problem is enough to make the symptoms of mitral valve prolapse seem easier to bear. However, if your symptoms are uncomfortable or disabling, some medications may be useful. Often cardiovascular drugs called beta blockers are used. Such drugs "muffle" the actions of the sympathetic nerves to the heart and are very effective in decreasing chest pain and regulating heartbeat. Apparently for the same reason that those with mitral valve prolapse appear hypersensitive to adrenaline, they also often appear hypersensitive to heart medications, so starting out with a low dosage is usually the wisest course. Your doctor may try different drugs before finding the most effective.

You may want to try sharply limiting your caffeine intake by avoiding coffee, tea, chocolate, and other caffeine-rich foods. Caffeine stimulates the production of adrenaline. Since women with mitral valve prolapse often appear to be oversensitive to adrenaline, eliminating or limiting your caffeine intake may prove a very good idea.

Also, don't neglect your physical condition. It's only natural, if you're suffering from such symptoms as fatigue and shortness of breath, to limit your physical activity. You may not even realize you're avoiding stairs, hopping into the car instead of walking, or parking closer to the stores when you shop. As a result, your body gets out of condition, which may make you even more tired and shorter of breath than you would be ordinarily. If your doctor has not placed any physical limitations on you, becoming more active will improve your general health.

Although learning that you have mitral valve prolapse is initially upsetting, there's another way to look at it. Unlike many women who neglect their hearts when they're young and develop heart disease, you're now more conscious of the importance of maintaining your heart's health. By developing heart-healthy habits now, you may even end up living a longer, healthier life.

If you have mitral valve prolapse:

· Avoid caffeine if you find it worsens your symptoms.
· Eat a nutritious diet.
· Improve your general cardiovascular fitness level.
· Learn to control your stress and anxiety.
· Discuss medication for disabling symptoms with your doctor.
· Contact your doctor right away if you develop shortness of breath with marginal exertion, change in your chest pain pattern, or frequent palpitations.

To sum up: Mitral valve prolapse is not a disease, but a condition which occurs commonly in women. Complications ensue only rarely. Treatment is usually not necessary unless symptoms are severe. In almost all cases, people with mitral valve prolapse can enjoy a normal, active life.

8
Congenital Heart Defects: Hidden Time Bombs

When my doctor told me I had a congenital heart defect, I stared at him in disbelief. I was forty years old! Whoever heard of a forty-year-old with a birth defect? I had always assumed that such defects were diagnosed when you were born, or certainly in childhood. Anxious for information, I called the local chapter of the American Heart Association to learn about congenital heart defects in adults. There was a long pause; then the voice on the other end apologetically said that the best they could offer me was a booklet written for parents. "Better late than never," I sighed, and handed the booklet over to my equally stunned mother.

I learned later that over half a million Americans are living with some type of congenital heart defect. Yet sometimes even doctors don't realize this. When my friend Pat, whose similar defect was diagnosed when she was thirty-six, told her children's pediatrician, he replied, "You can't have an atrial septal defect! You must have heard wrong." Not only had Pat heard right, but her mother was diagnosed with the same problem when she was in her late fifties.

Symptoms and signs of congenital heart defects are:

- Exercise intolerance
- A heart murmur
- Palpitations
- Symptoms of congestive heart failure
- Blood pressure irregularities

Before the era of open-heart surgery, babies born with serious congenital defects died at birth or shortly thereafter. If the defect was not severe, the child sometimes survived until adulthood, but often died young. Sometimes the reason for the death was mysterious—or it was said that the person had a "heart condition," although no one knew exactly what the problem was.

That's now ancient history. The correction of congenital heart defects is one of the most cheerful chapters in modern cardiology. Today, the vast majority of children born with heart defects are treated and go on to live out a healthy, normal life span. That holds true for most adults as well, since these defects are usually discovered in time. If they're not, however, serious heart problems can result.

If you have such a defect, you may very well have known about it for years. Perhaps it was diagnosed and corrected when you were a child. Or perhaps the defect is so mild it doesn't need correcting, and you visit a cardiologist for periodic checkups. If your defect is very mild, you may live out your whole long life this way.

But congenital heart defects can be sneaky. That's why we call them hidden time bombs: You can have one without knowing it for years; you remain completely oblivious as it inflicts serious damage on your heart.

WHAT IS A CONGENITAL DEFECT?

The word "congenital" means inborn or existing at birth. The heart begins to form from a single tubelike structure during the fourth week after conception. As the weeks progress, the tube lengthens, and eventually forms the chambers, dividing wall or septum, and valves which make up a functioning heart. If anything interferes with this development process during the first eight to ten weeks of pregnancy, a congenital heart defect is the result.

An estimated 8 out of every 1,000 babies born alive have some form of congenital heart defect. In general, congenital defects occur more commonly in females, although some types occur more frequently in male babies. In most cases, the reason for this gender difference is not known.

WHAT CAUSES CONGENITAL DEFECTS?

The reason for most congenital defects is not known, so there's no way to prevent them. Only about 10 percent of the time are these defects caused by genetic abnormalities; those include the heart defects commonly associated with Down's syndrome, which also causes mental retardation. Marfan's syndrome, discussed later in this chapter, is also an inherited defect.

In some cases, environmental factors also contribute to congenital defects, but again, the percentage is small. These include the mother's exposure to German measles (rubella), herpes simplex virus, influenza, or mumps. The heavy use of alcohol has been linked to birth defects as well, as has the use of some drugs, including some antidepressants, opiates, and some cardiovascular medications, including Coumadin, generically known as wafarin, a powerful anticlotting drug.

WHY DO ADULTS HAVE CONGENITAL DEFECTS?

Adults who have congenital heart defects generally fall into three categories:

· Those whose defect was discovered in childhood and surgically corrected. They are among the large number of adults who are living healthy, normal lives with their repaired hearts.
· Those who were told as children that they had a heart murmur or a congenital defect, and perhaps were even monitored by a pediatric cardiologist for a while. They were not bothered by any symptoms and eventually forgot about it. Now, as they

reach their twenties and thirties, they suddenly find themselves dragging. Particularly when they're active, they may become short of breath or experience palpitations.

· Those who assumed they were healthy until they learned, to their surprise, that they have a congenital heart defect. They may have gone to the doctor because they were experiencing symptoms. But more likely the problem was discovered through tests for another problem. With the sophisticated medical care we enjoy today, you might wonder how any baby with a cardiac defect could escape detection. But it still happens, although rarely. Most of the adults who today are discovered to be living with congenital defects were infants twenty or thirty years ago, when diagnosing such problems was much more difficult.

Most of the adults with congenital defects seen at the Cleveland Clinic's Adult Congenital Heart Disease Clinic fall into one of these two last categories, according to clinic director Dr. Daniel J. Murphy. "Some people have congenital heart defects which were not recognized by their family doctors, but there are probably just as many who knew they had a heart murmur or problem with a valve but they haven't seen a cardiologist since childhood," Dr. Murphy said. "So by the time they come here, they may have developed a lot of symptoms."

HOW CONGENITAL DEFECTS DAMAGE YOUR HEART

For your heart to properly perform its job, it's very important that all your blood flows through it in the correct direction, as noted in Chapter 2. A congenital defect can disrupt this flow. Many defects are structural problems which can result in some of your blood flowing back the wrong way. Or your heart valves may be malformed or narrowed, which prevents your blood from flowing unobstructed. Such problems damage your heart by forcing it to overwork. Over the years, your heart may become enlarged or weakened, and the blood pressure within your heart and lungs can build up. The eventual result can be heart failure.

Even if they are overlooked in infancy and childhood, most congenital heart defects are detected by the time people reach their twenties and thirties, sparing their hearts from irreversible damage. In many cases a damaged heart can still be repaired, but any damage already done may be irreversible.

HOW DO YOU KNOW WHETHER YOU HAVE A CONGENITAL DEFECT?

The answer is often that you don't. Congenital heart defects are not very common, and about 90 percent are diagnosed in childhood, Dr. Murphy estimates. This means that it's unlikely, though by no means impossible, that you've reached adulthood with an undetected congenital heart defect. Because these defects can be missed until adults are in their forties, fifties, and even sixties, some experts believe that the number of people with undiagnosed heart defects is larger than generally assumed. Symptoms of congenital defects are discussed below.

EXERCISE INTOLERANCE

This is the most common symptom of a congenital heart defect. Exercise intolerance manifests itself as fatigue and shortness of breath when you attempt to be active. But this is tricky to recognize. Exercise intolerance usually develops so gradually and insidiously that it can become quite severe before you realize anything much is wrong. Another problem is that people with congenital heart defects often don't even notice that they're growing less active.

I can certainly vouch for this. As an adult, I always seemed slightly short of breath. I attributed this to allergies. I was also puzzled because it seemed that no matter how hard I tried to exercise, I never built up any endurance. This I attributed when I was young to being on the plump side and later to growing older. My discomfort was so minor that the idea that anything could be seriously wrong with me would have struck me as perfectly ludicrous. According to Dr. Murphy, I fit the picture of an adult with an unrecognized congenital heart defect perfectly.

Not everyone with a congenital heart defect is inactive. Pat, for example, was a runner before her congenital heart defect was discovered. Since her surgery, though, she has noticed a big difference. "I was always frustrated by the fact that I was never able to put on any speed. It would drive me crazy that I was working so hard and never getting anywhere," she says. "So, after the surgery, I started checking my time, and I was really surprised. Overall, I've shortened my one-mile running time by quite a bit."

A HEART MURMUR

A heart murmur sometimes occurs with congenital heart defects and sometimes does not. It's not at all unusual for a girl to have a heart murmur, which she eventually "grows out of." Pregnant women often have heart murmurs as well, because of their normal increase in blood volume. The blood volume decreases after giving birth, and the murmur disappears.

If you're not pregnant and you have a heart murmur, you should ask your doctor to determine the reason. As an appropriate test, your doctor may suggest an echocardiogram, a noninvasive test which provides an image of your heart's structure. On the other hand, if your family doctor says it's nothing to worry about, be diplomatic but persistent. If your doctor declines to check further, consider going to a cardiologist, preferably one with experience in diagnosing and treating congenital heart defects. Sometimes because the patient sitting in front of him or her appears healthy, the doctor assumes a heart murmur is "innocent," or doesn't signify a problem. If your heart murmur does indeed turn out to be innocent, so much the better. This is far preferable to having a potentially serious problem overlooked.

PALPITATIONS

If your heart defect has gone undetected (or uncorrected) for a long time, you may begin to suffer from palpitations. Sometimes the pounding of your heart can become so severe it can cause fainting. Palpitations indicate a problem with your heart's electrical system and may indicate that your heart is suffering because of the defect. By the time palpitations appear, your heart has usually been overcompensating for quite a while. Unfortunately, even though your heart may benefit greatly from having the defect corrected, the problem leading to the palpitations may be irreversible.

SYMPTOMS OF CONGESTIVE HEART FAILURE

This serious syndrome rarely occurs in the case of congenital defects, but it can if the problem has gone undetected for years or even decades. These symptoms occur more commonly in people who are over fifty. Congestive heart failure (often referred to simply as heart failure) indicates that your heart has been overcompensating so long that it can no longer adequately perform its major function of supplying blood to your body. See Chapter 10 for symptoms of congestive heart failure.

BLOOD PRESSURE IRREGULARITIES

Often with congenital defects, blood pressure can remain normal as measured in your doctor's office, even though you may have developed pulmonary hypertension, which is high blood pressure within the right side of your heart and lungs. People with a certain type of congenital heart defect called coarctation of the aorta are found to have abnormal blood pressure readings. These people have high blood pressure in the upper body but low blood pressure in the legs. Most doctors do not routinely take blood pressure readings in both the lower and upper parts of the body, so they miss this highly suspicious sign.

♥ Lifesaving Tip: Having a blood pressure reading within normal range is not a guarantee that you don't have pulmonary hypertension. This dangerous condition can build up within your heart and lungs and cause damage even while your regular blood pressure reading remains normal or even low. It can be diagnosed during a physical examination and with the help of an electrocardiogram and an echocardiogram, both commonly performed cardiac tests.

DIAGNOSING CONGENITAL DEFECTS

If you suspect that you have a congenital defect, you should see a cardiologist, preferably one who has experience in congenital heart disease. Although it may seem odd for an adult to visit a pediatric cardiologist, this is the doctor with the most specialized training in this field. However, many pediatric cardiologists prefer not to see patients older than sixteen. If this is the case, seek out a cardiologist with special training in congenital heart defects. In many communities such a physician is difficult to find—in that case, consider choosing a general cardiologist who is experienced in treating adults with congenital defects.

The cardiologist will begin with a physical examination and, if there's reason to believe you may have such a defect, will recommend you undergo cardiac tests. Such tests would most likely include an electrocardiogram, chest X ray, echocardiogram, and possibly a cardiac catheterization. These tests are discussed in Chapter 6.

Types of congenital heart defects found in adults are discussed below.

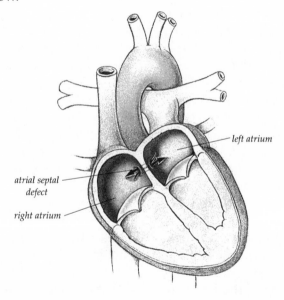

left atrium

atrial septal defect

right atrium

Atrial Septal Defect. The defect in the tissue separating the two upper halves of the heart results in a portion of the blood flowing improperly back through the heart.

ATRIAL AND VENTRICULAR SEPTAL DEFECTS (ASD AND VSD)

Septal defects, commonly referred to as holes in the heart, occur when the opening in the wall that divides the heart into left and right chambers fails to close before birth. They are among the most common forms of heart defects. Atrial septal defects (ASD's) occur in the upper chambers of the heart. Ventricular septal defects (VSD's) occur in the lower chambers.

If you have a significant septal defect, it should be corrected as soon as possible. If such a defect persists for too long, an irreversible and potentially deadly complication known as Eisenmenger syndrome can result. This problem occurs when the small blood vessels of the lungs are damaged by the prolonged high blood pressure that has built up within the heart and lungs. Symptoms of this problem include shortness of breath, fainting during exercise, and cyanosis (blue skin, lips, or nail beds caused by lack of oxygen in the blood). The damage caused by this complication is irreversible and will likely shorten your life, even if your septal defect is corrected.

While open-heart surgery is not 100 percent risk-free, the risk to an otherwise healthy adult is relatively low. A study published in 1990 reviewed the cases of 123 patients who underwent surgery at the Mayo Clinic some thirty years earlier. It was found that patients whose ASD's had been repaired before they'd reached the age of twenty-five lived the rest of their lives in excellent health. Patients whose surgery was performed later still enjoyed quite good results, but were more likely to develop heart problems as they grew older. Still, doctors today occasionally find adults whose congenital defects were diagnosed and should have been corrected years ago, but never were.

Typically, septal defects are corrected surgically. All the steps involved in this type of surgery are described in Chapter 12. Once you are placed on the heart-lung machine, the surgeon will repair the defect, using either a piece of pericardium (the cellophane-like sac covering the heart) or a synthetic patch to cover the hole. No matter which type of patch is used, the heart tissue soon grows over it, sealing it permanently. In uncomplicated cases, this procedure essentially eliminates the problem.

Research is now under way to gauge the success of using new nonsurgical techniques to fix such holes. As of this writing, such procedural devices have not yet received government approval, so they aren't generally available. For the time being, these techniques also hold more promise for children because they're used to close small holes; as people grow older, the holes apparently grow larger.

These nonsurgical methods involve small devices made of Dacron mesh or foam with stainless-steel ribs. One is shaped like a tiny umbrella, another like a tiny clamshell. Either device is delivered to your heart using a catheter, which is guided from outside your body through a vein. Once in position, the device is unfurled and blocks the hole. It's hoped that this procedure will eventually be perfected and approved, as it avoids open-heart surgery.

The day before I was to undergo open-heart surgery, I said to my cardiologist suspiciously, "Am I going to have this surgery, go home, and six months later read about a method which has made it obsolete?" "Oh, no," the cardiologist assured me, "that's years down the road." Just a few months later, these devices were being written up in general health magazines. Since then, I've been assured that they would not have been appropriate for me. But this story does underscore how fast medical progress can be made.

PATENT DUCTUS ARTERIOSUS

Every baby is born with a ductus arteriosus, an open passageway between the pulmonary artery and the aorta, the heart's two major blood vessels. Normally this passageway closes within a few hours of birth. If the passageway remains open, it creates a shunt, or pathway in which blood flows the wrong way, from the aorta back into the lungs, instead of out into the rest of the body. This problem, called patent ductus arteriosus, causes the heart to work too hard, and can result in serious complications. Patent ductus ateriosus occurs more often in females than in males. It can occur alone, or along with such other defects as a VSD or coarctation of the aorta.

Traditionally open-heart surgery was required to correct this defect. However, a new method using a special "double umbrella," similar to the device used to plug septal defects, shows promise. In this procedure, a catheter with one of these devices on the tip is inserted into a vein and pushed through the circulatory system until it is correctly positioned in the heart. Then one of the tiny umbrellas is opened on one side of the defect and the second is opened on the other side, blocking the abnormal passageway. This device is also undergoing study to win government approval.

AORTIC STENOSIS

The term "aortic stenosis" is somewhat misleading, as this problem can be a congenital heart defect, be the result of rheumatic heart disease, or be related to the normal aging process. When it occurs as a congenital heart defect, the term "bicuspid malformation of aortic valve" is more precise.

Normally your heart's aortic valve has three leaflets which open and close, enabling your heart to function correctly. People with bicuspid malformation are born with only two leaflets, which are often partially fused together. Instead of opening normally, the leaflets obstruct blood flow, making it more difficult for the heart to pump blood through the body. When this defect is severe, surgery is required, although under certain circumstances a procedure known as balloon valvuloplasty can be used. This is usually performed, though, on the very old or on those who are otherwise poor candidates for surgical repair.

Ninety-five percent of those born with this defect have only the valve problem. In about 5 percent of the cases, people born with the problem may also be missing one of the heart's coronary arteries.

PULMONARY STENOSIS

This congenital heart defect is also termed valvular pulmonary stenosis because it affects the pulmonary valve. In a normal heart, the pulmonary valve opens to allow the blood to flow from the right ventricle to the lungs, where it exchanges carbon dioxide and oxygen. If you were born with a malformed valve which is too narrow, it can partially or completely obstruct the flow of blood, causing your right ventricle to pump too hard. Over the years, this overcompensation causes the valve to become thickened and calcified, increasing the obstruction. Pulmonary stenosis can occur by itself or as part of a complex of heart defects called tetralogy of Fallot, which is explained below. Traditionally, surgery to repair or replace the valve was required, but this defect is now often corrected with balloon valvuloplasty.

COARCTATION OF THE AORTA

In people with this congenital heart defect, the aorta, the main artery which carries blood from the heart to the rest of the body, is pinched or constricted. This obstructs the flow of blood from the heart to the lower part of the body, including the legs. To compensate, the heart works harder, raising the blood pressure in the upper part of your body. This problem should be corrected as early in life as possible; otherwise the blood pressure may remain high after the coarctation is fixed.

If surgery is required, the surgeon reconstructs the aorta by removing the narrow segment and patching it with a portion of the blood vessel from the arm. Sometimes a graft made from synthetic material is used. Occasionally, years after such a repair, the segment can again become narrowed. In such a case, balloon angioplasty can sometimes be used to dilate it.

EBSTEIN'S ANOMALY

This is a defect in which the tricuspid valve of the heart is malformed, which leads to the valve's leaking badly. If you were born with this as a mild condition, you may not develop any symptoms for years. Open-heart surgery to repair or replace the valve is usually indicated. Often people born with this condition also have an atrial septal defect, which can be repaired at the same time.

TETRALOGY OF FALLOT

Tetralogy of Fallot is really a quartet of separate congenital defects. The two major components are a large ventricular septal defect and pulmonary stenosis. This narrowing of the pulmonary valve partially blocks the flow of blood into the lungs. In addition, the right ventricle is more muscular than normal, and the aorta is displaced, lying directly over the ventricular septal defect.

Tetralogy of Fallot is termed a cyanotic defect because it re-sults in cyanosis, a blue discoloration of the skin or, in mild cases, a ruddy complexion. This occurs because the blood being pumped through the body does not contain enough oxygen.

Surgery is required to fix the multiple defects associated with this condition. In most cases, surgery effects a cure; in some cases, however, the condition may result in a weakening of the right side of the heart or in heart rhythm disturbance, necessitating ad-ditional treatment.

MARFAN'S SYNDROME

Although it's not technically a congenital heart defect, Marfan's syndrome is an inherited congenital disorder that can manifest it-self in heart problems. Also, if mild enough, this problem can be overlooked, with sometimes fatal results.

If you follow sports you'll have have heard of Marfan's syn-drome. It was the cause of the unexpected death of Flo Hyman, one of the world's leading female basketball players. Some be-lieve Abraham Lincoln suffered from Marfan's as well. Marfan's syndrome is a fairly rare genetic disorder of the connective tis-sues, especially of the heart, eyes, and musculoskeletal system. One of every two children from an affected parent may inherit the syndrome. Recently the gene responsible for carrying the syn-drome was located, which may eventually result in a laboratory test to diagnose and, it's hoped, a way to correct it.

Marfan's can cause potentially serious eye disorders as well as changes in the musculoskeletal system which create a charac-teristic "Marfanoid" appearance. Often physical appearance pro-vides the main clue to the presence of Marfan's. People with Marfan's syndrome are often tall and thin, with slender, tapering fingers and unusually long arms and legs. However, appearances can be deceiving, and sometimes people who do not have out-ward physical characteristics of Marfan's can develop serious medical problems.

Marfan's usually threatens the heart in two ways: by affect-ing the aorta, the large artery that carries oxygenated blood from the left ventricle to the rest of the body, and by affecting the heart's major valves. The connective tissue in the aorta weakens and begins to stretch. By early adulthood, this swelling may develop into an aneurysm, a bubblelike formation on the aorta, which can cause the aortic valve to leak or even burst. About 60 percent of the people born with Marfan's also have a leaky mitral valve, which reduces their heart's ability to pump.

People with Marfan's require treatment as problems develop. Someone with a weakened aortic artery may need to avoid vigorous exercise. This is why diagnosing this ailment is particularly important when it occurs in young athletes.

♥ Lifesaving Tip: Marfan's syndrome can be a very dangerous "hidden time bomb." It may go completely unnoticed until the afflicted person dies suddenly of a ruptured aortic aneurysm. If one of your parents has Marfan's, you should be examined for it. You should also be examined if your family history includes an unusually large number of tall young men or women who died suddenly at a young age.

OTHER CONGENITAL HEART DEFECTS

There are other extremely unusual congenital heart defects. Although it's not impossible, it's doubtful they could remain undiscovered until adulthood. These include being born without a tricuspid or a pulmonary valve; transposition of the great vessels, in which the pulmonary artery and the aorta are reversed; or various absences or anomalies of the coronary arteries.

♥ Lifesaving Tip: A congenital heart defect can make your heart more vulnerable to infection. That's why if you have such a defect, even after it has been corrected, your doctor may recommend that you take antibiotics before dental cleanings and some other medical procedures. This is discussed in Chapter 10.

SURGICAL CONSIDERATIONS FOR CONGENITAL HEART DEFECTS

The correction of congenital heart defects has changed dramatically. Years ago, if your defect was very serious, you died at birth or shortly thereafter. After the development of the heart-lung machine, surgery became possible, but was risky. Over the past few decades, surgical techniques have become much safer.

Remember, though, that although the risks of open-heart surgery have fallen dramatically, such operations entail at least a 3 to 4 percent risk of death for women, the same as for a coronary bypass operation. However, the risk of suffering a stroke during surgery for correction of a congenital heart defect is slightly higher than that during a bypass because the chamber of the heart must be opened, increasing the possibility that air will get in, travel to the brain, and cause injury. While the danger of not having the surgery performed far outweighs the risks, if you must undergo such surgery, you should choose a surgeon experienced in the repair of congenital heart defects. Open-heart surgery is discussed in Chapter 12.

Am I too old to have my defect corrected? In the past, doctors subscribed to the belief that there was a cutoff age for the correction of congenital heart defects. This is no longer the case; studies have shown that very good results can be obtained in women well over the age of sixty, unless the defect has affected the heart to the extent that surgery would not be beneficial.

If a doctor says your congenital defect should be corrected but that you're too old for surgery, be certain that his or her conclusion is based on sound medical reasoning. Strongly consider getting a second opinion from a physician experienced in treating congenital heart defects in adults. You may have to seek out a major medical center, but often you can send your records ahead of time to learn whether further evaluation could help you.

What about cardiac rehabilitation? Cardiac rehabilitation traditionally has been seen as benefiting people who have undergone treatment for coronary disease or have suffered a heart attack. Increasingly its benefits are being seen in a broader context. Nowadays many cardiac rehabilitation programs have people trained to work with patients who have congenital heart defects. If you're in otherwise good health and you undergo surgery to correct your defect, you may not require such a program. If, on the other hand, you're in need of physical conditioning, you might benefit a great deal. For the program to be covered by your medical insurance, your doctor will have to attest that you need this type of therapy. Cardiac rehabilitation is discussed in Chapter 11.

If I have a congenital heart defect, should I become pregnant? If you have a defect, whether or not you should become pregnant, and how your pregnancy should be managed, depend generally on the seriousness of the defect and the condition of your heart. For more information on congenital heart defects and pregnancy, see Chapter 9.

♥ **Lifesaving Tip:** No matter what type of congenital heart defect you have, whether it is corrected or not, the best advice regarding pregnancy is "plan ahead." Discuss the possibility with your doctor before you become pregnant. If you're already pregnant, discuss your heart problem with your doctor as soon as possible. This is especially important if you're taking Coumadin or certain other cardiac medications.

Will my children's hearts be normal? If you were born with a congenital heart defect, you're probably concerned about the probability of passing the defect on to your children. The good news is that this is not very likely unless you have a defect with a strong genetic link, such as Marfan's syndrome. With other congenital heart defects, your risk of having a child with a heart defect rises slightly above normal, possibly to 3 or 4 percent, although in some cases the figures could be as high as 10 percent. Your risk is also slightly increased (about 2 to 5 percent) if you have diabetes, including gestational diabetes that develops during pregnancy. "There is no guarantee any time you have a child," says Dr. Daniel Murphy of the Cleveland Clinic. "For someone with a congenital heart defect, there is going to be an increased risk, but it is generally not significant."

Still, if you have a congenital heart defect, you should consider having a special diagnostic test called a fetal echo done after you've completed your sixteenth week of pregnancy. This test, which is identical to an echocardiogram, will usually show whether your baby's heart is developing normally. While such a test sometimes cannot detect a relatively minor heart defect, it can usually diagnose serious problems. In about 95 percent of the cases, the ultrasound will be negative, so, if you are very concerned about your baby's heart, this test can provide you with peace of mind. Some doctors question the value of the test, reasoning that if there is a defect which requires correction, this would be done after birth.

You should undergo a four-chamber sonogram if:

· You were born with a congenital heart defect.
· Your baby's father was born with a congenital heart defect.
· There is a strong history of congenital heart defects in either of your families.
· You have given birth previously to a child with a congenital heart defect.
· You have diabetes.

♥ Lifesaving Tip: Four-chambered sonograms have become routine. As with other diagnostic tests, they're only as good as the person interpreting them. Make sure your test is done in a hospital or clinic which specializes in fetal cardiology.

Still, for women with heart defects who do become mothers, the possibility that their child may have a similar defect lingers in their minds, even after they give birth to apparently robust babies. Even taking the youngster to a pediatric cardiologist and getting a clean bill of health doesn't always quiet the worry felt by women like Pat, who notes that her congenital defect was not discovered until she was in her mid-thirties.

Today, though, things are different. Thanks to sophisticated diagnostic tests, such defects are hard to miss. Dr. Catherine Neill, professor of pediatrics and cardiology at Johns Hopkins Hospital in Baltimore, says, "If the baby has a cardiac sonogram somewhere between the sixteenth and twenty-second weeks, and then the baby is checked again shortly after birth, I think the parents can be very confident that their child is normal."

Pat and I, and all the other women with congenital heart defects which were not diagnosed until adulthood, are, we hope, part of a vanishing group.

9

Pregnancy
and
Your Heart

"I learned I had heart disease when my son was two years old," says Sandra. "I didn't anticipate getting pregnant again. When I did, I was really scared. But my doctor said he was sure I could handle the pregnancy."

Sandra, who is thirty-seven, gave birth to her healthy daughter two years ago. Her pregnancy was complicated by two potentially serious problems. She had both coronary heart disease and mitral regurgitation, otherwise known as a leaky heart valve. Throughout her pregnancy, Sandra was watched by doctors skilled in treating high-risk pregnancies. Her heart was carefully monitored. Special ultrasound tests were also done to make sure her baby was developing properly. Was the result worth it? "When I look at my little girl and see how healthy she is, it's wonderful," Sandra says. "I just can't believe it."

Sandra is one of a growing number of women with heart problems who are able to carry a baby safely to term. Years ago, such women risked a further deterioration of their condition, or even death. Today, thanks to advances in cardiology, the probability that such a woman will enjoy a safe pregnancy and give birth to a healthy baby is much higher. "Generally, I'm very optimistic about pregnancies in women with heart problems," says Dr. Catherine Neill, of Johns Hopkins Hospital. "There are a small number of women with certain types of problems who can get into difficulties. But most women do very well in pregnancy."

Not every heart problem is cause for great concern during pregnancy, but most require some extra care. Just how much additional care you'll need depends on what type of heart problem you have, whether the problem is mild or severe, and whether it has damaged your heart. Only a few heart problems can endanger your life or the life of your unborn child, though the ones that can, can be deadly. After obstetrical causes, heart and cardiovascular problems account for the highest number of maternal deaths during pregnancy. Happily, most pregnancies of women like Sandra turn out well. With planning and careful consideration, you can help ensure that the outcome of your pregnancy will be a joyous one like hers.

BEFORE YOU BECOME PREGNANT ...

If you're concerned about your own health or a problem in your family's medical history, no matter how frivolous it seems, you should talk to your primary physician or obstetrician about it before you become pregnant, or as soon afterward as possible.

If you're aware that you have a heart problem, you should be evaluated by a cardiologist before you become pregnant. The more potentially serious your problem, the more important this is. Although you may initially be evaluated by a general cardiologist, it's important that the cardiologist following your case be experienced in treating pregnant women with your type of heart problem.

There are some key reasons that this prepregnancy evaluation is so important. During pregnancy, the sounds your heart makes differ from those it makes when you're not pregnant, rendering a problem found during pregnancy more difficult to evaluate. Also, when you're not pregnant, your doctor has the freedom to perform any type of diagnostic tests necessary without fear of harming the baby.

If you do have a heart problem, how closely you should be watched by a cardiologist during your pregnancy depends on the extent of the problem. Sometimes an evaluation before, during, and after your pregnancy is all that's needed. If you have a potentially dangerous problem, you may need to be closely monitored by a team which includes a cardiologist and an obstetrician very experienced in high-risk pregnancies.

You might seek out a super-specialist if you think your cardiologist may be unduly pessimistic about your chances for a successful pregnancy. According to Dr. Neill, this may happen, for example, to women with congenital heart defects. "I have had people call me and say, 'I went to see the doctor and he told me all patients who have my type of congenital heart defect shouldn't get pregnant,' when it turns out there is no basis for that at all. These are good, conscientious doctors, but they've probably had two or three patients do badly and they lump all patients with congenital heart defects together."

If you have a heart problem and you want to have a baby, but your general cardiologist is concerned about it, consider seeking a second opinion from a cardiologist at a major medical center who specializes in dealing with such pregnancies. That way, you'll be certain you have an accurate idea of the risks involved. If you live in a small town, you may have to travel to such a center, but you're well advised to do so—deciding whether or not to have a baby is one of the most important decisions you'll ever make.

♥ Lifesaving Tip: If you have a heart problem, besides seeing a cardiologist *before* you become pregnant, it's equally important that your heart be examined about six or eight weeks *after* you deliver your baby, to make sure it has returned to normal.

PREGNANCY AND THE NORMAL HEART

Everyone is familiar with the outward signs of pregnancy: You suffer bouts of morning sickness, your stomach expands to the size of a watermelon, and your feet swell. These signal the many changes going on within your body. During your pregnancy, your body must adapt to the changes involved in nurturing a developing baby. None of your body's organs is called upon to work harder than your heart.

Even if your heart is perfectly normal, pregnancy places a heavy burden on it. When you're not pregnant, your heart already must perform the Herculean task of pumping blood throughout your body day in and day out, without tiring. During pregnancy, several changes in your body make this already tough task even tougher. During pregnancy, you go through hormonal changes which apparently result in the retention of both salt and water. This accounts for a lot of your weight gain. By the fifth month of your pregnancy, your blood volume has increased by 40 to 50 percent. That represents a vast increase in the amount of blood your heart has to pump. Your heart also beats ten to twenty times more per minute than before you were pregnant, contracting more strongly with each beat.

During labor, the demands on the normal heart increase even more. With each uterine contraction, your heart's workload rises by about 25 to 30 percent. During delivery, your heart may be called on to work four to five times as hard as it did before you were pregnant. While the normal female heart can take this in stride (with some huffing and puffing, of course), such a workload can place a dangerous strain on a heart that is weak.

As your baby grows inside you, it needs more and more oxygen and nutrients. If you have a heart problem which makes it difficult for your heart to supply enough oxygen to your body, the problem only worsens when your heart is faced with supplying oxygen to your enlarging uterus and developing baby as well.

Also, in pregnancy, many women have a tendency to develop high blood pressure. Hypertensive disorders are among the most dangerous of pregnancy. If you have a heart problem, the probability that you will develop high blood pressure increases.

With all these biological changes going on, it's not surprising that pregnancy can place a burden on a heart which is not perfect. It's the type of heart problem you have, however, which determines how risky your pregnancy will be.

What is a "high-risk" pregnancy? A high-risk pregnancy poses dangers to you, your baby, or both. You will have to be monitored closely; you may have to undergo diagnostic testing, and your delivery may need to be scheduled in advance to make sure you're attended by the most experienced doctors and staff. In a high-risk pregnancy, such planning can literally mean the difference between life and death.

DIAGNOSTIC TESTING:
SAFE OR DANGEROUS?

The best way for a cardiologist to evaluate just how likely it is that your heart problem will endanger your pregnancy is with a thorough, up-to-date evaluation of your heart. If you consult the cardiologist about your plans before you become pregnant, all necessary diagnostic tests can be performed safely. But if you're already pregnant, the choice of tests is limited.

One reason that diagnostic tests don't pose the danger to your unborn baby that they formerly did is the development of echocardiography, which is discussed in Chapter 6. This type of imaging has amassed a strong safety record over several years. The version of an echocardiogram called a four-chamber sonogram can provide images of your unborn baby's heart.

In most cases, echocardiography can provide your doctor with most of the information required to evaluate your heart. Other diagnostic tests generally considered safe during pregnancy include monitoring your heartbeat by electrocardiogram or Holter monitor. Some other tests which may be indicated don't have such a safety record. For example, the radiation from a chest X ray can be hazardous to your unborn child during the first three months of pregnancy. In the later stages of pregnancy, a chest X ray can be safely performed if special precautions are taken, such as your belly being shielded with a lead apron.

Some tests used to evaluate your heart make use of radioactive isotopes, such as the thallium used in the thallium stress test, or the isotope called technitium used in a MUGA, or multiple-gated acquisition test. Whether or not these tests are safe during pregnancy depends on the type of isotope used, so talk to your doctor about it.

In rare cases, your doctor may want you to undergo a cardiac catheterization. Cardiac catheterization uses more radiation than a chest X ray, so ordinarily your doctor would avoid it during pregnancy. But in some cases the need for such a test may outweigh the risk to the baby. If your doctor suspects you may have a potentially life-threatening condition such as a clot in a coronary artery, the use of such radiation may be warranted. Such circumstances require careful discussion between you and your doctor.

CARDIOVASCULAR DRUGS DURING PREGNANCY

It was once believed that the placenta, the organ within the uterus through which a fetus receives its nourishment, protected the unborn baby from dangerous germs and chemicals. Today it's recognized that this is untrue, and that dangerous chemicals can reach your unborn baby. This is why pregnant women are advised not to take any drugs unnecessarily.

With some types of cardiac problems, you will be prescribed cardiovascular drugs. This is an area where much caution must be exercised. To gain FDA approval and be marketed in the United States, drugs must go through a rigorous testing process. However, there have never been any animal tests which could prove with certainty that a drug is safe for a pregnant woman. Since pregnant women are, quite rightly, barred from inclusion in such testing, there is a lack of information on safety, and sometimes a time lag: Some drugs once believed safe are later found to cause birth defects. A recent example was the discovery that angiotensin-converting enzyme inhibitors, known as ACE inhibitors, an important class of blood-pressure-reducing drugs, could cause serious birth defects. Until that warning was sounded, ACE inhibitors had been used by doctors to treat pregnant women with high blood pressure.

To be on the safe side, when you're pregnant you should take drugs only if they're absolutely needed. If you do require medication, there are many drugs now on the market which have established safety records, so your doctor will be able to recommend the right medication for you.

> ♥ **Lifesaving Tip: If you have a heart problem, you may be taking some medications which could prove unsafe for your unborn baby. Abruptly stopping some types of medications can also be risky. Contact your doctor for guidance.**

TYPES OF HEART PROBLEMS WHICH CAN OCCUR DURING PREGNANCY

One type of heart disease that occurs during pregnancy involves heart problems you've had since before you became pregnant, but of which you may or may not be aware. These include congenital heart defects and cardiac problems caused by rheumatic heart disease. Other heart problems can occur in pregnancy whether you have a preexisting heart problem or not. These include blood pressure disorders which occur only during pregnancy, and peripartum cardiomyopathy, a rare disease of the heart muscle.

Every woman is an individual and every pregnancy is different. The information in this chapter is designed to give you an idea of what to expect when you have a certain type of heart problem, and the kinds of treatment available.

CORRECTED CONGENITAL HEART DEFECTS

Over the years, an estimated 300,000 women in the United States have been treated for congenital defects, and many of them are now in their childbearing years. If your heart defect has been corrected, you should still discuss your plans to become pregnant with your doctor. The vast majority of the time, your corrected heart defect won't present any problem at all. If you've had surgery for a very complex problem, such as tetralogy of Fallot, you may still have a residual problem, such as a heart valve which is leaky, or perhaps a tendency to develop irregular heart rhythms.

UNCORRECTED CONGENITAL HEART DEFECTS

A congenital heart defect may or may not pose a problem during pregnancy. This generally depends on the type and severity of the defect and whether it has compromised the function of your heart. Congenital heart defects are not commonly discovered during pregnancy, but sometimes the extra load on your heart can result in your experiencing cardiac symptoms or exhibiting clinical signs for the first time. Congenital heart defects are discussed further in Chapter 8.

♥ **Lifesaving Tip: In adults, a heart murmur may indicate a heart problem, such as a congenital heart defect.**

However, it is not uncommon for pregnant women to develop heart murmurs. If your heart murmur appears during your pregnancy and doesn't go away after delivery, it should be checked by a cardiologist.

Whether or not your heart defect should be corrected during pregnancy depends on what type of defect it is and its severity. Today, even open-heart surgery can be performed safely on a pregnant woman, but usually less risky measures can be used.

Congenital heart defects which are unlikely to cause problems during pregnancy, even if they have not been corrected, are:

- Small, uncomplicated ventricular septal defects
- Uncomplicated patent ductus arteriosus
- Mild to moderate pulmonary stenosis

The following uncorrected congenital heart defects may cause problems during pregnancy. Again, their impact depends on their severity. If they're not severe enough to cause symptoms during pregnancy, it's unlikely they will cause problems during pregnancy. But you should be watched by doctors familiar with this type of defect in pregnancy.

- **Atrial septal defect.** An atrial septal defect (ASD) is a "hole" in the atrium, between the upper chambers of the heart, and is one of the most common congenital heart defects found in women. Most of the time, an ASD does not pose problems during pregnancy. On rare occasions, complications can develop, particularly if you have a large "shunt" or abnormal blood flow through your heart, allowing a significant amount of blood to wash back into your lungs. Extremely serious problems can develop if your atrial or ventricular septal defect has caused you to develop Eisenmenger syndrome, a condition in which blood pressure on the right side of the heart becomes greater than the left, shunting oxygen-depleted blood into the major organs of the body. This problem is discussed in Chapter 8.
- **Coarctation of the aorta.** If you have coarctation of the aorta, part of your aorta is too narrow. Whether or not it will cause complications depends on how severe the narrowing is. Your doctor may recommend you have it surgically corrected before pregnancy. If you don't, your blood pressure may become very

difficult to control during pregnancy and delivery—particularly during labor. If your defect is not corrected, your doctor may want to induce delivery before your due date.

- **Cyanotic congenital heart defects.** Some congenital heart defects are known as cyanotic because they can cause your lips and the beds of your fingernails and toenails to take on a bluish tint. This means that the blood going to your skin has a lower than normal amount of oxygen in it because of your heart defect. Congenital heart defects which cause such problems include tetralogy of Fallot, transposition of the great arteries, and Ebstein's anomaly.

These defects are referred to as cyanotic because they also result in the formation of a shunt, a pathway by which some of your blood flows in the wrong direction. This is dangerous because the abnormal blood pathway prevents your body's vital organs from receiving enough oxygenated blood. When you're not pregnant, your heart can compensate for this deficiency by increasing the number of oxygen-carrying cells in your blood. Because of the changes in your blood which occur during pregnancy, your body is no longer able to compensate. As your heart struggles to delivery oxygenated blood both to your body's organs and to the baby, it can become overworked and weakened.

If your defect is mild, it probably will not cause a problem during pregnancy. If it's severe enough to cause symptoms either before you become pregnant or early in your pregnancy, this is a forewarning that you may experience problems during your pregnancy. These are not generally the serious types of problems which can doom a pregnancy, but they do require that your pregnancy be very carefully monitored by doctors skilled in handling high-risk pregnancies.

Will my baby inherit my congenital heart defect? Congenital heart defects are very uncommon, and the chances of your baby's inheriting your defects are slim. Some types of congenital heart defects, however, do tend to run in families. For more information, see Chapter 8.

HEART VALVE PROBLEMS IN PREGNANCY

Most women with valve problems in the United States are past the age of childbearing. Their problems usually result from aging or from rheumatic heart disease, but there are heart valve problems which can affect younger women; they're discussed below.

MITRAL VALVE PROLAPSE

Mitral valve prolapse, an anomaly commonly found in women, generally causes no problems during pregnancy. Indeed, the increase in your blood volume during pregnancy may result in the temporary disappearance of symptoms. Such symptoms usually reappear within a few weeks to a few months after the baby is delivered. Rarely, women with mitral valve prolapse develop a complication called mitral regurgitation, which is discussed below. For a further discussion of mitral valve prolapse, see Chapter 7.

RHEUMATIC HEART DISEASE

There is a faulty belief that rheumatic fever is an old-fashioned disease that has gone the way of high-button shoes and bustles. This is only partly true. While it's becoming less common for women of childbearing age to exhibit signs of rheumatic heart disease, which is often the aftermath of rheumatic fever, it's not impossible to find it, particularly in women who have immigrated to the United States from countries where rheumatic fever is still prevalent.

Most commonly, women who have suffered rheumatic fever develop either mitral stenosis (blockage) or mitral regurgitation (leakage), or a combination of both. Frequently women with such problems can also develop atrial fibrillation, a type of heart rhythm irregularity which can lead to serious problems. Atrial fibrillation is discussed in Chapter 10.

MITRAL STENOSIS

Mitral stenosis, a stiffening and thickening due to calcification of the heart's mitral valve, can be very worrisome in pregnancy, particularly if it has heretofore remained undetected. Symptoms of mitral stenosis include shortness of breath and bodily swelling.

If you have a mild version of this problem, you may need to do nothing more than follow a salt-restricted diet and possibly take a diuretic, or "water pill," to avoid retaining fluid during your pregnancy. If your valve is considerably damaged, however, you could develop major problems such as congestive heart failure or pulmonary edema, a dangerous buildup of fluid in your lungs. In this case, your doctor may recommend valvuloplasty, a nonsurgical method of widening the valve. Even during pregnancy, open-heart surgery can be done to replace your heart valve, but it's obviously not the first choice if other options are available.

AORTIC STENOSIS (CONGENITAL OR RHEUMATIC)

A normal aortic valve has three valvular cusps, which enable it to function properly. If you were born with this defect, you have one or two cusps, which prevent the valve from working properly. Damage to your heart valve caused by rheumatic heart disease can also prevent it from working properly. This valve problem means that your heart must work extra hard to pump enough blood through your body. During pregnancy, this can cause your heart to become very seriously overburdened.

If your defect is mild and you have no symptoms, the chances are good you won't experience problems during pregnancy. However, fainting, chest pain, or symptoms of congestive heart failure portend significant problems during pregnancy. In this case, your cardiologist may advise you to have your aortic valve replaced early in your pregnancy. If you're in the later stages of pregnancy, your doctor will take measures to reduce the demand on your heart, such as ordering bed rest and prescribing cardiovascular medications.

What if I need a heart valve replaced? If you have a valve disorder that may eventually require surgical repair, your doctor may recommend that you have the surgery before you become pregnant. If you're in the early stages of pregnancy and in urgent need of a valve replacement, your doctor may recommend open-heart surgery. If you're in the later stages of pregnancy, your doctor will probably recommend that surgery be postponed until the baby is delivered. Eventually, though, you'll probably face valve surgery.

Cardiac valve replacement in women of childbearing years raises difficult issues. If your heart valve needs to be replaced, the major question is whether or not you plan to have more children. Your decision has a direct bearing on the type of valve replacement you choose.

Two types of heart valves are currently available. One type, called a biological valve, is made from animal tissue, most often taken from a pig. The other is a mechanical valve. Biological valves deteriorate fairly quickly and need to be replaced, sometimes only after several years; some experts believe they wear out even more quickly during pregnancy. Because they last longer, mechanical heart valves are generally the choice for younger people. Although the mechanical valve would seem the logical choice, this is not true in women who plan to become pregnant. Mechanical valves are more vulnerable to the formation of blood clots, so those who have them must take the powerful anticlotting drug called wafarin, known popularly under the trade name Coumadin, which has been linked to birth defects and other complications.

Hence the dilemma: If you have a biological valve implanted while you're still young, there's a strong probability it will need to be replaced before long. Most cardiovascular surgeons don't balk at the prospect of performing the operation to replace a biological valve once, but consider having to do the surgery twice or more increasingly hazardous. If you need a valve replaced, your surgeon may advise you to have a biological valve because it poses less risk to your unborn child should you become pregnant. However, if you want more children, you'll probably also be advised to have your family quickly so that when your biological valve wears out, it can be replaced with a mechanical version.

In some cases, it may be possible to repair the aortic valve. This type of "plastic" surgery of the valve is commonly performed on the mitral valve and is being found suitable for some patients with aortic valve problems. Repair has fewer of the problems associated with either mechanical or biological valve replacement. Since you still have your own "native" valve, blood clots rarely form after surgery, so you don't need to take powerful blood thinners. Also, the durability of the repaired valve probably exceeds that of a valve made from animal tissue.

What if I already have a replaced valve? Most women whose valves have already been replaced usually suffer no problems during pregnancy. If you become pregnant and you have a mechanical valve, your doctor will want to switch you from Coumadin, which is taken orally, to a safer blood thinner, most likely heparin, which you must inject yourself. This underscores why, if you have such a problem, you should be cared for by a doctor experienced in treating it. Such a physician will have staff who can teach you to inject the heparin.

CARDIAC ARRHYTHMIAS DURING PREGNANCY

In pregnancy, women sometimes develop arrhythmias, or abnormal heart rhythms. Usually this doesn't signify anything worrisome. However, arrhythmia which develops during pregnancy should be evaluated; if it's caused by an underlying heart problem, it may require treatment. In a few cases, an arrhythmia may be life-threatening.

Treatments for arrhythmias vary depending on the type of rhythm disturbance. Most methods for treating arrhythmias, such as drugs, pacemakers, low-frequency radio wave ablation, and even portable defibrillators have been used successfully in pregnant women.

If an antiarrhythmic medication is indicated, your doctor should try to choose one that has been on the market long enough to acquire a safety record when given to pregnant women. This is an area where you should expect your doctor to be cautious, as some antiarrhythmic medications can be dangerous. (Also see Chapter 10.)

MARFAN'S SYNDROME

Marfan's syndrome technically is not a congenital heart defect but a disease of the connective tissue. If you have Marfan's but have not experienced problems, you most likely will have no complications during pregnancy. However, if before becoming pregnant you experience cardiovascular problems, they can become life-threatening during pregnancy. Such problems can include dissection or tearing of the aorta, a dangerously leaky mitral valve, or congestive heart failure. And there is a 50 percent risk of passing Marfan's to your children. Under these circumstances, whether or not to have a baby is a difficult decision. Before deciding, consider consulting a genetic counselor.

PULMONARY HYPERTENSION

Pulmonary hypertension, or high blood pressure which builds up in the vessels that carry the blood from your heart to your lungs, is a threatening condition for both you and your unborn baby. This condition should not be confused with ordinary high blood pressure.

Sometimes pulmonary hypertension occurs for no underlying reason, but at other times there is a medical cause, such as Eisenmenger syndrome, which was discussed earlier. If you have pulmonary hypertension, your doctor may advise you not to become pregnant or to consider terminating the pregnancy. If you choose to continue your pregnancy, you and the fetus will have to be closely monitored, and you may spend most of your pregnancy in bed and possibly on oxygen. The baby will be delivered as soon as it's judged safe to do so.

Pulmonary hypertension is by no means a common disease, but it does tend to afflict women more than men. The average age of women when they're diagnosed is thirty-five. If you have pulmonary hypertension, you may be able to bear a child successfully, but you should consider yourself at extremely high risk and seek out highly expert medical care.

PERIPARTUM CARDIOMYOPATHY

Peripartum cardiomyopathy is a rare but very serious disease which results in heart failure. It may appear for no apparent reason during the last month of pregnancy or shortly after delivery. Estimates vary, but it's thought to occur once in every 1,300 to 4,000 deliveries. Although it seems to appear for no apparent reason, an unrecognized underlying cardiac disorder often becomes evident.

Signs and symptoms of peripartum cardiomyopathy are:

· Inability to breathe comfortably without being propped up
· Coughing
· Palpitations
· High blood pressure

Peripartum cardiomyopathy appears most frequently in:

· Older women
· Black women
· Women who have given birth before
· Women who are carrying multiple babies
· Women who experience high blood pressure disorders in pregnancy
· Women who develop high blood pressure after giving birth

There have been cases in which, with careful management and sheer good fortune, women have given birth to healthy children. If you develop the disease before you go into labor, however, the baby may be stillborn. There is also a 25 to 50 percent chance that you will die during pregnancy. The causes of death include congestive heart failure, blood clots, and infection. Sometimes after delivery a woman recovers completely and her heart apparently returns to normal. But if she becomes pregnant again, the condition can return, with even more disastrous results. This is the reason that doctors generally advise women who have had peripartum cardiomyopathy not to have more children.

♥ **Lifesaving Tip: Although peripartum cardiomyopathy develops during pregnancy, its symptoms may only show up in the several weeks after delivery. If you experience such symptoms, contact your doctor immediately.**

ENDOCARDITIS

This potentially deadly inflammation of the heart is rare during pregnancy, which is fortunate because it can be very difficult to treat. If your heart is already weakened, this disease can push you into congestive heart failure. The drugs used to treat it must be chosen with care because of potential harm to the unborn baby. The best precaution is to guard against developing endocarditis if you have a heart problem that puts you at risk. (Also see Chapter 10.)

HEART ATTACKS

Because coronary artery disease more commonly occurs after menopause, heart attacks are unusual in women of childbearing years. Heart attacks appear to be occurring more frequently, however, particularly in pregnant women who are older, smoke, or have hyperlipidemia, a metabolic disease which causes abnormally high cholesterol levels. Heart attacks can also occur in women who have mitral stenosis, whose heart valves have been replaced, and who have certain types of heart rhythm disturbances.

While suffering a minor heart attack during pregnancy does not necessarily pose a danger to either mother or unborn baby, it can be dangerous if it occurs during labor, or delivery.

HIGH BLOOD PRESSURE DISORDERS IN PREGNANCY

Hypertensive disorders are not directly heart-related, but are a major type of cardiovascular disorder in pregnant women. Because of the cardiovascular changes pregnant women undergo, such problems are not uncommon. Whether high blood pressure is pregnancy-induced or not, it can be very dangerous to a woman and her unborn baby.

PREGNANCY-INDUCED HYPERTENSION (PIH), PREECLAMPSIA AND ECLAMPSIA

Hypertensive conditions in pregnancy used to be called by one name, "toxemia." Today the terminology is a little more complicated. Some researchers like to classify hypertensive disorders of pregnancy into three distinct, progressive stages: pregnancy-induced hypertension, preeclampsia, and eclampsia. Others prefer to use "pregnancy-induced hypertension" as an umbrella term. Whatever the term used, such hypertensive disorders can mean serious problems for a woman and her unborn baby. The risk mounts in each progressive stage of hypertension.

An estimated one-quarter of all women who give birth in the United States develop abnormally high blood pressure, or pregnancy-induced hypertension (PIH), by the end of their pregnancies. Between 6 and 7 percent of women with PIH go on to develop preeclampsia, and about 5 percent of that group develops eclampsia. This is the most severe stage and can result in seizures, coma, and even death.

A substantial list of factors is considered to put women at increased risk of developing this problem. Women at risk include:

- Teenagers and women over the age of thirty-five
- Black women (although some studies do not show this)
- Women who are having their first pregnancy
- Women who have high blood pressure, diabetes, or kidney disease
- Women who have heart problems
- Women whose mothers had a hypertensive disorder in pregnancy

Any high blood pressure disorder is dangerous during pregnancy because the heart must work harder. This results in the blood vessels' becoming constricted, which lessens the amount of blood and nourishment the unborn baby receives. Hypertensive disorders also cause the body to manufacture less blood than it requires, which can make blood loss during delivery dangerous. For the unborn child, the chance of premature birth is greatly increased, as well as the chances of life-threatening disorders which can lead to death or severe permanent disabilities.

If you have pregnancy-induced hypertension, you probably won't notice any symptoms. The diagnosis is made by a combination of a high blood pressure reading and a finding of protein in the urine. If you're at risk for hypertension, your doctor may recommend that you monitor your blood pressure at home.

Among the many mysteries of pregnancy, none is more baffling to doctors than the reason that some women develop such hypertensive disorders and others do not. Current speculation is that the cause is an abnormality which occurs as the placenta is being formed. Genetic factors are also being studied.

Preeclampsia is a very serious disorder during pregnancy, and at present there is no treatment for it, notes Dr. Valerie M. Parisi, director of the maternal fetal medicine division at the University of Texas Medical School in Houston. According to Dr. Parisi, if a woman develops preeclampsia late in her pregnancy, the ideal treatment is to deliver the baby. If the disorder occurs too early in pregnancy for this to be considered, bed rest is often prescribed. While bed rest is not considered a treatment for preeclampsia, it may (with the emphasis on "may") potentially retard the disease's progression. Bed rest is also ordered for another reason, Dr. Parisi says: By lying in a certain position, the mother maximizes the flow of the blood to the baby.

Since the cause of such hypertensive disorders is not known, there is no certain way to prevent it, Dr. Parisi notes. However, several studies have shown that low doses of aspirin may prevent the development of such problems in women who are at high risk. The results of these studies are still preliminary, so a pregnant woman should discuss the pros and cons of such aspirin use with her doctor.

> ♥ Lifesaving Tip: If you're at risk of developing a hypertensive disorder in pregnancy, make sure your blood pressure and urine are tested frequently and regularly. If you develop this condition, even if you feel fine, follow your doctor's instructions to the letter. This condition, if untreated, can worsen, gravely endangering both you and your unborn baby.

A WORD ABOUT SMOKING AND PREGNANCY

There are plenty of excellent reasons to quit smoking if you're not pregnant. If you are pregnant, your need to quit becomes even more urgent. Besides the hazards cigarette smoking presents to you, babies of mothers who smoke are more likely to be born prematurely. Such babies are in danger of being born with such life-threatening lung conditions as respiratory distress syndrome and hyaline membrane disease. In addition, scientists have also found a possible link between mothers who smoke and sudden infant death syndrome. Studies have shown that children of smoking parents have health problems as well, such as respiratory illness.

Many women find pregnancy a strong motivation to quit smoking. If that's true in your case, congratulations. You may find it useful to consider how you'll handle life without smoking after the baby is born, so that you'll be less likely to turn to cigarettes if you're under stress or find yourself in a situation where you're accustomed to smoking.

IF YOU'RE ADVISED NOT TO HAVE CHILDREN

It's very rare for a cardiologist to advise a woman that because of her heart problem she should not become pregnant or that a pregnancy should be terminated. If you should receive such advice, make certain the cardiologist is very experienced in dealing with your particular heart problem.

In closing ... If you have a heart problem, you may be concerned that it will cast a shadow on the family you've been hoping for. But in the vast majority of cases, women with complicated heart problems who years ago could never hope to safely bear a child now can. It's very likely you're among them.

10
Other Heart Problems

This chapter is designed to provide you with information on many different problems which can befall your heart. The topics are arranged in alphabetical order. Problems which are relatively common in women, such as coronary artery disease and heart attacks, are dealt with at greater length than rarer problems, such as cardiac tumors.

ARRHYTHMIAS

"It's like a hummingbird fluttering in my chest," Joan, a woman in her late thirties, says, describing the feeling which was disrupting her life. Often the flutter escalated into a terrifying panic. A doctor gave her tranquilizers, which helped some. One night, she felt a crushing pain in her chest. She was hospitalized, but was told the tests showed nothing. "The doctor was very patronizing. He gave me a pat on the head, in essence, and told me, 'Go home and don't be such a nervous girl.'"

Joan struggled with her symptoms, frustrated because she couldn't find a doctor to take them seriously. It wasn't until she went to the Cleveland Clinic for cosmetic surgery that the mystery was solved. Since the cosmetic procedure required an anesthetic, Joan was hooked up to an electrocardiogram. The results sent the surgeons scurrying for a cardiologist. Some simple tests were performed which found that Joan suffers from Wolff-Parkinson-White syndrome, a type of arrhythmia, or irregular heartbeat.

Joan is not alone. Heartbeat irregularities are a common reason that many women end up in the offices of cardiologists.

Symptoms and signs of arrhythmias are:

- Palpitations (a pounding, fluttering, skipping, thumping, or racing heartbeat)
- Lightheadedness or fainting
- Chest pain
- Shortness of breath

Often such heartbeat irregularities aren't serious, but they can be truly frightening. As James Thurber once observed, the little innocent things that we hear in the darkness of night are always magnified by our imagination. So it is with the "pounding" or "jumping" that people frequently notice in their chests. This sensation, also often described as "stopping," "flopping," "bumping," or "racing," is collectively referred to by doctors as palpitations. It usually represents some irregularity of the heartbeat.

On the other hand, some types of arrhythmias can be very serious, even deadly. This is especially true if your heart is already weak from coronary disease or cardiomyopathy, a disease of the heart muscle. Cardiac rhythm disturbances associated with these problems account for the sudden death of about a thousand Americans every day.

The number of people with some type of arrhythmia appears to be increasing, particularly of those with arrhythmias after heart attacks. Ironically, this is because of improvements in cardiac treatment. "More people are surviving with coronary disease. More people are not dying because of heart attacks," notes Dr. Lynda E. Rosenfeld, a staff cardiologist at Yale–New Haven Hospital. "They are surviving, but are living on with problems associated with having had a heart attack. One such problem is arrhythmias."

♥ **Mindsaving Tip:** Having palpitations doesn't mean you have heart disease. Palpitations can have non-cardiac causes such as a too-active thyroid or a sensitivity to caffeine. Arrhythmias can also occur after a chest injury or open-heart surgery, or as a side effect of some drugs. Fatal heartbeat irregularities can also be caused by using cocaine.

WHAT CAUSES ARRHYTHMIAS: THE ABC'S OF PAC'S AND PVC'S

Although it's referred to as a pump, your heart actually consists of two pumps attached to one another side by side: a right one which pumps blood to the lungs, where the blood absorbs oxygen, and a left one which pumps this oxygen-laden blood to all the organs of the body. The upper chamber of each side is called the atrium; each bottom chamber, the ventricle.

Your heart's electrical system controls this pump function. This system has its own "timers" and "wiring" which stimulate it to contract a hundred thousand times per day on average. Each heartbeat originates in a specific area of the right atrium called the sinoatrial node. This is often referred to as your heart's intrinsic pacemaker.

But all the tissue of your heart is capable of originating heartbeats. When this occurs, and the beat comes from tissue in the atrium other than the sinoatrial node, or when signals echo and reenter the atrium, a premature heartbeat occurs. This is called a PAC, or premature atrial contraction. When a similar event occurs in the ventricle, it's called a premature ventricular complex (PVC). Virtually all of us experience PAC's and PVC's every day. Why some people are aware of even one or two a day and others tolerate several hundred an hour remains a mystery.

TYPES OF ARRHYTHMIAS

Your heart beats an average of 60 to 100 beats a minute, with most people's averaging about 72. An arrhythmia is a significant deviation from the normal range. There are two basic types of arrhythmias: tachycardias and bradycardias.

Tachycardias are arrhythmias in which your heart beats too fast. Types of tachyardia include atrial flutter, atrial fibrillation, paroxysmal supraventricular tachycardia (PSVT), Wolff-Parkinson-White syndrome, runs of premature ventricular contractions, ventricular tachycardia, and ventricular fibrillation.

Each of these arrhythmias has different characteristics, such as the rate of the heartbeat, whether it beats in a pattern or is chaotic, and whether the irregularity originates in the atrium or the ventricle. Wolff-Parkinson-White syndrome, for example, is caused by the development of an abnormal pathway in the heart which conducts electricity and can produce very fast heart rhythms.

Bradycardia is a heartbeat slower than sixty beats per minute. The hearts of well-conditioned athletes often beat more slowly than this. In practical terms, a slow heartbeat becomes abnormal when it results in too little blood flowing to the body, causing symptoms such as fatigue, shortness of breath, and even fainting spells.

HEART BLOCK

This is a disorder of the heart beat caused by an interruption in the passages of impulses through your heart's electrical system. Depending on the degree of the heart block, it can cause dizziness, fainting, or even strokes. Although heart block can occur at any age, it's primarily found in older people. Causes include coronary disease, hypertension, myocarditis (an inflammation of the heart muscle), and aging. It can also be caused by an overdose of heart drugs, such as digitalis. Mild cases do not require treatment. In the case of fainting, a pacemaker may be used. Medication is also sometimes prescribed until the person can be treated with a pacemaker.

♥ **Mindsaving Tip: Sometimes an arrhythmia which causes a number of symptoms can be harmless, while one which you may not even be aware of can be dangerous. Your doctor should diagnose any arrhythmia you have.**

FAINTING SPELLS

Some arrhythmias result not in palpitations but in fainting spells, or in a combination of the two. When such fainting spells occur, they may be harmful, even potentially deadly. If you suffer from unexplained fainting spells, you should definitely see your doctor. Several noncardiac causes of fainting are discussed in Chapter 5.

TESTING FOR ARRHYTHMIAS

The decision whether to treat an arrhythmia depends on what kind it is and whether you have any other heart problems. A strong, healthy heart can withstand an arrhythmia that might push a weakened heart into cardiac arrest.

If you're a healthy woman who experiences only an occasional palpitation, your doctor will probably tell you not to worry about it. If, on the other hand, you experience severe palpitations that interfere with your activities, or if you have other heart problems, your doctor will recommend that you undergo diagnostic tests. These tests are explained in Chapter 6.

If your test results are normal, then your arrhythmia probably is not serious, and unless it's very bothersome you'll probably prefer not to be treated for it. Sometimes such reassurance is all you need to live with minor flutters. Eliminating caffeine, tobacco, and alcohol, which can cause palpitations, can also help. However, if your arrhythmia requires treatment, the treatment will depend on the kind of heartbeat irregularity you have.

TREATING ARRHYTHMIAS

Over the past few decades, tremendous strides have been made in the treatment of arrhythmias. Doctors now can choose among several types of procedures or a combination of methods. Thus, it's especially important that your particular arrhythmia be evaluated by a cardiologist who specializes in electrophysiology (your heart's electrical system) and has access to up-to-date hospital facilities.

♥ **Lifesaving Tip:** If you suffer from a serious arrhythmia, particularly if it manifests itself as an episode of "sudden death," or cardiac arrest, you should be taken to the nearest hospital for immediate medical attention. After the crisis is over, consider getting a comprehensive evaluation of your heart by a cardiologist who specializes in arrhythmias.

DRUG TREATMENT   Antiarrhythmic drugs are responsible for saving hundreds of thousands of lives each year. Most of these drugs work by reducing the irritability of the heart cells responsible for the rhythm disturbances. These are strong drugs and should only be taken under close supervision by your doctor. You may also have to undergo periodic testing to make sure your medication is working properly.

RADIO WAVE ABLATION   In the past few years, this technique has shown excellent results in providing permanent relief for certain types of tachycardias, or fast heartbeats. Some specific arrhythmias it is used to treat include Wolff-Parkinson-White syndrome, AV nodal reentry tachycardia, and atrial fibrillation.

Radio frequency ablation does not require surgery. Dr. Deborah Williams, a cardiologist at the Cleveland Clinic, recalls attending a conference a few years ago at which surgery was presented as the only definitive treatment for Wolff-Parkinson-White. Today ablation has emerged as the treatment of choice. "That just shows you how fast things are changing," says Dr. Williams.

Radio wave ablation is a nonsurgical method in which thin wires are threaded up to your heart by way of your femoral vein, the accessible vessel near your groin. The catheter is advanced slowly and positioned within your heart, and radio waves are aimed at the heart tissue which is causing the problem. The procedure can last two to ten hours, although the trend is toward a shorter period to avoid excessive exposure to radiation. With these kinds of arrhythmias, ablation is proving more effective than medication; drugs typically work for a while, but then the arrhythmia reappears.

One complication is that in some cases the radio waves destroy not only the abnormal tissue, but also the specialized tissue which acts as your heart's intrinsic pacemaker system. How often this occurs depends on the type of arrhythmia treated. With Wolff-Parkinson-White, it occurs only rarely, an estimated 5 percent of the time. For AV nodal reentry tachycardia, it occurs about 15 percent of the time. When ablation is used for atrial fibrillation, however, a pacemaker is always required because, in order to eliminate the arrhythmia, the area of the heart which controls the heartbeat is damaged and heart block occurs.

♥ **Lifesaving Tip:** If you're planning to undergo radio wave ablation, you should understand that for certain rhythms you may require a pacemaker afterward. Try to minimize this possibility by asking the physician how often patients undergoing these types of procedures require pacemakers. If the figures are significantly higher than those mentioned here, you may want to consider consulting another doctor.

Radio wave ablation also has been used in cases of ventricular tachycardia, but with mixed results, usually a 40 to 50 percent success rate. If it fails, however, ablation with a higher energy frequency (DC ablation) is often successful in eliminating the problem.

People who have suffered with arrhythmias for years find great relief after ablation. "Before this technique, I remember seeing patients who weren't doing well on medication," says Dr. Williams. "They didn't feel well and their quality of life was not that great. Nowadays, there is a terrific difference, because the day they walk out after having the ablation, we can say, 'You're cured.' "

Undergoing the ablation procedure is very similar to undergoing balloon angioplasty; however, because of the length of the procedure, you're usually sedated a bit more. Though you're not unconscious, you'll probably sleep during at least part of the procedure. According to Dr. Williams, patients are most bothered by having to lie on their back for the several hours of the procedure. Eventually ablation may become an outpatient procedure, but currently an overnight stay in the hospital is routine.

♥ **Lifesaving Tip:** Ablation is *not* considered safe if you are or may be pregnant.

PACEMAKERS   Artificial pacemakers, small devices used to re-place the heartbeat, were introduced some twenty-five years ago. Over the years, they've become smaller, lighter, and more stream-lined. Once the size and weight of a can of tuna fish, they're now about the diameter and twice the thickness of a half-dollar.

Who are pacemakers for? Different types of rhythm distur-bances can result in your needing a pacemaker. One type is heart block. Another is bradycardia, which causes your heart to beat too slowly. An example of bradycardia is "sick sinus syndrome," which results in a very slow heartbeat or even very short periods of cardiac arrest. Pacemakers are also used to treat certain types of tachycardias known as "refractory." This means that, although your heart is beating very quickly, only some of these beats are functional and the rest are just beats which "echo," so for func-tional purposes, your heartbeat is actually very slow.

Besides the fact that it's a serious medical problem, the symptoms caused by a bradycardia can be frightening. A pace-maker may seem a very welcome alternative to being so tired that you can't even drag yourself around or fearing that you may pass out any minute. "If you're walking around with a heart rate of twenty beats, you don't feel very good," says Michelle Tobin, a nurse clinician who works with pacemaker patients at the Cleve-land Clinic. "You don't have a lot of energy, you might feel light-headed. A pacemaker can make a big difference."

It's more common for older women to require pacemakers, but not too rare for younger women to need them. Sometimes these women require a pacemaker after surgery for the correction of a congenital heart defect.

How do pacemakers work? A pacemaker is, in essence, a "chronostat." The device not only regulates the timing of your heartbeat (*chrono* is the Greek word for time), but it also works like a thermostat. A thermostat is designed to be set at a certain temperature and to be activated when the temperature falls be-low that. A pacemaker works much the same way; it's designed to start up automatically if your heartbeat falls below a certain point.

Over the years, the image of the pacemaker wearer has changed dramatically. Once the word "pacemaker" engendered images of the elderly, but they are worn by people of all ages. Over the years, different types of pacemakers have been developed to suit different needs. Some work constantly, providing the heart with a constant, regular beat. Others work "on demand," providing beats only when needed. Dual-chambered pacemakers, which replicate a normal heartbeat which starts in the atria and stimulates the ventricles, can vary the heart rate, enabling the wearer to enjoy vigorous exercise. Once implanted, a nurse, using a radio transmitter, can reprogram the pacemaker to adjust the heartbeat automatically for various activities. Once reprogrammed, you'll have the correct rhythm whether you're sleeping, exercising, or even having sex. Some pacemakers can even provide your doctor with diagnostic information over the telephone.

If you need a pacemaker, talk to your doctor about the one best suited for you. There are plenty of choices.

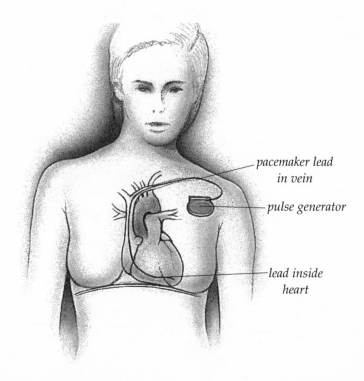

pacemaker lead in vein

pulse generator

lead inside heart

Cardiac Pacemaker. A pacemaker consists of a pulse generator containing the "brains" and the system's battery, as well as an insulated wire (a "lead") that maintains the flow of electricity from the pulse generator to the heart muscle. The lead is inserted into the heart through a vein located underneath the collar bone. The pulse generator is slipped into a small pocket created between the skin and the muscle of the upper chest.

How is a pacemaker inserted? If you're going to have a pacemaker inserted you'll probably check in to the hospital the day of the procedure and stay over for a day or two, so that you can rest and so that your pacemaker can be tested to make sure it's working properly.

For the procedure itself, you're conscious, but heavily sedated. A local anesthetic is used. An incision of about two inches is made below your collarbone. Using a device similar to those used to insert a catheter, the wires of the pacemaker are inserted through a vein into your heart. The pacemaker's generator, the coin-sized unit, is connected to a wire and is implanted where the incision was made. The procedure, which takes about three hours, is usually performed by a surgeon or cardiologist.

What will the pacemaker look like when it's in? How a pacemaker will look once it's implanted is a concern of some women. Though pacemakers have gotten much smaller and lighter, the device can still be noticed when you wear a bathing suit or low-cut evening gown, and you can feel it if you brush your fingers over your skin. Talk to your doctor to make sure the pacemaker is implanted as unobtrusively as possible.

> ♥ **Mindsaving Tip: If you're very self-conscious, ask your doctor about the possibility of implanting the pacemaker in an area where it will be completely hidden. You may need to consult a plastic surgeon in addition to the doctor. Don't be surprised if this notion is not greeted with enthusiasm. Doctors sometimes resist deviating from their normal procedures. But if it's important to you, it's worth pursuing.**

What happens afterward? You can go home from the hospital within a few days after the pacemaker is inserted. You may feel fatigued at first. There will also be a period of adjustment lasting about six weeks, when you're becoming accustomed to having a pacemaker nestled beneath your skin. Over this period, the pacemaker's wires will grow into your heart tissue so that the pacemaker is less likely to be dislodged. During this time, you'll need to be careful. Your doctor will probably give you permission to drive, but strenuous activities which involve you using your arms a lot, such as golf or tennis, are out. So is most housework and lifting anything heavier than ten pounds—including children and grandchildren!

Your new pacemaker also may need to be adjusted so that it provides you with the right heart rhythm for your activities. If your heartbeat is too slow, for example, you'll never have the oomph you need to do aerobics or even take a brisk walk. At the Cleveland Clinic, pacemaker nurses go to great lengths to make sure you're happy with your pacemaker. They can put you on a treadmill and adjust your pacemaker's function properly, to make sure your pacemaker is providing you with enough zip.

"We've even had patients make beds here," says nurse clinician Michelle Tobin. "One woman told us, 'Every time I make a bed and rustle the sheets just so, I feel funny.' So we had her do it here. Sure enough, we were able to adjust her pacemaker so she'd feel fine."

There may be other, more subtle adjustments as well. If your heart rate has been very slow for a while, you may need some time to become adjusted to your new, quicker one. Although you can't hear your pacemaker, you may be very conscious of your heart beating, especially at night, before you fall asleep.

Some women have difficulty adjusting at first to a pacemaker because they feel as if a device, not they, is in control of their heart. "A woman thinks she is invincible, and now she is relying on a device," says Betty Ching, a pacemaker nurse at the Cleveland Clinic. "I've found that men seem to handle that a bit better than women do."

Invariably, that feeling subsides when women discover that the pacemaker enables them to do things they haven't done in a while. Sometimes, Betty Ching says, the change can be very dramatic. She recalls a forty-one-year-old woman who worked for a local company. She had a heart rhythm problem which caused her to pass out several times a day. While the rhythm problem itself was not considered medically serious, it was, for all practical purposes, ruining her life. "This woman used to faint four or five times a day," says Ching. "Every time she'd stand up, she'd gray out, and all of a sudden, she'd be down. You can't live your life like that. With her pacemaker, she's feeling so much better. She's back at work. She's not afraid to go out anymore."

♥ **Mindsaving tip: Some people are unable to become psy-chologically adjusted to their pacemaker, but this is ex-**

tremely rare. It's much more likely that before long, you'll become so used to your pacemaker it will feel as if it was always a part of you.

Here are some common questions about pacemakers.

How long do pacemakers last?

Pacemakers generally don't wear out, but their batteries do. You can expect your pacemaker battery to last at least five years. However, if your pacemaker is the "on demand" type and is rarely needed, it could last years longer. When the battery does wear out, the unit needs to be replaced. No one looks forward to this, but since pacemakers are always being improved, this may provide you with an opportunity to be fitted with one which suits your needs even better.

How do I know whether the battery is wearing down?

You don't need to worry about it. These days, a nurse or technician at the hospital periodically checks on the strength of the battery by using a special device over the phone.

With a pacemaker, can I do all the activities I normally do?

Absolutely! Once the incision is healed and the pacemaker is firmly in place, it's not likely to dislodge, so you can perform all the activities you normally did.

When pacemakers were first developed, people had a lot of misconceptions about them. Some would be laughable if they hadn't been so worrisome. For example, nuclear-powered pacemakers were once available until they were replaced by the lithium-cell-powered devices which are now favored. One patient a few years ago was delighted when her nuclear pacemaker was removed. "Can I take my honeymoon now?" she asked. The poor woman had waited twenty years to take the trip because when her nuclear-powered pacemaker had been implanted, she had been warned not to leave the state without notifying the Atomic Energy Commission. She had tried to call the commission without success, not knowing it had been dismantled!

How do I know my pacemaker is working okay?

Problems with pacemakers, and the wires which connect them to your heart, are uncommon, but they can occur. If you experience the symptoms which resulted in your getting a pacemaker, call your doctor. Sometimes, you may not have experienced anything more than subtle symptoms; if so, ask your doctor to review with you symptoms which indicate that your pacemaker or its wiring may not be working right. You'll be taught to take your pulse; usually minor pulse irregularities don't indicate a problem, but if, for example, your pacemaker is set to give you 70 beats per minute, and you carefully check your pulse and discover it has fallen below 60, this could indicate a problem. Likewise, if while you're resting your pulse consistently stays over 100, this may indicate your pacemaker is not working properly, and you should call your physician.

♥ Lifesaving Tip: Problems with pacemakers are uncommon. However, if you've suffered a fainting or near fainting spell, or you have other reasons to believe your pacemaker is not working properly, contact your doctor immediately. In most cases, whether or not the pacemaker is working properly can be determined over the telephone.

If you have a pacemaker, you're wearing a piece of artificial material in your heart, which can make you more vulnerable to bacterial endocarditis, discussed later in this chapter. Some doctors recommend taking antibiotics as a protective measure, but others don't believe it's warranted. Discuss this with your doctor.

Over the years, there have been other misconceptions about pacemakers. Here are the most common:

· **If you wear a pacemaker, your permanent won't hold.** A pacemaker has no effect on your hairstyle.
· **You can't go through the metal detector at an airport without setting it off.** Again, untrue. But pacemaker wearers are issued identification cards, so if you're concerned about metal detec-

tors, you can show your card to the security guard in airports or stores.

- **A garage-door opener can turn off or reprogram my pacemaker.** Not true, though a lot of people worry about this.
- **If I'm wearing a pacemaker, it's unsafe to use an electric blanket or heating pad.** It's perfectly safe for you to use any home electrical appliance while wearing your pacemaker.

♥ Mindsaving Tip: The most widely held myth about pacemakers is that you must not go near a microwave oven if you're wearing one. Modern pacemakers are well shielded, so you can approach and operate a microwave (unless it's a really old model) without a second thought.

IMPLANTABLE DEFIBRILLATORS Among the most dangerous of heart conditions is the type of arrhythmia which can cause cardiac arrest, usually when the heart goes into such a quick erratic rhythm, it can no longer pump blood effectively. The result is "sudden death," or cardiac arrest. In cases such as these, a device called an implantable cardioverter defibrillator (ICD) is implanted in the body. It uses an electric shock to restart the heart rhythm.

This device, which became available in the late 1980s, is made up of electrodes connected to a sensing unit implanted in the abdomen. The electrodes are actually implanted in or on the heart. A typical ICD senses arrhythmias in ten to thirty-five seconds, then delivers an electric jolt to the heart. ICD's are used in cases of life-threatening arrhythmias that don't respond to other types of treatment.

While most people adjust to wearing a pacemaker quite easily, the ICD is significantly larger, about the size of a portable cassette player, and heavier as well. The sensing unit (the "brains" of the unit) is implanted under the skin of the abdomen, where it can be seen and felt, especially in slim or petite patients. But implant techniques can minimize this.

"Less than twenty years ago, pacemakers were the size of defibrillators and now they're the size of a tiny eyeshadow case," says Dr. Lynda Rosenfeld, a cardiologist at Yale–New Haven Hospital. "That's what's going to happen to defibrillators. They've already gotten smaller." Until then, she is experimenting with different positioning to conceal ICD's as well as possible.

Obviously, if you're concerned about your appearance, an ICD is an issue. But it's worth remembering that, if you have been revived after an episode of cardiac arrest, the chances are very great that it could occur again, this time with deadly results. So the ICD, cumbersome as it seems, is truly a lifesaver, and any cosmetic considerations should truly be secondary.

SURGERY   Today, open-heart surgery is rarely used to correct arrhythmias; it's resorted to mainly when other types of treatment have failed, or when a person is slated for heart surgery for another reason and such treatment for an arrhythmia at the same time is deemed beneficial.

Different surgical procedures are used for various types of rhythm disturbances. Sometimes surgery is done following a heart attack. In this case, the surgical procedure involves cutting away, or even freezing, the area of scar tissue which may be causing a ventricular arrhythmia. In the case of atrial fibrillation, when all else fails, another type of surgery may be used. This radical operation is called a maze procedure in which the atrium is actually taken apart and reassembled. In general, though, other techniques discussed earlier in this chapter, such as radio wave ablation, have largely supplanted surgery for many other arrhythmias.

♥ **Lifesaving Tip: If your doctor is talking about surgery before other techniques have been tried, consider getting a second opinion. It's preferable to correct an arrhythmia nonsurgically, if possible.**

♥ **Mindsaving Tip: If you have a rhythm disturbance which requires treatment, but that's your only heart problem, medication or a device such as a pacemaker or ICD may benefit you greatly. But if your heart has been damaged or greatly weakened by coronary disease, such devices can be helpful, but are not a cure-all.**

BACTERIAL ENDOCARDITIS

Throughout this book you'll find many references to bacterial endocarditis. This is because bacterial endocarditis (also referred to simply as endocarditis) is a potentially deadly heart infection that many people with heart problems are at risk of contracting. Although it is easily prevented, endocarditis is difficult to treat, and can result in death or a seriously damaged heart. Even procedures used to correct a heart problem, the most noticeable example being an artificial heart valve, can make your heart vulnerable to endocarditis.

WHAT IS ENDOCARDITIS?

Endocarditis is an inflammation of the endocardium, your heart's internal lining. The infection is often caused by bacteria which normally reside safely in your mouth, respiratory system, or gastrointestinal tract. Such bacteria are dangerous if they escape into your bloodstream and enter organs which are usually bacteria-free, such as your heart and brain. Usually your body's immune defenses destroy such bacteria almost instantly, but if a bacterium lodges in the tissues of your heart's lining or valves, and evades your body's natural defenses, serious damage can be done. If you have certain types of heart problems, you're at risk for this potentially fatal and difficult to treat ailment.

Although it's not known why some people get endocarditis while others don't, if your heart is structurally abnormal or damaged, you're at particular risk for the disease. This is because the bacteria which cause endocarditis are attracted to areas of the heart which have been damaged or where there is exposure to a turbulent blood flow. If you have a leaky heart valve, or your heart valve has been replaced, just such conditions exist. The bacteria can then lodge in your heart, begin to grow, and cause damage.

SYMPTOMS OF ENDOCARDITIS

Endocarditis can be insidious. The infection can cause symptoms immediately or can remain undetected for months. Acute bacterial endocarditis comes on suddenly. Symptoms include:

- Severe chills
- High fever (102 to 104 degrees) or, in some cases, low fever (102 degrees or less)
- Shortness of breath
- Rapid, irregular heartbeat

Endocarditis can also develop slowly, over a period of weeks or even a few months. Symptoms include:

- General malaise, fatigue, weakness
- Low-grade fever
- Loss of appetite
- Night sweats
- Muscular aches and pains
- Painful joints
- Headache
- Pallor

♥ **Lifesaving Tip: Sue Dehner, a Cleveland Clinic nurse who educates cardiac patients about endocarditis, says that too often a person may develop endocarditis but think she has only the flu. Bear this in mind if you're at risk for developing endocarditis.**

HOW IS ENDOCARDITIS TREATED?

When endocarditis is discussed, the focus is usually on prevention, because this ailment is proof of the adage, "An ounce of prevention is worth a pound of cure." Treatment for endocarditis often involves a lengthy hospital stay, perhaps six weeks or even longer, while the patient is given strong antibiotics by injection.

♥ **Lifesaving Tip: Endocarditis is diagnosed by blood culture, but the results may take several days. If your doctor seriously suspects you do have endocarditis, you'll probably be hospitalized even before the results of the blood culture are received so that treatment can begin.**

Even though endocarditis is sometimes difficult to treat with even the strongest antibiotics, it's fairly easy to prevent. If you're at risk for endocarditis, you should take antibiotics *before* undergoing procedures which could introduce the bacteria into your bloodstream. The American Heart Association recently updated its guidelines on how and when antibiotics should be used. If you're at risk, ask your doctor for a list of the procedures before which penicillin should be used, or contact your local chapter of the heart association. The procedures range from a dental cleaning to more elaborate medical procedures.

♥ Lifesaving Tip: If you're at risk for endocarditis, keep in mind that although antibiotics protect against endocarditis quite well, no method is 100 percent effective. Call your doctor immediately if you have symptoms of endocarditis.

CARDIAC TUMORS

When we were working on the final chapters of this book, I had a visit from my friend Henry, whom I had not seen in nearly twenty years, and his wife, Shirley, whom I had never met. When we discussed my experiences, Shirley, who is forty-two, mentioned that she had had a heart murmur years before which had not signified any problem. Our conversation stuck in her mind, though, and she decided to have an echocardiogram. The test did show that her heart murmur was nothing to worry about. But then the doctor added, "I'm really glad you came in. The echocardiogram showed you have a mass growing in your heart." Shirley turned to him, shocked. "That's impossible," she said. "I feel fine."

Improbable, yes. Impossible, no. Shirley had a benign cardiac tumor. Within a month, she had undergone open-heart surgery, the tumor had been removed, and she was well on the road to recovery. She was very lucky, the doctor told her; though benign, the tumor might have proved fatal.

The good news about cardiac tumors is that they're rare and most often benign. In fact, about 75 percent of primary tumors are benign, and myxomas make up about half of this group. Although a myxoma can occur in either sex, it's most commonly found in women between the ages of thirty and sixty. Benign tumors can also occur in the pericardium, the heart's inner lining.

A myxoma, which can be most easily described as similar to a polyp, is a benign tumor which grows on a stalk and is comprised of mucuslike tissue. It is more common for a myxoma to develop in other parts of the body, such as under the skin in the limbs or neck, or less commonly in the abdomen, bladder, or bone. More rarely, it can develop in the heart, usually occurring in the left atrium, the upper chamber on the left side of the heart.

Although myxomas are benign, it's generally recommended that they be removed. They can grow quite large, sometimes to the size of a golf ball or even larger. A myxoma often grows on a stalk and can flop back and forth, seriously disrupting the normal flow of blood through the heart, causing such cardiac symptoms as fainting, breathlessness, coughing, palpitations, chest pain, and fatigue (although sometimes, as in Shirley's case, the myxoma manifests no symptoms at all). While it's very unlikely that such a tumor will become detached, in an estimated 50 percent of the cases, a bit of material can break off and may travel to the brain, resulting in a stroke. Open-heart surgery is required to remove a myxoma, and usually results in a complete cure. It's often possible to remove other primary tumors which occur in the heart as well.

Tumors such as myxomas which occur in the heart are called primary tumors. Sometimes secondary tumors appear in the heart as well. These are tumors which have metastasized, or spread, from malignancies located elsewhere in the body. These are usually not considered curable, but are shrunk with radiation and chemotherapy.

The diagnosis of a cardiac tumor usually comes as a shock to both doctor and patient because these tumors occur so rarely. In medical parlance, in fact, my friend Shirley is known as a "zebra." This comes from the old diagnostic saying, "If you hear hoofbeats in the average American town, it's a horse, not a zebra." For a doctor, this means that if a relatively young woman is experiencing symptoms such as chest pain or palpitation, the diagnosis is probably something common, like mitral valve prolapse, not a cardiac tumor. Being known as a "zebra" probably wouldn't comfort Shirley, but it does explain her doctor's surprise.

CONGESTIVE HEART FAILURE

"Congestive heart failure" is one of those terms which sounds drastically worse than it may actually be. This is not to say that it doesn't denote a serious heart problem. But "congestive heart failure" (and the equally frightening term "heart failure") sounds as if the heart could stop beating at any moment, which is only rarely the case. The term simply means that the heart is too weak to adequately perform its pumping function.

Unlike the other cardiac problems discussed in this book, which can occur independently, congestive heart failure is always a manifestation of an underlying cardiac disease. It's a common malady; some 2 million Americans have congestive heart failure, and 250,000 new cases are diagnosed each year. It's particularly common in people over the age of seventy, but with proper treatment, individuals who have it can often lead reasonably normal lives.

WHAT IS CONGESTIVE HEART FAILURE?

In congestive heart failure, pressure "backs up" in the pulmonary veins, where the blood loses fluids to the lungs and tissues of the legs, causing telltale shortness of breath and bodily swelling. The inefficient pumping of blood can also result in low cardiac output which, in turn, causes fatigue, especially with exertion. As the heart strives to compensate for these problems, it usually becomes enlarged and thickened, and the problem grows progressively worse.

Sometimes congestive heart failure is caused by a problem not specifically related to the heart, such as severe lung disease, severe anemia, or hyperthyroidism (overactivity of the thyroid gland). But it's most commonly caused by heart problems, such as coronary disease (damage from a heart attack), a faulty heart valve, cardiomyopathy (a destructive disease of the heart muscle tissue itself), bacterial endocarditis, or undetected congenital heart defects. Although congestive heart failure most commonly occurs in the elderly, it sometimes appears in younger people, often caused by an undiagnosed heart ailment.

Symptoms of congestive heart failure are:

- **Shortness of breath.** This can occur with exertion, or when you're lying flat in bed. You may feel unable to catch your breath. When you go to bed, you find you sleep more comfortably propped up against pillows. During the night, you may wake up panting or gasping for breath.

· **Profound fatigue.** Simply walking up a flight of stairs can leave you winded and exhausted.
· **Coughing.** In the early stages of congestive heart failure, the cough can be nonproductive; later on, you may bring up bloody or frothy sputum.
· **Rapid weight gain and/or bodily swelling.** This is caused by an accumulation of fluids in your body, usually in the legs and ankles.
· **Rapid heartbeat.**

If you've been diagnosed with a type of heart problem which can lead to heart failure and you experience one or more of these symptoms, it's an important signal that your condition may have worsened. Call your cardiologist right away. If you don't have any heart problem of which you're aware, symptoms such as these suggest that a visit to your family doctor or internist is in order. If you suspect you may have a heart problem, and you don't believe your doctor is giving the possibility adequate consideration, consider requesting a referral to a cardiologist.

HOW IS HEART FAILURE TREATED?

Congestive heart failure is treated in two main ways. In an estimated 5 to 10 percent of cases, the underlying disease causing the symptoms can be cured. Otherwise, the symptoms of the disease are a major focus of treatment. The milder the symptoms, the better the outlook.

To treat heart failure, your doctor will prescribe drugs, sometimes in various combinations. If you're in an advanced state of heart failure, you may have to be hospitalized. The medications used to treat congestive heart failure include digoxin (Lanoxin), which increases the heart muscle's ability to pump, and diuretics, to help rid your body of excessive fluid. Recently, ACE inhibitors, a type of vasodilator (which helps relax the arteries), have shown promise in preventing the onset of symptoms as well as being a major new therapy for heart failure itself. Cardiovascular drugs are discussed in more detail in Chapter 11.

♥ Lifesaving Tip: The cardiovascular drugs used to treat heart failure are powerful, so periodic follow-ups with your doctor are necessary.

If you have congestive heart failure, you should take care to avoid contracting infections. You should also try to maintain your ideal weight, not smoke, and eat a low-salt diet. Following these guidelines can prevent the condition from worsening and ensure that you have many productive years ahead.

♥ Mindsaving Tip: Many people lead active lives long after their congestive heart failure problem has been diagnosed. Although you may not be aware of it, some of the people you see at work or in your neighborhood every day may be living proof that it's possible to lead a reasonably normal life with congestive heart failure.

CORONARY ARTERY DISEASE

Lindsay, a pretty woman of thirty-six with shoulder-length dark hair which framed her heart-shaped face, sat in a chair in an examining room at the Cleveland Clinic. She nervously twisted her hands in her lap. By her side sat her husband, Pete. Like Lindsay, he looked worried. For the past three years, Lindsay had been having pains in her chest, which were now radiating to her shoulder blades as well. Two doctors had brushed her worries aside. "They told me I was too young to have heart disease." But Lindsay was not inclined to believe them.

"Virtually every relative on my father's side has had heart disease," she said. "I just lost an uncle last November to a heart attack, and my dad's had heart surgery. I even have a cousin who's a year younger than me; she has chest pains too. Her father died of a heart attack, and he was only fifty."

As her test results showed, Lindsay did indeed have coronary artery disease, although it had not yet become advanced. If she had listened to those first doctors and ignored her chest pains, she might eventually have had a heart attack. Now her disease can be treated, and she may avoid the need for more drastic measures, such as angioplasty or coronary bypass surgery, possibly forever.

WHAT IS CORONARY ARTERY DISEASE?

Coronary artery disease is commonly referred to as heart disease, but that's like referring to all kinds of cancers simply as cancer. Coronary artery disease refers to a particular type of ailment characterized by the formation of fatty deposits, known as plaque, on the walls of the three major coronary arteries. These three vessels deliver oxygenated blood to your heart, and it's this oxygen your heart needs to survive. When the arteries are narrowed by atherosclerosis, the result may be angina pectoris, or chest pain from coronary artery disease. If the arteries suddenly become completely blocked, the result is a heart attack.

RECOGNIZING CORONARY ARTERY DISEASE

Because women tend to develop coronary artery disease several years later than men, it was once believed that it was not a danger for women at all. In the past few years, this attitude has greatly changed, but some doctors may still be practicing with this outdated and dangerous viewpoint.

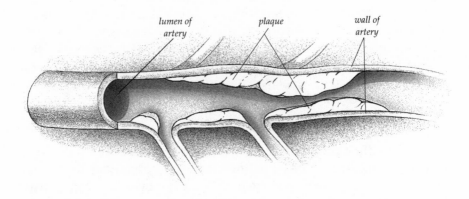

lumen of artery   *plaque*   *wall of artery*

Atherosclerotic Artery. Fatty deposits called atherosclerotic plaque narrow the artery, impeding the flow of blood to the heart and possibly causing a blood clot which may result in a heart attack.

TREATING CORONARY ARTERY DISEASE

Not so long ago, little could be done for coronary artery disease. The comedian George Burns, in his best-selling book *Gracie*, wrote movingly about the death from heart disease of his beloved wife, Gracie Allen: "Her heart was bad and there was nothing we could do about it. This was long before they started doing bypass operations. In those days, when your heart stopped, you died."

Over the decades, coronary artery disease has changed from a disease you died of to a problem you lived with. Today the viewpoint is that it's not only a problem you can live with, but under some circumstances, you may even be able to beat it. Currently, there are four major methods of treatment. One of them, or a combination, can be your key to conquering this once fatal disease. They are:

- Lifestyle changes
- Cardiovascular drugs
- Angioplasty and atherectomy
- Coronary bypass surgery

In Lindsay's case, it's hoped that changing her lifestyle will be sufficient to slow, or even stop, the progression of coronary artery disease. The changes she can make are discussed in this chapter. The other treatment alternatives are discussed in Chapter 11.

If I have heart disease, won't I need surgery? When Lindsay was waiting for her test results, one of the thoughts that gnawed at her was that she might need coronary bypass surgery. But over the years, other effective treatments have been developed. The best plan for you is an individual one which should be determined by you and your doctor, taking such factors as these into consideration:

- **Your age.** Once it was unusual for a coronary bypass to be done on people over sixty-five, but this has changed. The surgery is now successfully performed on people in their seventies and even their eighties.
- **Your overall health,** including whether you have other conditions such as high blood pressure. If you have high blood pressure, for example, you may be a good candidate for certain cardiovascular drugs, since some work on both problems.
- **Which of your coronary arteries is affected and to what extent.** This can determine whether lifestyle changes and medica-

tion are enough, or whether you need angioplasty or bypass surgery.

· **Your preferences.** Sometimes the best way to proceed is evident. Often, though, there may be more than one "right" method, and choices can be made. Your informed decision should be the last word.

Since Lindsay's test results showed that her arteries were only moderately narrowed, she and her doctor hope that lifestyle changes will do the most to halt the progression of the disease. Her test results suggested that the likely cause of her problem is an exceedingly high blood cholesterol level. To lower it, she's been told to lose about thirty pounds, follow a diet low in saturated fat and cholesterol, and do regular aerobic exercise. In about four months, she'll return to the clinic for another cholesterol test to see whether the changes are working. If her cholesterol level is still dangerously elevated, she'll be given a drug to lower it.

If you have coronary artery disease, it's likely you'll have to take one or more cardiovascular drugs. These drugs are discussed in Chapter 11.

What about exercise? If you have coronary disease, another major component in your strategy to beat it is most likely to be exercise. This may seem startling: Years ago, the prescription was just the opposite. In fact, even the suspicion of heart problems turned many healthy people into semi-invalids. Today doctors advocate regular physical exercise for coronary patients. Your doctor may recommend that you undertake an exercise program on your own, or join a cardiac rehabilitation program. This is a terrific way to add exercise to your life and also get help in making other changes, such as improving your diet and quitting smoking. Cardiac rehabilitation is discussed in Chapter 11.

> ♥ Lifesaving Tip: If you have coronary artery disease, or any other type of heart problem, exercise may be an important part of your therapy, but <u>never begin any exercise plan without first consulting your doctor.</u>

REVERSING CORONARY ARTERY DISEASE

When doctors first began studying atherosclerosis, the process by which coronary arteries become clogged, they believed it was irreversible. They thought that once your arteries had begun narrowing, nothing could be done to reverse it.

Over the years, some have disagreed, maintaining that lifestyle changes alone can accomplish such a reversal. The first of these mavericks was Nathan Pritikin, author of the well-known Pritikin Diet. He suffered a mild heart attack in 1955 and was found to have a very high cholesterol level. Over the next thirty years, Pritikin followed a special low-fat, low-cholesterol diet and became an avid runner. His cholesterol level dropped dramatically, and, after his death from cancer, his autopsy showed that his coronary arteries were unusually clear.

More recently, the work of Dr. Dean Ornish, a San Francisco–based cardiologist, has become widely known. Dr. Ornish not only designed a package of lifestyle changes, but also provided proof that they could indeed reverse arterial blockages in a group of twenty-eight heart patients. There is a catch, however. Dr. Ornish's program calls for lifestyle changes, particularly in diet, which might seem fine for some people but too drastic for others. His book does make for intriguing reading. If you have coronary disease and want to follow the program, you should first discuss it with your doctor.

HEART ATTACK

On a November morning, Helen drove down the highway in her yellow school bus filled with kids. At the age of forty-five, Helen knew her blood pressure and her cholesterol were "on the high side," but she'd been feeling pretty satisfied with her health lately. She'd quit smoking a few years ago and, feeling stressed out, had just cut back on her work hours. Just in time, too; it was two days before Thanksgiving, and Helen had a big dinner to cook.

Suddenly a car swerved into her lane, nearly colliding with the bus. The scare left Helen with a sudden cramping in her chest, but it quickly disappeared. Greatly relieved over having avoided an accident, Helen finished the route and went home for lunch. After eating, she recalls, "I had this gassy sensation I thought was indigestion." By dinnertime, she was feeling worse. She figured it was "an unusually severe gas attack." But nothing she did would relieve it. She cooked dinner, but was feeling worse and worse. "By this time," she remembers, "I'm realizing there's more to this than I'm admitting to. I was beginning to feel pain creeping up into my neck and my jaw."

Helen's son and daughter begged her to call a doctor. Helen refused, and they got into a fight. Helen grabbed her purse, stormed out of the house, and jumped into her new car. "Then I came to my senses and thought to myself, 'What are you doing? If you don't kill yourself, you could kill somebody else.' " She slipped back into the house, unnoticed, and lay down on her bed. But no matter how much she tossed and turned, the pressure bearing down on her chest would simply not let up. Finally she emerged from the bedroom. "My daughter said to me, 'Ma, I only wanted to know what was the matter,' and I said, 'It hurts.' And then I started to cry. They called 911, and the ambulance came."

On the way to the hospital, Helen was still insisting nothing was wrong. Even as the emergency medical technician was giving her oxygen, she told him, "I don't know what everyone is making such a fuss about; it's only gas." Helen was admitted to the hospital. The next day, when her doctor arrived to tell her she'd suffered a heart attack, she burst into tears. "I just about lost it right there in the bed. I was hysterical. I yelled at the doctor, 'I don't have time for this!' "

Helen's reaction is not unusual. Despite all the publicity about the importance of people's seeking help if they suspect they may be having a heart attack, both men and women often deny it. In fact, studies have shown that women delay even longer, with dangerous consequences.

Medically known as a myocardial infarction (MI), a heart attack occurs when the blood flowing to your heart is cut off completely. Your blood carries oxygen, among other important things, which your heart needs to survive. Thus, a lack of oxygen results eventually in injury to your heart muscle. When your heart muscle is damaged severely by one large or by several of these attacks, your heart cannot pump the oxygenated blood to the rest of your body efficiently.

That women delay seeking medical attention may stem from the fact that they've been led to believe that men are much more likely to suffer heart attacks. If women experience chest pain or pressure, they may attribute it to other causes, like heartburn or even anxiety. But the fact is that of the approximately 500,000 Americans who will die of heart attacks this year, nearly half will be women.

Another reason that women tend to put off getting help is that they apparently experience heart attack symptoms differently than do men. "Men, when they come to the hospital, come in and talk about severe pressure in the middle of their sternum," says Dr. Eric Topol, head of the Cleveland Clinic's cardiology department. "Women, on the other hand, tend to have more nausea or other nonspecific signs."

People who are less sensitive to their bodily sensations, and thus less likely to recognize or correctly interpret symptoms, also delay getting medical help, and this goes for both men and women. A study of 103 patients at a Detroit hospital in November 1991 found those who recognized their symptoms still took about four hours to seek help, while those who were less perceptive took longer, up to thirteen hours. Such a delay can have enormous implications in the case of a heart attack.

Women, like men, are sometimes unwilling to seek help because they simply believe they can't take the time to be sick. Like Helen, they try to ward off a heart attack with sheer willpower. If you ignore heart attack symptoms, you're not only risking your life, you're also forfeiting the possibility that prompt emergency treatment will minimize the damage to your heart. Not long ago, once a heart attack began, nothing could be done to affect its course. Today there are treatments which can halt and, in some cases, even lessen the damage to your heart. But to benefit, you must get to the hospital quickly.

WHAT CAUSES A HEART ATTACK?

Coronary artery disease is the most common cause. A heart attack usually results when a blood clot blocks the flow of blood in coronary arteries already narrowed by disease. A less common cause is a sustained coronary spasm which pinches off the blood flow in arteries that appear otherwise healthy.

A "silent" heart attack is one you have without even realizing it. Usually you become aware of it when the results show up on a cardiac test. If you've suffered a silent heart attack, you're at greater risk of suffering a heart attack again. Diabetic women are particularly prone to missing the important sign of chest pain because their bodies sometimes misinterpret pain messages.

♥ **Lifesaving Tip: If you're at high risk for heart attack, have suffered one, or have had a "silent" heart attack, you should have an emergency plan worked out so that you can get to the hospital or summon help without delay.**

How do women fare after a heart attack? On this question, studies have shown conflicting results. An often-quoted 1991 Israeli study found that women did not fare as well as men after a heart attack: 23.1 percent of the 1,524 women studied died during their initial hospitalization, compared with 15.7 percent of the 4,315 men. More women than men died after the first year, and women were more likely to suffer a second heart attack as well. A Massachusetts study found women faring a little better, but still not as well as men. However, a 1992 study of heart attack patients at nineteen Seattle-area hospitals showed that although the death rate for women was higher, after adjusting for the fact that the women were older, the gap disappeared.

♥ **Mindsaving Tip: If you do have a heart attack, the odds are great that you'll survive. Every day, women suffer major heart attacks and go on to recover fully.**

How do I know if I'm having a heart attack? Sometimes there is no way to be certain. You may suffer chest pain so severe that it couldn't be anything else. But often the symptoms of a heart attack are subtler, such as annoying chest discomfort, pressure, and nausea. Such symptoms can come on suddenly, or you may have been feeling out of sorts for some time.

"Recognizing symptoms and getting to the hospital is very important," says Charles Maynard, Ph.D., a research scientist at the University of Washington who is involved in a major study of Seattle-area heart attack patients. "Especially if women are elderly, they may get their symptoms confused with other health problems they have." Since symptoms in women are often misdiagnosed, having a doctor who's familiar with you and with whom you can talk freely increases the possibility that your heart attack will be accurately diagnosed and treated, Dr. Maynard says.

Fifty-eight-year-old Roberta, a psychiatric nurse, was feeling, as she puts it, "lousier and lousier." She thought it was indigestion. One night her symptoms got worse; she had pressure and burning in her chest, and felt unable to breathe. The next morning, awakening, she walked into the kitchen and fainted. The previous night, while she paced back and forth worrying about her discomfort, she had actually been suffering a heart attack. "My first husband died of a fatal heart attack," she says. "It was just like a heart attack you see in the movies; he clutched his chest and fell right to the floor. Since that didn't happen to me, I assumed I couldn't be having a heart attack."

You may be having a heart attack if:

- Chest pain comes on suddenly over a minute or two and builds in intensity.
- The pain occurs near the center of your chest.
- The pain lasts at least twenty minutes and is not relieved by rest or by changing position.
- The pain ranges from mild to severe and usually feels like tightness or heaviness.
- The pain radiates into your jaw, into your back, or down your left arm.
- You experience nausea, shortness of breath, or a sense of impending doom.

♥ **Lifesaving Tip: These signs of a heart attack are the most common ones in both men and women. But studies have shown that women often experience more subtle symptoms: indigestionlike discomfort or difficulty breathing.**

GETTING HELP

If you think you may be having a heart attack, call for an ambulance. Do not attempt to drive yourself. Besides the fact that you're risking an accident if you drive, emergency measures that could save your life can be started right away in the ambulance. In their book, *The Female Heart*, Dr. Marianne Legato and Carol Colman advise women not to be vague or uncertain in describing their medical history and symptoms. Because in the past women have not been recognized as being at risk for a heart attack, it is important you state your concerns clearly when you arrive at the emergency room.

After you're initially evaluated at the hospital, if it appears that you may be having a heart attack, you'll probably be taken to a special intensive care unit, in some places called a coronary care unit. During a heart attack, your blood pressure can shoot too high or fall too low. The internal electrical system which regulates your heartbeat can go haywire, sending your heart racing irregularly or slowing it down too much. Today's coronary care units have equipment and staff to counteract such occurrences and stabilize your condition.

You will also undergo further tests to determine whether you are indeed having a heart attack. Your heartbeat will be monitored continuously—although even in the midst of a heart attack the heartbeat may appear normal. The diagnosis of a heart attack may not be definite for several hours—until the results of a particular blood test are available. When you're having a heart attack, a portion of your heart muscle is injured. As the muscle is damaged it produces an enzyme called creatine kinase, or CK. After a few days, that enzyme level drops. But while it is present in high levels in your bloodstream, it's a telltale indicator of a heart attack.

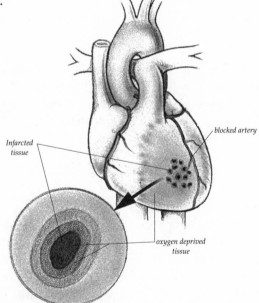

Heart Muscle Damaged by Heart Attack. "Infarcted" tissue (irreversibly injured heart muscle) resulted from the loss of coronary blood flow for too long. Surrounding the area of injury is muscle with varying degrees of oxygen deprivation, which can recover if blood circulation is restored.

Your heart muscle, however, is not the only muscle that gives off creatine kinase; the enzyme is present in some of your other muscles as well. Let's say you spent the day playing tennis and then began suffering chest pains. At the hospital, tests may show an elevated level of CK in your blood. If your doctor suspects you did not have a heart attack, another test can be ordered to determine whether the CK enzyme was produced by the muscles involved in the physical exertion or came from damage to your heart muscle.

♥ Lifesaving Tip: Should you arrive at the hospital only to learn later that you did not suffer a heart attack at all, don't be embarrassed. It's far better to assume the worst and find out the problem isn't serious than to underestimate it and risk serious damage to your heart or even death.

CLOT BUSTERS

Not long ago, if you suffered a heart attack, lifesaving measures could be administered, but nothing could be done to prevent damage to your heart. Happily, this is no longer true. Thanks to a group of drugs commonly known as clot busters, damage to your heart can be stopped and, in some cases, even lessened. These powerful drugs act to dissolve the clot, enabling the flow of blood to resume.

Miraculous as these clot busters seem, they're useful only when administered within a few hours after the heart attack begins. "The early time frame is important," says Dr. Eric Topol, who has pioneered this type of therapy, known formally as thrombolytic therapy. "That is, the earlier we get to patients, the more chance there is that we can do something positive."

But although studies have shown that these drugs work equally well in men and women, that message may not be getting through to doctors. According to Dr. Charles Maynard, the Seattle study showed that only 14 percent of the women received this type of therapy, compared to 26 percent of the men. Some of the difference may be due to the fact that women's heart attacks are more difficult to diagnose and that the women in the study were older; doctors may have been reluctant to use the medicine, fearing it might cause strokes. But some doctors might be too cautious, says Dr. Maynard. "Thrombolytic therapy has been shown to be a very effective means of affecting mortality, and my concern is that women are being undertreated."

There are different types of clot dissolvers. Tissue plasminogen activator, or tPA, is a genetically engineered drug. Another popular clot buster is called streptokinase. Both drugs have been at the center of controversy because a single dose of tPA costs about $2,000 while streptokinase costs about $300.

If you've had streptokinase during a heart attack before, it should not be given again. Streptokinase contains trace substances which are potentially sensitizing, meaning that a second administration of the drug could result in a severe allergic reaction. In this case, tPA or another clot dissolver would be the drug of choice.

There's another consideration as well. If you're black, your blood tends to clot more readily than if you're white, raising the threat of heart attack or stroke. While both tPA and streptokinase are effective in blacks and in whites, research has shown tPA to be more effective in blacks. In fact, according to Dr. Topol, if you're a black woman, the probability of your blood clot's being dissolved with tPA is about 90 percent, compared to about 75 percent if streptokinase is used.

Some research questions the practice of following the administration of clot busters with balloon angioplasty, a procedure in which narrowed arteries are dilated. At the American Heart Association's annual meeting in 1992, a study done on 122 patients at two North Carolina hospitals found that when balloon angioplasty was used on patients who had received streptokinase, they suffered significantly higher complication rates. A 1992 study by Cleveland Clinic cardiologist Stephen G. Ellis found similar results at six medical centers. He recommends balloon angioplasty not be done on heart attack patients who were in stable condition after having been treated with clot busters, unless there is evidence that remaining undamaged heart muscle is at risk.

By the way, breaking up clots with clot busters is just the first step in treating a heart attack. You may be placed on a blood thinner like aspirin or Coumadin on a long-term basis after your heart attack.

♥ Lifesaving Tip: Clot busters are powerful drugs which can cause serious bleeding complications, so they are only administered under a doctor's supervision. In several communities, administration of these drugs is being done by specially trained paramedics.

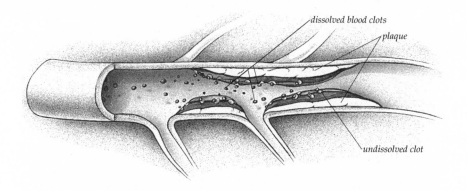

dissolved blood clots

plaque

undissolved clot

Clot Busters. Blood clots normally form and dissolve naturally in all of us. However, when a blood clot causes a heart attack, a type of drug therapy called thrombolysis may be used to break up the clot.

Are women heart attack victims treated differently? Since some studies have shown that women heart attack victims do not fare as well as men, any differences in the way men and women are treated are important. A major study done in Seattle, known as the MITI study (Myocardial Infarction Triage and Intervention Registry) looked at 4,891 patients, 34 percent of whom were women. The study found that women were less likely to be given clot busters and less likely to undergo cardiac catheterization and balloon angioplasty.

The study found that cardiac catheterization, a critically important test to determine the presence of narrowed or blocked coronary arteries as well as to determine what can be done to correct them, was performed in 40 percent of the women, as compared to 58 percent of the men. Since that test is required before balloon angioplasty, a procedure in which narrowed arteries are dilated, it was not surprising that only 14 percent of the women underwent that procedure, compared to 22 percent of the men.

The study also found that women and men who underwent catheterization were referred for angioplasty or bypass surgery equally.

Dr. Maynard speculates that sometimes gender bias may be involved. "Cardiologists, when they talk to a guy, say, basically, 'You've gotta have this thing done.' With women, I think there may be a reluctance. It's a cultural, subtle thing which is very hard to study. But I've heard too many cardiologists say that the men are stronger than women and more able to withstand the rigors of the procedure when, medically, that assumption is not always warranted."

On the other hand, a study published in 1992 looked at 2,473 patients who had been treated for heart attacks at Boston's Beth Israel Hospital. The researchers found that the 1,350 men and 1,123 women were generally treated equally, with the women as likely as the men to undergo balloon angioplasty. And although the women were less likely to undergo coronary bypass, once the study's results were adjusted to reflect the women's greater age and milder coronary disease, these results were only of borderline significance.

Another area of concern is the time it takes to transfer heart attack patients who suffer complications to larger treatment centers where they can get more advanced treatment. A 1992 study found that of 264 patients transferred from community hospitals, men were transferred after an average of 2.4 days and women after 4.5 days. In interviews with the women, Jane Sherwood, a research nurse who coordinated the study, attributed the delay to the women's reluctance to inconvenience their families, their loyalty to the community hospital, or their lack of realization of just how sick they were. While not all heart attack patients need to be transferred to more sophisticated facilities, this tendency may result in some women not receiving the treatment they need.

The debate over whether there is a gender bias in the treatment of men and women after heart attacks will continue. It's worth noting, however, that cardiac catheterization is an expensive, uncomfortable, and sometimes risky procedure which is not always necessary. As with men, when a woman has had a heart attack, sometimes a carefully selected program of other cardiac tests may provide all the information required for her proper diagnosis and treatment. The important thing for women, and their doctors, to keep in mind is that when a woman has a heart attack, she is entitled to a careful, thorough evaluation to meet her individual medical needs, and her standard of care should not be any lower than that afforded to a man.

ON TO RECOVERY

If tests confirm that you have suffered a heart attack, you can expect to spend the next few days in the intensive care unit, being monitored and undergoing diagnostic tests. These tests will seek to determine the cause of your heart attack, how severely your heart was damaged, and what steps need to be taken to ensure your full recovery. This may involve balloon angioplasty or coronary bypass surgery, depending on your individual case.

Years ago, total bed rest for several weeks was the rule for treating heart attack patients. How times have changed! Once you're transferred to a regular room, you'll rest, of course. But before long you'll be encouraged to begin taking care of your personal needs. At first a nurse will be on hand to assist you, but soon you'll be doing your personal care yourself.

You'll probably be amazed to learn how quickly you're expected to make exercise part of your recovery plan. You'll be taught exercises to do at first in bed and while sitting down. Before being discharged, you'll probably undergo a short form of an exercise stress test to make certain your heart is strong enough to deal with the demands of living outside the protective walls of the hospital. About six weeks later, you'll probably return for a regular exercise stress test, which gauges the amount of activity your heart is capable of performing safely. Not only does this provide your doctor with information about your medical condition, but it also provides you with confidence that you can depend on your heart to get you through the daily work of living.

ONCE YOU'RE HOME

"Recuperation? What recuperation?" hoots Helen. "When I went home, my doctor told me, 'I want you to go home and do what you've done here,' which was nothing but walk the halls. He gave me a schedule which said, 'Next week, you can dust the furniture, and the following week, you can sweep the floor, and four weeks down the road, you can run the vacuum cleaner.' I said,

'Fine,' but what I was thinking to myself was, 'Are you out of your mind?' "

Just how much you try to do when you return home will depend, of course, on how you feel. If you're an elderly woman, it may take much longer for you to begin getting back even a small portion of your energy. But no matter what your age, you must take care of yourself. Your heart needs time to mend, and you must provide it. Leaving the protected environment of the hospital for home will take preparation. Your recuperation will be similar to that of patients recovering from open-heart surgery; that topic is covered in Chapter 12.

> ♥ **Mindsaving Tip: When a man returns home from the hospital, he may have nothing to do but rest. If you're a woman, you may be a homemaker and a mother and may feel that all the responsibilities of the world are on your shoulders. You need to treat the challenge of recuperating seriously.**

RIDING THE EMOTIONAL ROLLER COASTER

Although your heart suffers the attack, your emotions receive an enormous jolt as well. After a heart attack, many women feel as if they're on an emotional roller coaster, feeling lucky to be alive one moment and nearly in tears the next. Some women continue to deny the heart attack, like Helen, who two years later says she still has a difficult time believing her attack ever happened. Others, though, find themselves in one of the most emotionally charged times of their lives.

> ♥ **Mindsaving Tip: Right after a heart attack, it's normal to be keenly aware of every flutter of your heart and every stab of pain in your chest, heart-related or not. You may very well feel that your heart, which you always depended on without a thought, has betrayed you, and have trouble imagining yourself living a normal life. That feeling usually fades with time.**

HEART ATTACKS AND DEPRESSION

A catastrophic event such as a heart attack, the need for heart surgery, or even the diagnosis of coronary artery disease, can depress the most cheerful of women. But while some depression is normal, some women may experience a serious depression from which they cannot emerge without help.

Just ask Lucinda, who at forty-seven was divorced, had grown children, and worked full time. But juggling home and a job never seemed to bother her; in fact, she seemed to thrive on it. She seemed to have it "all together." At least until she suffered a heart attack.

"I was always the iron woman of my family. I was never sick. I worked all the time. I was very productive. I don't imagine anyone takes a heart problem lightly, but I never expected it. All of a sudden, from a very healthy woman I went to being a heart patient. Everything in my life had changed. It was too much to handle."

As a result, she drew into herself. "When I was in the hospital, I didn't want to talk to people, I didn't answer the phone, I didn't see anyone outside of my immediate family. I didn't want to hear people say, "How are you doing?" or "How are you feeling," or, especially, "I know how you feel." That expression, "I know how you feel," just sent a shiver down my spine, because they didn't know how I felt. Only I knew how I felt."

When she returned home from the hospital, Lucinda felt even worse. "I wasn't eating. I wasn't sleeping. When my friends called, I wouldn't answer the phone. I didn't care about anything. It just got progressively worse."

Finally, at the urging of her family, Lucinda decided to see a psychiatrist. She was put on an antidepressant and went for counseling. Now, the future no longer looks bleak. "I have days which are difficult, but days which are also joyous. I won't lie to you and say things changed overnight. But I am feeling better," she says.

"One of the important things about both depression and heart disease is that they are poorly diagnosed in women and not always treated appropriately. Sometimes, physicians pick up on the anxiety or depression but minimize the heart complaints. And the opposite can happen as well," says Dr. Susan J. Blumenthal, chief of the Behavioral Medicine Program at the National Institute of Mental Health and clinical professor of psychiatry at Georgetown School of Medicine.

Certainly some sadness or worry is normal after a heart attack or heart surgery. But if you're unable to shake feelings of anger, worthlessness, distance from others or despair, or if you have persistent sleep and appetite problems or thoughts of suicide, it's important to seek help from your doctor, a therapist, a hospital social worker or a psychiatrist. Sometimes people fail to realize that cardiac medications themselves can cause symptoms of depression. In the past, women have also been treated too often with tranquilizers instead of antidepressants. Getting appropriate treatment for your depression can make a world of difference in your recovery.

Signs of depression include:

· Sleep and appetite disturbances
· Feeling your life is hopeless and not worth living
· Feelings of fatigue or agitation not related to your physical condition
· Loss of interest in usual activities
· Trouble concentrating or making decisions
· Suicidal thoughts

There are many ways to treat depression in women who have heart problems. Sometimes just talking to someone can make you feel better. But if you're seriously depressed, antidepressant drugs can be very effective, as can psychotherapy or their combination. The important thing is to get help.

♥ Lifesaving Tip: If you're depressed, you may lack the energy or resolve to try to do something about it. But it is very important that you talk about it to someone who can facilitate your getting help, be it a family member, a nurse, or your doctor.

RESUMING SEX

"After I had my heart attack, my husband treated me as if I was breakable. I was afraid, and so was he. It did not make for a passionate sexual encounter," Roberta says. When asked if she talked about the problem with her doctor, she shrieks with laughter.

"My doctor! He's just a baby! He's the same age as my daughter. I could never talk to him about sex!"

Roberta's dilemma is not unusual. Some doctors make it a point to bring up the subject of sex. If your doctor doesn't, you do it. If your doctor is male and you feel uncomfortable, perhaps you can talk to your doctor's nurse or change to a female doctor. What you need is the reassurance that resuming sexual activity will be no more stressful to your heart than other activities you're able to do. In fact, you should be able to resume passive sex with your usual partner safely if you can climb one flight of stairs without becoming short of breath or feeling chest pain. If you plan to be the active partner, or are having sex with someone new or anticipate becoming especially excited, being able to climb two flights of stairs without breathlessness or chest pain is the rule of thumb.

Some of the most common reasons for sexual problems after a heart attack or heart surgery are depression and fear. Depression can manifest itself as a loss of sexual desire. And it's understandable that either partner may fear that intercourse itself will overstress your heart.

Above all, be frank. "What was most helpful to me was that my husband and I were able to discuss it," Roberta says. "We knew what the problem was; we knew we were both scared, and that gave us the opening to talk about it."

> ♥ **Mindsaving Tip: Some cardiovascular drugs or medications used to combat depression can result in a loss of sexual desire or ability to reach orgasm. If you think this may be true in your case, talk to your doctor.**

A WORD ABOUT FAMILY AND FRIENDS

In a crisis, nothing can count more than the support of family and friends. But if you've had a heart attack, some of their reactions may surprise you. "After my heart attack, I found some of my friends seemed to back away from me, almost as if I'd done something wrong," says Helen.

Helen found help from a heart support group. The leader explained to her that this response was not uncommon. "She made me realize my friends were scared. That they thought, if I, a relatively young woman, could have a heart attack, they could, too. It's taken some time, but now everything is back to normal."

Having a heart attack is a very frightening experience. But many women, to their surprise, later discover that they have emerged from the experience feeling stronger than before.

HEART VALVE PROBLEMS

Bernice is a "snowbird," a retiree who winters in Florida and flies home to summer up north. A few years ago, in preparation for her annual southern trip, she stopped in to see her doctor for a routine physical. She felt fine but her doctor detected a heart murmur and sent her for tests. They showed Bernice's aortic valve was becoming stiff. That year Bernice's doctor bid her *"Bon voyage."* But when she returned the next year, the usually energetic, cheery Bernice was tiring easily and becoming short of breath. "Can't I just go to Florida for the holidays?" she asked. "No way," her doctor responded, "not before you have that valve replaced." Bernice did as her doctor instructed. The following year, she was winging her way back to Florida.

Your heart has four valves (tricuspid, pulmonary, mitral, and aortic), and all four must function properly in order to circulate blood effectively through your heart. The right atrium and ventricle of your heart receive oxygen-depleted blood as it arrives from your circulatory system and pump it into your lungs, where it is replenished with oxygen. Then this oxygenated blood flows into the left side of your heart, where it is pumped back into your circulatory system and to the rest of your body. That process is repeated over your entire life. For it to work smoothly, all of the blood must flow in one direction. The efficient opening and closing of your valves keep it that way. But problems can arise with your valves.

Years ago, if you had valve problems, little could be done for you. These days, valve surgery accounts for one-third of the open-heart surgeries in the United States. Not only are surgeons replacing valves at a record pace, but they're also discovering new ways to repair valves.

A heart valve can fail in one of two ways. The valve can become stiff, no longer opening and shutting freely. When such

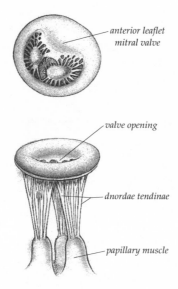

*anterior leaflet
mitral valve*

valve opening

dnordae tendinae

papillary muscle

Mitral Valve. Blood flows down through the opening of the valve past the chordae tendinae, which support the valve leaflets. The fingerlike protrusions of the heart muscle, the papillary muscles, connect the cordae tendinae to the interior of the heart's muscular pump.

stiffening occurs in the aortic valve, it is called aortic stenosis. When it occurs in the mitral valve, it's called mitral stenosis.

The other type of failure occurs when a valve becomes "leaky" and allows blood to flow backward, in the wrong direction. This happens more commonly in the mitral valve and is called mitral regurgitation or mitral insufficiency. This problem can also occur as a complication of mitral valve prolapse, and is discussed in Chapter 7.

Stiffening and leaking can occur in more than one valve, and both conditions can also occur in the same valve. If this sounds confusing, just think about a house you might have lived in, a summer cottage, perhaps, which had an old screen door. If the door was repainted several times, the paint would build up. Eventually the door wouldn't shut tightly enough. In fact, it would be both hard to open (stiff) and hard to shut (leaky). This is a useful analogy when considering how these seemingly opposite problems can occur in the same heart valve.

No matter which type of valvular disorder you have, the result is the same: Your heart is forced to overcompensate. The result is an enlarged, weakened, and eventually failing heart. An abnormally functioning valve also makes you vulnerable to a heart infection, and can lead to the formation of blood clots which can cause heart attacks and strokes.

CAUSES OF HEART VALVE PROBLEMS

Most female valve patients are older, like Bernice. But young women are not necessarily immune. You can be born with a heart valve abnormality, or you can develop such a problem at any age.

Heart valve problems can be caused by:

- **Coronary disease or a heart attack.** Either can result in damage to one or more of your heart's valves.
- **Congenital defects.** You can be born with a heart valve abnormality, which may be discovered when you're young, or not until you're an adult. For more information, see Chapter 8.
- **Aging.** As we age, our heart valves sometimes stiffen. With more women living longer, often well into their eighties, it's not surprising that this problem is among the fastest-growing type of heart disease among women in this country.
- **Rheumatic heart disease.** Years ago, rheumatic fever caused a large proportion of valvular heart problems, particularly in women. Today, that threat is seen as the vestige of a bygone era by some, but not by cardiologists, who have noted an increasing number of patients among new immigrants.
- **Mitral valve prolapse.** In the vast majority of cases, mitral valve prolapse poses no serious threat to the heart. In about 5 percent of those who have it, however, it can develop into a "leaky" mitral valve.

SYMPTOMS OF VALVE PROBLEMS

Some people with a valve problem experience no symptoms and don't know about the problem until it's discovered during a physical examination. Others experience exhaustion, shortness of breath, dizziness, fainting, lung congestion, irregular heart rhythms, or chest pain.

DIAGNOSING VALVE PROBLEMS

Sometimes a problem with a heart valve is noticed first by a physician who, on listening to your heart with a stethoscope, notices a heart murmur and orders an echocardiogram, which shows the structures of your heart. Cardiac catheterization is often performed as well. These tests are discussed in Chapter 6.

Will I need valve surgery? A few decades ago, if you had a bad heart valve, often not much could be done for you. Your heart, forced to overextend itself, would gradually weaken and eventually fail. But those days have vanished. The development of the heart-lung machine marked the advent of modern valvular heart surgery. Such surgery can restore those with failing valves to an active, healthy life.

If you have a valve problem, you may only need to be monitored regularly by a cardiologist. But if you begin to suffer from symptoms or tests show that your heart is overworking, surgery may very well be the recommended course.

VALVE REPAIR

Both valve replacement and valve repair necessitate open-heart surgery. The goal of valve repair is to improve the function of the valve you already have. Valve repair is usually done in the case of "leaky" valves, either aortic or mitral. The more commonly repaired valve of the two is the mitral valve. The surgeon accomplishes the repair with a combination of trimming, sewing, and reinforcing the valve. Repairing a leaky aortic valve is much more unusual, so it may be very difficult to find a hospital where it is being done. This type of surgery is done only at a few major heart centers.

If you've been told you have a valve problem which must be corrected, be sure to select a surgeon who's comfortable with both replacement and repair. If at all possible, it's preferable to retain your own heart valve. Valve repair has fewer of the problems associated with most types of valve replacement. Since with repair you retain your own "native" valve, blood clots rarely form after surgery. Also, if the repair works, the durability of the repaired valve will probably exceed that of a valve made from animal tissue.

Sometimes repairing a valve is not feasible. Experienced cardiologists and surgeons can usually make an accurate evaluation from the findings of the echocardiogram, but this decision will sometimes have to be made during surgery.

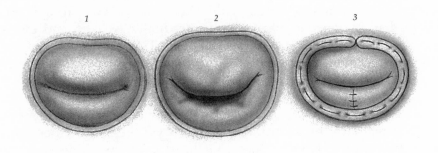

Mitral Valve Repair. The first sketch represents a normal closed mitral valve. The second shows an abnormal valve where the leaflets don't close properly. The third shows the repaired valve with leaflets that now come together tightly.

♥ Lifesaving Tip: If the surgeon you select rules out the possibility of repair on the grounds that he or she is not familiar with performing it, you have a good reason to seek a second opinion. At the very least, you want the possibility of valve repair to be considered.

The two alternatives to valve repair are balloon valvuloplasty and valve replacement.

BALLOON VALVULOPLASTY FOR MITRAL VALVE PROBLEMS

With balloon angioplasty becoming increasingly useful in the widening of coronary arteries without surgery, it's not surprising that this technique should also be used to help open valves which have become stiff, or "stenotic," without the need for open-heart surgery. The balloon valvuloplasty procedure is very similar to the angioplasty procedure. You're given a sedative to make you drowsy and relaxed. A catheter tipped with two balloons is inserted through your right femoral vein, near your groin. Once that is accomplished, the balloons are inflated to open the heart valve.

Valvuloplasty is usually *not* recommended:

· For the aortic valve, as there is a 50 percent chance of reclosure.
· If the valve is too thickened or stiff.
· If you're at risk for blood clots.
· If you have a leaky valve which requires correction as well.

But even if balloon valvuloplasty is not useful in all cases, it's worth exploring. The preparation, procedure, and recuperation are similar to what you would experience with balloon angioplasty, which is described in Chapter 11.

VALVE REPLACEMENT

If you have a problem which requires valve replacement, you'll want to give careful consideration to the type of valve used. There are two categories. The first is a "biological" valve, usually taken from a pig; surprisingly, a pig's circulatory system is very similar to a human's, and the pig valve is used intact. (Rarely, a heart center may use a valve from a human cadaver.) The second category is a mechanical valve, made from metal, plastic, and carbon fibers.

The main argument in favor of using a biological valve is that if you have this type of valve, you probably won't need to take a powerful anticlotting drug such as Coumadin. Because this medication can cause bleeding, the amount you take must be very precisely measured, and you must undergo regular blood tests to monitor it. The main drawback of a biological valve is that it does not generally last as long as a mechanical valve. The average life span of a biological valve is about ten to twelve years. If you're a younger woman who undergoes biological valve replacement, it's likely that your new valve won't last as long as it would if you were older. Although it's not known precisely why, biological valves tend to wear out more quickly in younger people.

In quite elderly people, the decision to opt for the biological valve is usually easy. If you're a middle-aged woman, the mechanical valve would seem the logical choice. But if you're a woman of childbearing years, the choice becomes more complicated. This issue is discussed in Chapter 9.

Can a mechanical valve break? Although this is not likely, it can occur. The replacement valves used today have a track record of at least several years, but there's no way to make 100 percent certain that a manufacturer's defect will not occur. A case in point is the well-publicized problem with a type of heart valve manufactured by Shiley, Inc. While not all Shiley valves were defective, studies in the United States and abroad have found that the wire frame of some Bjork-Shiley Convexo-Concave (CC) valves occasionally fracture without warning. The valve was withdrawn from the market in 1986, but as of this writing, this model valve had cracked in 461 people, killing more than 300. A controversy rages over whether leaving the valve in outweighs the risk of undergoing a new operation. If you have this model valve, you should discuss the matter with your doctor. (If you have a mechanical valve but don't know the type, your doctor should be able to tell from your medical records and a chest X ray.)

VALVE SURGERY

The preparation and most of the recuperation for a valve procedure are essentially the same for as open-heart surgery; this is discussed in Chapter 12.

After the heart-lung machine has taken over the functions of the heart and lungs, the surgeon gently opens the pericardium, the membranous sac around the heart, to expose the muscle of the heart. The surgeon cuts through the muscle to enter the heart and expose the valves. If the valve is not repairable, the surgeon carefully cuts the old valve away. Then the new valve, either a mechanical or a biological one, is sewn into place using numerous stitches, and the process of taking the patient off the heart-lung machine begins.

As for what you do after the surgery, every single doctor and nurse who works with heart valve patients stresses this command: Protect yourself from future infection! Whether you've had a valve repaired or replaced, you must vigilantly guard yourself against valvular infection for the rest of your life. Even if it has only been repaired, your heart now includes material which is foreign to your body, making it a target for infection. Bacterial endocarditis, an infection which can be life-threatening, was discussed earlier in this chapter.

♥ Lifesaving Tips: When you first have a new heart valve, you may be overly conscious of it. In time that feeling will fade. It may then be tempting to forget about the valve completely, but this can be dangerous. There are some important things to keep in mind.

If you have a mechanical valve, know the type of valve, manufacturer, and the serial number of the valve. Although it's unusual, malfunctions and recalls do occur. If this happens, it doesn't necessarily mean you'll have to have the valve replaced, but there may be important medical information you need. Also, if you experience dizziness, shortness of breath, or fainting, contact your doctor immediately.

If you have a biological valve, remember that they don't last forever. If you start feeling the way you did before your own valve failed, experiencing such symptoms as chest congestion, chest pain, unusual fatigue, fainting, or shortness of breath, contact your cardiologist. If your cardiologist is not available, make sure the doctor you see is aware you have a biological valve. Make sure a valve problem is ruled out. If your symptoms persist, consider getting a second opinion.

HYPERTENSIVE CARDIOVASCULAR DISEASE

Untreated high blood pressure can lead to a serious problem known as hypertensive cardiovascular disease, a leading cause of congestive heart failure in adults. This deadly problem is preventable.

One reason that high blood pressure is so dangerous is that over time it can lead to changes in your coronary arteries which make them more vulnerable to atherosclerosis, the deadly buildup of fatty deposits and other materials which narrow the vessels and can impede the flow of blood. But high blood pressure can also lead to hypertensive cardiovascular disease. When this occurs, the high blood pressure, besides accelerating the damage to the coronary arteries, can also damage the heart itself by causing the heart's muscular walls to thicken. The resulting stress on the heart can cause it to dilate, eventually leading to heart failure.

Thirty or forty years ago, hypertensive cardiovascular disease was a very common cause of heart failure. Today, with the emphasis on the importance of having high blood pressure diagnosed and treated, this ailment is found less often, but it's still far from uncommon. Marie was a sixty-two-year-old woman whose electrocardiogram showed changes indicative of hypertensive cardiovascular disease. She'd been increasingly short of breath and suffered other symptoms of congestive heart failure, too. "I was diagnosed several years ago with high blood pressure, and I took medication for a while," she recalls. "But it seemed to go away. So I stopped taking the medicine and assumed everything was fine." Since high blood pressure usually has no symptoms, Marie did not realize that her high blood pressure had come back. She felt fine, so she stopped going to her doctor as well, and had no way of knowing her blood pressure had started climbing again.

Fortunately, if a person with hypertensive cardiovascular disease has not yet experienced heart failure, the cardiac changes from this problem can be largely resolved when the person goes back on the proper medication for high blood pressure. Damage from hypertensive cardiovascular disease is not irreversible as is damage to the heart muscle caused by a heart attack.

♥ **Lifesaving Tip: Until it causes heart failure, hypertensive cardiovascular disease has no symptoms. The best way to prevent this complication is to take your blood pressure medication as prescribed.**

STROKE

What is a section on stroke doing in a book about your heart? The answer is that heart problems and stroke are very closely linked.

A stroke is a form of cardiovascular disease that affects the brain. Some forms of stroke have many similarities to heart disease. For example, a heart attack is a form of cardiovascular disease that damages the heart muscle. A stroke is similar, but it causes damage to the brain. Your brain, like your heart, needs oxygenated blood to thrive. If for any reason the blood supply to the brain is cut off, the result may be a stroke.

Possible symptoms of stroke are:
- Sudden weakness or numbness of the face, arm, or leg on one side of the body.
- Sudden difficulty speaking or understanding others.
- Sudden dimness or impaired vision in one eye.
- Loss or near loss of consciousness.
- Confusion.
- Unexplained dizziness or sudden falls, especially along with any of the above symptoms.

TIA's OR "MINI-STROKES"

A stroke can have warning signs, just as can an impending heart attack. Before a heart attack, a person may suffer attacks of angina pectoris, the chest pain of coronary artery disease which signals that the heart muscle is temporarily not getting enough oxygen. Similarly, a person who is in danger of suffering a stroke may suffer what is called a TIA, a transient ischemic attack. This is also sometimes called a mini-stroke. The symptoms are the same as those of a stroke, but their duration is brief, usually from several minutes to a half hour.

TYPES OF STROKE

Strokes can come at any age, but most commonly they occur in elderly people or those who have high blood pressure or certain types of heart problems, such as valvular heart disease. As with a heart attack, damage, from very mild to devastating, can occur.
    There are three types of stroke:

- **Cerebral thrombosis.** This is most analogous to coronary thrombosis, another name for a heart attack caused by a blockage in the coronary arteries. In this case, the blockage is due to a thrombosis, or clot, that has built up on the wall of a neck or brain artery. Often this is due to atherosclerosis, the same gradual narrowing of the artery that occurs in coronary artery disease. Since it's uncommon for a person's arteries to be narrow in just one place, a person with coronary artery disease may very well have such narrowing in the arteries of the brain as well. Thrombosis accounts for most strokes.

· **Cerebral hemorrhage.** A stroke can occur as the result of the rupture of a blood vessel in or near the brain. People who have high blood pressure or congenital abnormalities of certain blood vessels of the brain are predisposed to this type of stroke.

· **Cerebral embolism.** This type of stroke occurs when a clot, or embolus, carried in your bloodstream from elsewhere in your body is swept into an artery of the brain and causes a blockage in the blood flow. Causes of this type of stroke include coronary artery disease and valvular disease. For example, a blood clot may form in the inner lining of a heart which has been previously damaged by a heart attack and may travel in the bloodstream to the brain.

Another major cause of this type of stroke is cardiac valvular disease. Your heart has four cardiac valves, all of which must function well for your heart to pump blood properly throughout your body. For various reasons, such as aging or rheumatic heart disease, one of your valves may become stenotic, or stiff. This can result in your blood's flowing too sluggishly through the valve, which can lead to the blood's thickening and forming a clot. Atrial fibrillation, a type of heartbeat irregularity, can make it more likely that a clot will form as well.

These types of strokes can also occur during or after open-heart surgery. Rarely, a tiny bubble of air enters the bloodstream during the procedure and travels to the brain, often with devastating consequences.

A stroke occasionally signals an undiagnosed heart problem. Mona, a sixty-four-year-old woman, suffered a stroke. When she underwent diagnostic tests, it was discovered that after a bout of rheumatic fever when she was a young girl, she had developed a diseased mitral valve. The mitral valve had grown stiff, interfering with the blood flow through her heart, enlarging the left atrium and setting the stage for her future stroke.

How are strokes treated? The way strokes are treated bears some similarity to the treatment of heart attacks. Since, as with heart attacks, most strokes are caused by blood clots, the same anticlotting drugs are often prescribed. Because a stroke can damage the brain, leading to weakness and inability to function, rehabilitation also plays a very important role in treatment. The outlook for recovery depends on how much damage occurs. About half of patients recover fully, or nearly so, from their first stroke, and many people who are paralyzed learn to walk again.

♥ Lifesaving Tip: As with heart attacks, the key to successful stroke treatment is getting to the hospital early. This can minimize the damage caused by a stroke. A 1992 study showed that people suffering a stroke who called the emergency number 911, rather than calling their physician, arrived at the hospital sooner.

11

Treating Coronary Heart Disease

Over the past few decades, vast strides have been made in the treatment of heart problems. Thanks to such advances, many cardiac problems considered hopeless are now treatable, and some are even curable. What follows is the latest information on treatment techniques.

THE CARDIOVASCULAR MEDICINE CHEST

If you've been told you need to go on cardiac medication, you may not welcome the news. Remember, though, that it's because of such drugs that many people are now enjoying life despite having once-untreatable heart problems. You may have to take cardiovascular drugs for a short period or indefinitely. You may be put on a single drug or a combination. Even if you undergo balloon angioplasty or coronary bypass surgery, you'll probably still be put on one or more cardiovascular drugs.

There are currently several books on the market which can help you sort through the many cardiovascular drugs in more detail. Some are listed in the "Recommended Reading and Resources" section.

ANTIANGINAL DRUGS

These drugs relieve angina pectoris, the chest pain which often accompanies coronary disease. These medications include nitrates, beta blockers, and calcium-channel blockers.

NITROGLYCERIN: "AN OLDIE BUT GOODIE"

Almost everyone with coronary artery disease has taken nitroglycerin or nitrates in some form. They're some of the oldest heart medicines. Nitrates provide temporary relief from chest pain by dilating your blood vessels. They can be taken during an attack as a small pill dissolved under the tongue (Nitro-Stat). Longer-acting capsules or pills and Band-Aid–style patches are also available. Some brand names of nitroglycerin include Nitro-Bid, Isordil, Nitro-Dur, and Transderm.

♥ **Mindsaving Tip: Most doctors prescribe nitro tablets for under-the-tongue use. A product called Nitrolingual Spray is more expensive but is more rapidly acting and easy to use even in the dark. The spray is easier if you have arthritis in your hands or if you are wearing gloves.**

BETA BLOCKERS

Beta blockers block the effects of adrenaline, lowering your heart rate, reducing the squeezing of your cardiac muscles, and lowering your blood pressure. There are twelve or fifteen types of beta blockers on the market. (Brand names include Lopressor, Tenormin, and Blocadren.) Propranolol (Inderal) was one of the earliest available and is still frequently prescribed because it has more than just cardiovascular effects; some people report that it reduces anxiety.

CALCIUM-CHANNEL BLOCKERS

Calcium-channel blockers interfere with the movement of calcium through specialized channels in the cell membranes of your cardiac and vascular muscles. These drugs affect the squeezing of your heart and cause your blood vessels to relax. Because of this, calcium-channel blockers, like beta blockers, are excellent drugs for lowering high blood pressure also. Calcium-channel blockers are also useful in regulating erratic heart rhythms. Calcium-channel blockers include diltiazem (Cardizem), verapamil (Isoptin, Calan), and nifedipine (Procardia, Adalat).

DIURETICS

For years doctors prescribed diuretic drugs ("water pills") for high blood pressure. Today experts no longer believe that diuretics are the best first-step therapy for most people with high blood pressure. The development of new drugs—beta blockers, calcium-channel blockers, and angiotensin converting-enzyme inhibitors (ACE inhibitors)—has diminished their role. Now diuretics are used more often as backup drugs when other medications fail, or in combination with other antihypertensive agents. However, diuretics are still commonly used to treat heart failure and fluid retention.

> ♥ **Lifesaving Tip: Some diuretics, such as furmosemide (Lasix) and bumetamide (Bumex), are extremely powerful and can cause potassium loss, so you may need to take a potassium supplement in addition to the diuretic. Other less powerful diuretics may not require such a supplement, especially if used in combination with another diuretic that causes potassium retention. They include Dyazide, Aldactazide, and Maxzide.**

ACE INHIBITORS

Angiotensin converting-enzyme inhibitors, commonly called ACE inhibitors, have been found effective in treating different types of heart problems. ACE inhibitors lower blood pressure by blocking the formation of an enzyme that is a powerful retainer of salt in the kidney. They are another line of defense against heart failure and high blood pressure. Also, because they may cause potassium retention, you may not need a potassium supplement if you're on a combination of an ACE inhibitor and a diuretic. ACE inhibitors include enalapril maleate (Vasotec), lisinopril (Zestril, Prinivil), and captopril (Capoten).

CARDIAC STRENGTHENERS

Some drugs are used to strengthen the heart muscle and improve its squeezing action. Digoxin (Lanoxin) is the only such drug that can be taken orally. In the past, the effectiveness of digoxin for people with heart failure was questioned, but research shows it helps many. It's also used to control certain types of heart rhythm disturbances. Dobutamine (Dobutrex) also improves the heart's squeezing, but can only be administered intravenously, so it's usually reserved for hospital use, though special home programs are becoming available.

BLOOD THINNERS

Two common types of blood thinners, or anticoagulants, are used to prevent strokes or heart attacks in some people. One kind prevents blood platelets from clumping together to form a clot. The most popular type of drug in this class is aspirin.

The other common blood thinner, wafarin (Coumadin and others), interferes with your blood's normal coagulation. Wafarin is commonly prescribed for people whose heart valves have been replaced with mechanical valves, or to prevent stroke in those who suffer from atrial fibrillation, a type of heartbeat irregularity. Wafarin is a very powerful blood thinner. If you're taking it, your blood must be tested periodically, and eating green, leafy vegetables like spinach or drinking alcohol can alter the test results. Heparin is a stronger blood thinner used when quick action is needed. It can be given only by injection.

♥ **Lifesaving Tip:** When you take blood thinners such as wafarin, internal bleeding after an injury could prove especially dangerous. You should consider avoiding such potentially dangerous activities as horseback riding, motorcycle riding, and climbing ladders.

RHYTHM STABILIZERS

These drugs correct an irregular heartbeat or slow one that's too fast. Over the past five years, the thinking about when to administer such drugs, especially after a heart attack, has changed dramatically. It has been discovered that using stabilizers to treat the heartbeat irregularities known as premature ventricular complexes (PVC's) may be more dangerous than the PVC's themselves. Studies also show that people treated with antiarrhythmics after a heart attack may not fare as well as people whose heartbeat irregularities are not treated.

Beta blockers are the only rhythm-stabilizing drugs that seem to lower the probability of dying after a heart attack. Other medications such as procainamide (Procan, Pronestyl), Quinidine (Quinidex, Quinaglute), propafenone (Rhthmol), and amiodarone (Cordarone) are used judiciously. Today, treatment with antiarrhythmics is usually reserved for patients with severe ventricular rhythm disturbances. If you have a much-weakened heart and potentially deadly rhythm disturbances, your doctor may ask you to consider being fitted with the device called an implantable cardioverter defibrillator (ICD).

> ♥ Lifesaving Tip: Many cardiovascular drugs are powerful and may have side effects, such as fatigue, depression, fainting, dizziness, and loss of sexual desire. If you experience such side effects, contact your doctor. If the medication is causing the problem, the dose or schedule may need to be changed, or you may need to be switched to another drug. It's very important that you never start or stop taking a cardiovascular drug without your doctor's approval.

ASPIRIN

One of the oldest drugs in your medicine cabinet, aspirin is also one of the most useful. Over a hundred years after its discovery, new uses are still being discovered for the familiar tablet. Some of the most exciting developments are in the area of cardiovascular disease.

Over the past few years, studies have shown that taking aspirin on a regular basis can protect men from heart attacks. Recent studies indicate that aspirin benefits women as well. In the 1991 Nurses' Health Study, 87,678 female nurses who took aspirin regularly cut their risk of a first heart attack by 30 percent. Taking aspirin seemed to benefit most women at the highest risk for heart disease, such as those over fifty, especially if they were also smokers or diabetic.

The standard adult aspirin dosage to prevent blood clotting is 325 milligrams (coated) every other day, or daily, if you find that easier to remember. "Baby" aspirin is a tiny 80-milligram tablet that, taken daily, works as well as the adult dosage taken every other day.

♥ **Lifesaving Tip:** Although aspirin is likely to be the most familiar item in your medicine chest, taking it is not risk-free. An anticlotting agent, aspirin protects against heart attack and stroke, but taking it daily can be dangerous if you're already on anticlotting drugs or have other risk factors for bleeding. Ask your doctor first.

BALLOON ANGIOPLASTY AND RELATED PROCEDURES

Nina sat propped up comfortably in her hospital bed at the Cleveland Clinic. Her shoulder-length brown hair fanned out on the pillow behind her, her eyes sparkled, and her smile broadened in response to a visitor's inquiry as to how she was feeling this morning. "Fine, I'm really feeling fine," Nina said. "I wasn't expecting to feel this good."

Less than twenty-four hours earlier, Nina had been lying on an imaging table. Although awake, she was sedated. On a screen above her feet were displayed X-ray images of her arteries. Nina's coronary arteries (like yours) resemble a large river which divides into branches, then tributaries. Normally the blood flows through this network smoothly, but Nina's left main coronary artery, which supplies most of the blood to her heart, was almost completely blocked. If nothing was done, Nina almost certainly would suffer a heart attack.

Working quickly but with great care, Dr. Russell E. Raymond, an interventional cardiologist, began a procedure that within an hour had removed the blockage. The blood flow to Nina's heart returned to normal and the threat of an impending heart attack virtually disappeared. What's amazing about the procedure is that Dr. Raymond accomplished it without picking up a scalpel. Known formally as percutaneous transluminal coronary angioplasty (PTCA), more commonly as balloon angioplasty, this procedure can widen blocked coronary arteries without subjecting your body to open-heart surgery.

If you have a blocked or narrowed coronary artery, angioplasty may be preferable to coronary bypass surgery. It can be a lifesaver for patients considered too frail to survive open-heart surgery, and has spared hundreds of thousands of others from the rigors of this surgery. It is also a safe, effective means of treating coronary artery disease. But as a woman, you need to keep a few points in mind.

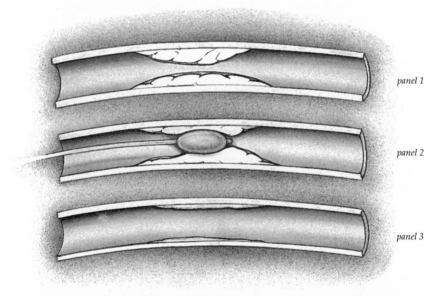

panel 1

panel 2

panel 3

Balloon Angioplasty. The first panel shows an artery narrowed by atherosclerotic plaque. In the second, a special balloon-tipped catheter is inserted into the artery and inflated. In the third panel, the balloon has been removed and blood flow largely restored.

Although this procedure has been embraced by the cardiologic community, it is performed far less often on women. In fact, figures released by the American Heart Association in 1992 showed that out of 259,000 angioplasties done, only 82,000 were performed on women.

In the early years of angioplasty, the procedure was riskier and less successful when used on women. A study published in 1985 which reviewed over 3,079 patients found that 12 of 705 women died, compared with only 7 men out of 2,374. Tearing of the coronary artery, a complication, occurred more frequently in women as well.

During those early years, use of a balloon that was possibly too large for a woman's smaller arteries was considered the culprit. Today smaller balloons are used and the overall complication rate for women has decreased, although women still tend to have a slightly higher death rate and also experience more complications, particularly from bleeding, which may not be life-threatening, but can result in a longer recuperation. Still, the differences in complications with balloon angioplasty between men and women are disappearing, notes Dr. Paul Casale, a cardiologist at the Cleveland Clinic who is an angioplasty expert. He noted that, in a study of angioplasty procedures done from 1980 to 1986 at the Cleveland Clinic, 4 out of 969 women died as a result of the procedure, compared to 3 out of 2,727 men. Although the death rate for women was slightly higher, it was still under 1 percent for both genders.

WHO IS ANGIOPLASTY FOR?

Balloon angioplasty is not for everyone, but the procedure is now performed in many instances in which it would have been advised against just a decade ago. Originally the procedure was used if the patient had only a single vessel narrowed by a single, easily accessible blockage. But times have changed, and angioplasty procedures are now performed even on women with multiple blockages in two vessels.

Because angioplasty is so much less stressful to the body than bypass surgery, most doctors are inclined to at least give it a try if it's likely to be successful. Balloon angioplasty is sometimes also performed as an emergency procedure to open clogged coronary arteries after a heart attack. In the case of "three-vessel disease," in which all three coronary arteries are narrowed, coronary bypass surgery is still the procedure of choice, because it is likely that one or more vessels would eventually reclose, necessitating repeat angioplasty procedures.

♥ **Lifesaving Tip:** To find out whether you're a good candidate for angioplasty, you should be evaluated by a cardiologist who has considerable experience in performing the procedure on women.

BEFORE YOUR ANGIOPLASTY: CARDIAC CATHETERIZATION

If you've been told you're a candidate for angioplasty, you've already had a cardiac catheterization. Sometimes the angioplasty is done at the same time as the catheterization. Often, though, catheterization is done first and the patient returns at a later time for the angioplasty. Catheterization is discussed in Chapter 6.

♥ **Mindsaving Tip:** It's normal to feel anxiety about any cardiac procedure. Talking with women who have undergone angioplasty can make you feel better. Visiting a heart support group before the surgery can ease your mind.

WHO DOES THE ANGIOPLASTY?

According to the American College of Cardiology and the American Heart Association, the doctor who does your angioplasty, known as an interventional cardiologist, should have performed at least 125 coronary angioplasty procedures, serving as the primary operator in at least 75. In some large medical centers, angioplasty is performed by a team, and you don't necessarily get to pick the person who will perform yours. In that case, make certain all the team members meet this minimum qualification.

It's important that you choose the hospital where you undergo your angioplasty with the same care you would use if you were having open-heart surgery. Although the vast majority of angioplasties go smoothly, sometimes emergency surgery is required. You should only undergo your angioplasty in a hospital which is equipped to perform open-heart surgery. "Some hospitals are doing angioplasty without open-heart surgery backup, but use a hospital nearby to cover them," says Dr. Anita Arnold, an interventional cardiologist at Olympia Fields Osteopathic Hospital and Medical Center. "In the event of an emergency, you should never have to be transported to a different building."

YOUR ANGIOPLASTY

An angioplasty begins very much as a cardiac catheterization does: In fact, many of the steps are identical. Just as for the catheterization, you're heavily sedated; the doctor makes a tiny puncture in your femoral artery, which leads from your groin to your coronary arteries. Once that's accomplished, the doctor maneuvers a thin guide wire along your arteries just past the point of the blockage. Then a special catheter with a balloon on its tip is threaded over the guide wire and pushed along until it reaches past the area of the blockage. The balloon is then inflated and held in that position from several seconds to several minutes. It may be reinflated a couple of times to maintain patency (the opening). The procedure usually takes about two hours, depending on the number and severity of the blockages.

AFTER YOUR ANGIOPLASTY

Your sedation will not wear off right after the procedure, so you'll probably sleep for a while. Heavy pressure will be applied to your groin to stop any bleeding. You'll probably sleep until the next morning. When you wake up, your groin area will be a little sore, but probably not as sore as you expect. You'll be encouraged to get up, and before long you'll be walking around the hospital floor. If no problems occur, you'll be discharged the next day. You'll be closely watched to make sure no chest pain or cardiac symptoms occur.

Once you're home:

- If you have a car with a standard transmission, you should probably skip driving it for a few days to rest your leg.
- You won't have any other restrictions related to this procedure, but you'll probably want to take it easy for a few days.
- If you work primarily at a desk job, you can return to work almost immediately. If you work at a job where you use your leg a lot, or do bending or lifting, you should stay out of work at least a few days longer.
- You'll probably be asked to return after six weeks for an exercise EKG. This is not only done to make sure that your arteries have remained open, but also furnishes results which can be

used for comparison if you have any chest pain or other symptoms later on.

♥ **Lifesaving Tip: Once you're home, if your chest pain or other cardiac symptoms return, contact your doctor immediately.**

THE PROBLEM OF RESTENOSIS

If you're thinking that balloon angioplasty sounds too good to be true, in one respect you're right. When balloon angioplasty achieves lasting results, it really can seem like a miracle. However, the arteries sometimes become narrowed again, a process called restenosis.

In a sense, restenosis occurs because your body does too good a job of repairing itself. When your doctor uses a balloon or other instrument to press against or widen your arterial walls, your body may mistake this attempt to help as an injury and set about trying to repair itself. Restenosis, the reclosing of the newly narrowed artery, is the undesirable result.

Restenosis occurs in an estimated 15 to 30 percent (although some doctors peg it as high as 40 percent) of cases. Although it usually occurs for no apparent reason, studies show that it's more likely if you're an insulin-dependent diabetic. Although 30 percent may seem high, it doesn't usually deter doctors from recommending angioplasty once, or suggesting that it be repeated if restenosis occurs. Sometimes two angioplasties are needed to achieve lasting results, and you'll still be spared open-heart surgery.

However, restenosis can take an emotional toll on you. Hope underwent angioplasty four times (on two different blood vessels) over a nine-month period. "After the third angioplasty, I was ecstatic. I thought I had absolutely licked it," she recalls. "Then I began having chest pain again, and the angiogram showed the blockage had returned." Hope may be part of a small minority of women whose arteries have a tendency to become reclogged no matter what. For her, coronary bypass surgery may provide the only long-term solution.

♥ **Mindsaving Tip: Even though your first angioplasty will probably be your last, you should be emotionally** prepared in case it doesn't turn out that way. Restenosis can occur no matter how good a job the doctor did or how model a patient you were.

THE PROS AND CONS OF ATHERECTOMY

Because of the restenosis problem, doctors have been seeking ways to improve on angioplasty. While the alternative called atherectomy appears to have reduced the incidence of restenosis, the risks of death and complications from this newer procedure and its variations are slightly higher for women. However, those new tools are also proving very useful in treating blockages that may be too hardened or inaccessible for balloon angioplasty.

An atherectomy is similar to angioplasty, except that instead of a balloon compressing the fatty deposits against the walls of your arteries, special instruments are used to remove plaque. These include:

- **Extraction atherectomy.** This procedure uses a tiny rotating blade which works in much the same fashion as the cutter on a food processor to whisk away blockages inside the artery wall at a rate of up to 1,200 revolutions per minute.
- **Rotational atherectomy.** This procedure uses a high-speed diamond-tipped drill to penetrate fatty deposits and is particularly useful on hard, calcified plaque.
- **Directional atherectomy.** This procedure uses a device that is a combination of a balloon and a shaving blade. The cutting device, usually located on the side, is run back and forth and shaves the deposits away.

In a study published in 1992, Dr. Paul Casale of the Cleveland Clinic found that while these newer techniques were largely safe for women, they did have higher rates of major complications as compared to men. Fine-tuning the technology may resolve some of these problems, Dr. Casale believes. If an atherectomy is the right procedure for you, this study underscores the need to carefully choose the doctor who performs your procedure.

♥ **Lifesaving Tip: The interventional cardiologist who evaluates your case should also be experienced in these** newer, similar techniques. Some are designed for cases in which the blockages are considered inaccessible or resistant to the balloon methods; but if they're not practiced by your doctor, you won't be offered them. Hence, you may be slated for bypass surgery without learning whether these newer procedures might have worked for you.

LASERS: "ZAPPING" BLOCKAGES

The use of lasers has always intrigued cardiologists, but presents some problems. A laser beam shoots straight ahead and is unable to follow the winding course of your coronary blood vessels. However, newer techniques use the laser beam at the tip of a catheter, which is then beamed at the blockage with pinpoint precision. The laser shows promise in reaching blockages which would be inaccessible in traditional angioplasty-like procedures. Lasers may be important in the future for treating heart disease, but currently this technology is used primarily for treating peripheral vascular disease, such as blockages in the leg. It's use in heart disease is very experimental.

Intravascular ultrasound, a technology that combines echo with catheterization, may have a significant effect on making this therapy a reality. Dr. Steven Nissen, a cardiovascular imaging specialist at the Cleveland Clinic, believes this technique will revolutionize coronary artery intervention by permitting ultrasound guided therapies. It is the equivalent of having a camera on the tip of a catheter providing clear images of the presence and extent of atherosclerotic blockage, allowing more precise targeting of angioplasty, atherectomy, and laser technique. "This capability is going to change how we diagnose and treat coronary artery disease, and by the end of the 1990s," predicts Dr. Nissen, "diagnosis and therapy will be combined."

A WORD ABOUT RESEARCH

If you're approached to become a subject in a research study, you should seriously consider it. Throughout this book, we often note that information on women's health problems is lacking because they have seldom been included in major research studies. Even when research projects are formulated specifically for women, it can be difficult to find enough female volunteers.

If you're asked to participate and don't wish to, just say no. No one at the hospital will think any less of you, and your care won't suffer in any way. But there are some good reasons to say yes.

First, patients who participate in experimental studies get special care. They're very carefully followed according to strict protocols established by committees "watchdogging" the experiment. Second, these studies usually give you the opportunity to receive therapies that won't be generally available for several years. While they're called "experimental," these therapies have been carefully screened for safety. Dr. Michael Cressman, director of the Cleveland Clinic's lipid research and referral clinic, puts the key reason for participating in research studies this way: "Clinical trials need to be performed because there is no way to determine whether or not new treatments are actually improved treatments. Unfortunately, there is no way to tell whether or not a new treatment is actually an improved treatment unless you carefully compare them. That's the bottom line."

Medical science has made tremendous strides over the years in treating cardiac problems, including many formerly considered hopeless. As of this writing, though, that symbol of the bionic age, the artificial heart, remains out of reach. Perhaps that should serve to underscore the tremendous importance of taking good care of the hearts with which we were born.

BEAR IN MIND . . .

When angioplasty and similar procedures work, and in the majority of cases they do, they certainly can seem like a miracle. But these procedures don't correct the underlying condition which caused your coronary arteries to become narrowed in the first place. Because angioplasty is a relatively brief and painless procedure, you can be lulled into thinking you're now cured and don't have to do the hard work of changing your lifestyle. Before you know it, you're back to work, managing your household and dealing with the other pressures of daily life. It's easy to slip back into old habits. If you do, you could end up back in the hospital, this time as a heart attack victim or a bypass surgery patient.

To get yourself on the right track, consider participating in a cardiac rehabilitation program. Such a program may have been introduced to you in the hospital, or you may have to inquire about it yourself. Joining a support group for people with heart problems can also provide you with an emotional bulwark and help you make the necessary lifestyle changes.

> ♥ **Lifesaving Tip:** Adopting a healthy lifestyle, which includes quitting smoking, eating a low-fat diet, and undertaking a regular program of exercise, is as important for those who have angioplasty as for people who undergo coronary bypass surgery.

CORONARY BYPASS

It was a chilly, wet autumn and Beverly was having trouble shaking what she thought was bronchitis. That nagging problem was the only shadow cast on her happy, energetic life. She had a wonderful marriage, had raised two adoring sons, and loved her job as a customer representative for a telecommunications company. At the age of fifty-six, she was mildly diabetic, but considered herself otherwise healthy. Her only concern was this respiratory problem. But as the days wore on, Beverly was finding it harder and harder to breathe.

"I went into congestive heart failure around Thanksgiving time, although, of course, I didn't realize it," she remembered. "When I went to the doctor and was literally gasping for breath, my doctor told me, 'You're in heart failure. I'm sending you to a cardiologist.'"

At first, the cardiologist thought a virus had attacked and weakened Beverly's heart. But tests showed her problem was caused by coronary heart disease. When we interviewed her, only a few months after coronary bypass surgery, Beverly was doing fine.

WHAT IS CORONARY BYPASS SURGERY?

Coronary artery bypass surgery, known informally as bypass grafting (and even more informally among doctors as CABG, pronounced "cabbage"), is a type of open-heart surgery. The procedure involves taking a vein or artery from another part of your body and grafting it onto the vessels of your heart. This grafted vessel provides an alternative route for blood to reach the heart muscle, literally providing a bypass around a clogged vessel which has been narrowed by coronary disease.

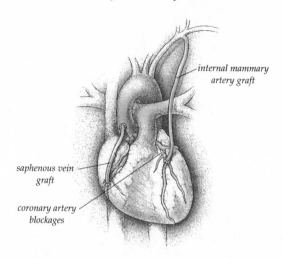

*internal mammary
artery graft*

*saphenous vein
graft*

*coronary artery
blockages*

Coronary Bypass Surgery. This procedure uses "grafts" to route blood around areas of serious blockage. If a leg vein is used as a graft, it is inserted into the aorta on the one end and anchored past the obstruction in the coronary artery on the other end. If an internal mammary artery is used, only the end is freed from the chest wall and attached to the blocked coronary artery, bypassing the obstruction.

When it was developed in the 1960s, this surgery was considered miraculous. Skeptics, however, viewed it as only the latest in a parade of procedures devised to counter the devastating effects of coronary disease. Many of those procedures had been hailed as breakthroughs but had later been abandoned. Over the years, however, studies have proved that bypass surgery, although no longer considered a miracle cure, is a very effective treatment. One major study showed that 87 percent of patients with severe narrowing in their three coronary arteries survived at least another five years after bypass, while only 59 percent were alive after being treated with drugs. Besides prolonging the life of certain patients, bypass surgery also has been shown to relieve the debilitating chest pain of coronary disease when it doesn't respond to medication.

When it comes to women, another type of controversy has arisen. Today bypass surgery is among the most common of operations, and some question whether the surgery is being performed too often. But this is not the worry for women. According to the American Heart Association's 1992 report, only one-quarter of 368,000 bypasses were performed on women. This has raised the concern that bypass surgery is not being performed on women often enough.

BYPASS RISKS FOR WOMEN

Although coronary bypass surgery is considered, by and large, a safe procedure, after twenty-five years it remains riskier for women. A major study of Cleveland Clinic cases from 1967 to 1981 found that overall 2.9 percent of the women died, compared to 1.3 percent of the men. A study of bypass cases between 1982 and 1987 at Cedars-Sinai Medical Center in Los Angeles also found that the women had a significantly higher mortality rate, 4.6 percent compared to 2.6 percent for men. The authors of the Los Angeles study attributed the higher death rate for women to the fact that they tended to be referred later for the surgery and so were sicker.

Most studies attribute the higher mortality rate for women to the fact that they more often undergo the surgery during an emergency, which makes it riskier, and that they're very often older and more likely to have other complicating conditions such as high blood pressure and diabetes. Yet even when these factors are adjusted for, women still remain at a slightly higher risk. Part of this problem is attributed to women's having smaller, more delicate coronary arteries, which makes the surgery more difficult. The size of the coronary vessels varies according to height.

"A small woman, say, one who is four feet, eleven inches or five feet tall, can have very, very small coronary arteries and it can be technically difficult to do a good job," says Dr. John A. Elefteriades, a heart surgeon at Yale–New Haven Hospital. "I've done bypasses on women who were five feet, ten inches or so, and their arteries were just as big as a man's."

If you're a petite woman and in need of a bypass, this doesn't mean you shouldn't go ahead. You should, however, consider yourself at higher risk. "We don't turn a patient down on the basis of body size," Dr. Elefteriades says. "We proceed and do it if there is an important need for it. We worry more about it, and it's definitely more common to have problems."

Since women do run a higher risk during bypass, it's extremely important that you choose your surgeon and hospital wisely. Studies have shown that death rates for bypass vary widely according to these factors. For guidelines in making these selections, see Chapter 12.

TREATMENT, NOT CURE

Doctors now know that bypass surgery does not halt the progression of coronary disease. Over the years, the remaining native arteries can become blocked by disease, as can the newly grafted vessel. This means that after a bypass:

- You may still need to take cardiovascular drugs.
- You *must* make lifestyle changes.
- You *must* quit smoking. Cigarette smoking has a profoundly negative effect on new grafts, and greatly increases the probability they will eventually close up. Dr. Elefteriades even tells patients, "If you cannot decide right here and now never to smoke another cigarette, don't have the operation. It's not worth it."

SHOULD YOU HAVE A BYPASS?

Ever since bypasses were first performed, the question of which patients benefit most has been hotly debated. Recently the American College of Cardiology and the American Heart Association issued joint guidelines which show that the patients who benefited most from coronary bypass were those with the worst prognosis. Whether or not a bypass is your best course should be decided by you and your doctor. Nevertheless, here are some examples of situations when a bypass is clearly the best therapy. You may be a candidate for CABG if:

- Tests show a critical narrowing of your left main artery, the channel which supplies most of the blood to the main portion of your heart.
- You suffer from severe angina, the chest pain of coronary artery disease, which does not respond to medication in adequate amounts.
- You suffer from three-vessel disease, which is characterized by

blockages affecting your three major coronary arteries. In such cases, bypass is often preferable to angioplasty because, with so many vessels to be opened, there is a great likelihood that one or more of them will reclose, necessitating a repeat procedure.

· You've had angioplasty repeatedly and the vessels have closed again.

· You underwent bypass years ago and the graft has become clogged.

♥ Lifesaving Tip: The final decision to undergo bypass surgery can only be made by you. If you have any doubt, by all means seek a second opinion, or even a third. Coronary bypass is serious surgery which requires serious consideration. Likewise, you should consider getting a second opinion if you're told you need a bypass but for some reason are an unsuitable candidate.

ARE YOU A HIGH-RISK PATIENT?

Just by being a woman, you're at a slightly higher risk of dying or suffering a serious complication, but being female alone does not mean you're a high-risk patient. If you're in otherwise good health, a community hospital with a well-experienced cardiovascular staff may provide satisfactory care. On the other hand, if you have additional risk factors, you'd be wise to seek out a medical center which specializes in heart surgery. For a list of factors which may indicate you are at high risk for open-heart surgical procedures including CABG, see Chapter 12.

WHAT TYPE OF BYPASS GRAFT: LEG VEIN OR CHEST ARTERY?

Traditionally, in many hospitals most coronary artery bypass operations were done using a vein graft taken from the legs. Most recently, surgeries which use the internal mammary artery, taken from the chest wall, are gaining in general popularity, having been previously performed only in a handful of centers. Such grafts are much less likely to develop future disease, and studies show that using the internal mammary artery greatly reduces the possibility the graft will soon become narrow again.

Since most coronary bypasses today are done to replace more

than one artery, even when the internal mammary artery is used, a vein from the leg is also used. The internal mammary artery is used for the most important graft.

Surgeons differ in their preferences, and some very highly regarded surgeons still maintain that the internal mammary artery is too difficult to use routinely. If your surgery is done on an emergency basis, you probably won't have a choice. If it's elective surgery, however, you should make certain your surgeon is willing to consider using your mammary artery. Whether or not the internal mammary artery is suitable for use can usually be determined by cardiac catheterization. Sometimes using the internal mammary artery can result in some pain around the incision or an increased risk of infection, especially if you're diabetic.

CABG ITSELF

Whether you're undergoing open-heart surgery for a bypass or for another type of heart repair, many of the preliminary steps are the same, including hooking you up to the heart-lung machine. They're covered in Chapter 12.

If the bypass is to be done with your leg vein, that vein is removed after you've been put to sleep. Then the surgeon makes an opening in your aorta, which is your main artery, and another in the narrowed artery beyond the blockage. The surgeon sews one end of the grafted vein to each opening, creating a new route along which the blood from your aorta can flow. This procedure has been likened to sewing on spaghetti. If the surgeon is using your internal mammary artery, he or she frees that vessel from your chest wall, then sews the end of that artery below the blockage in the affected artery.

♥ **Mindsaving Tip: Don't worry about missing either your leg vein or your mammary artery. You can get along without either. In the case of your leg, other veins will take over its circulation. In the case of your mammary artery, you were born with duplicate circulation and can easily spare it.**

Although it's by no means minor surgery, coronary artery bypass is very frequently done today, and many women in your circle of friends may already have gone through it. For our tips on recuperating, see Chapter 12.

CARDIAC REHABILITATION

With her masses of red hair, it was impossible to overlook Hope. Clad in black stretch pants and a purple-and-lavender over-blouse, she pedaled away on her stationary bike to the beat of the jazz classic "In the Mood." She was in a mirrored room filled with exercise bikes and treadmills. The scene could have been any health club, but Hope was happily pedaling away in the Out-patient Cardiac Rehabilitation Center at the Cleveland Clinic.

If you have a heart problem, probably your first fear is that you will die. Your second fear is mostly likely to be that you will become an invalid. Though once firmly rooted in reality, these are now misconceptions.

WHAT IS CARDIAC REHABILITATION?

Cardiac rehabilitation (referred to usually as "cardiac rehab") is a specially structured program of exercise, education, and support designed to strengthen your heart's ability to perform exercise and return you to normal health—or better. If you've been hospi-talized with a heart problem, your program may get under way while you're still in your hospital gown. At the Cleveland Clinic, for example, cardiac patients are given a notebook with an exer-cise program that begins in the hospital and continues once they've gone home. Cardiac rehab is seen as an integral part of virtually every heart patient's treatment.

NEW FRIENDS

A good cardiac rehab program provides you with more than just exercise; you also get a circle of new friends, friends who know what you're going through because they've been there. "After my heart attack, I got very depressed," says Roberta, the fifty-eight-year-old psychiatric nurse. "Part of it was dealing with the reality that I might have died. I got very low. One of the things which really helped was signing up for the cardiac rehab program. It meant getting up, going out, and meeting people who'd also had this experience. I learned that I really wasn't alone."

Cardiac rehabilitation may benefit you if:

· **You have chest pain (angina pectoris) from coronary disease.** By exercising, you condition your body to handle greater physical activity, so you experience less chest pain. You'll also learn ways to make the necessary lifestyle changes.

· **You've had a heart attack.** Studies have shown that cardiac rehabilitation can reduce the likelihood of your suffering a second heart attack and decrease the likelihood that you'll become disabled because of your cardiac problem.

· **You've undergone heart surgery or angioplasty.** Whether you've had a bypass, valve replacement, or any type of cardiac procedure, such programs can benefit you. Studies show that you can experience a 90 percent improvement in your ability to exercise after four months in such a program.

· **You're at high risk for developing coronary artery disease.** You don't need to have suffered a heart attack or had bypass surgery to benefit from cardiac rehab.

· **You have an irregular heart rhythm, a pacemaker, or a weakened heart.** Once people with such problems were not considered suitable for cardiac rehab. But new studies have proved otherwise. Although it depends on your individual case, cardiac rehab may improve your condition.

· **You've had surgery to correct a congenital heart defect.** Cardiac rehabilitation has not traditionally been viewed as necessary for patients with congenital heart defects because most patients recover well without it. However, if your heart defect has interfered with your ability to exercise for some time, you may be in poor physical condition or unsure about your own exercise ability.

♥ Lifesaving Tip: Cardiac rehabilitation has been found to benefit people with a whole range of heart problems, but there are some situations in which exercise is dangerous. No matter what your heart problem, you should check with your doctor before starting any exercise program.

FINDING A GOOD CARDIAC REHAB PROGRAM

A good cardiac rehab program must meet important standards to provide you with a safe environment in which to exercise. Your doctor or local hospital can refer you. Here's a list of things to look for:

· A good cardiac rehab program conforms to guidelines of the American Heart Association, the American College of Cardiology, and the American Association of Cardiovascular and Pulmonary Rehabilitation.
· The program should be supervised by a cardiologist or otherwise qualified physician.
· A qualified nurse should be on hand at all times.
· The exercise instructors should have a college degree in physical fitness or a related field and should also be trained in cardiac rehabilitation.

♥ **Mindsaving Tip: If you've been diagnosed with a cardiac problem, you may suddenly feel very fragile. A cardiac rehab program provides you with a safe environment in which you can improve your strength and endurance to a point you never expected to achieve.**

WHAT'S THE PROGRAM LIKE?

There are several phases of cardiac rehabilitation. These are the same whether you've had a heart attack, surgery, or angioplasty. The first phase begins while you're in the hospital, where you'll be visited by a rehabilitation therapist, who will teach you exercises to do while still in bed or sitting down. The exercise pace will be slow, but by the time you're discharged, you should be able to get around at home. The second phase begins when you're discharged. You'll be given a program to continue at home, which will probably include warm-up exercises and walking. Before you know it, you'll probably be walking a couple of miles a day. You can also exercise in a group setting, at an outpatient rehab center, and become comfortable with such exercise devices as stationary bikes and treadmills. Phases two and three focus on the intensity of your exercise and the amount of supervision and monitoring, which will decrease as your physical condition and confidence improve. Phase three often takes place in an outpatient center, which may be at the hospital, or a community gym, YMCA, or health club—any setting is fine as long as the program meets high cardiac rehab standards.

After you "graduate" from phase three, you may choose to exercise at home or continue your program at a health club or exercise facility. While you will no longer need the medical supervision you once did, many people find they miss their friends from cardiac rehab. Some programs are structured so that you can continue indefinitely. Charlene, for example, has been attending cardiac rehab faithfully since she had her heart attack seven years ago. "It's not just an exercise group, it's a support group," she says. "We talk over our problems and exchange recipes or articles. If one of us is in the dumps, we pull ourselves out of it. That's the real important benefit."

> ♥ **Mindsaving tip: As part of cardiac rehab, you may be told to walk extra on your own. If it's cold or inclement, try your walking in an indoor mall. Some malls even sponsor walking clubs.**

CARDIAC REHAB REAPS BIG BENEFITS

The benefits of cardiac rehabilitation are many. They include an improvement in cardiovascular function, an increased ability to exercise, and added confidence. An important component of a good rehab program is the educational sessions: lectures, group discussions, and fireside chats which are held regularly. Here you can get support in making your lifestyle changes—low-fat cooking tips, ideas on quitting smoking—and share ways to deal with the emotional issues that arise for people with heart problems.

CARDIAC REHAB AND WOMEN

As good as cardiac rehab programs are for women, they appear to have some drawbacks. Studies have shown that women are less likely to join and more likely to drop out. Much as Hope enjoys her program, such studies don't surprise her. At the moment, she's the only woman in her group. "Sometimes it's hard being the only woman here," she says. "I like the guys, but I miss having a woman to talk to."

Part of the reason for that, of course, is that more men than women are currently undergoing hospital procedures for their heart problems. The cardiac rehab educator may focus the lectures and materials on men's needs and erroneously assume that any woman present must be a spouse, not a patient. Single women like Hope sometimes feel even more like outsiders. Also, while doctors usually don't hesitate to refer men to cardiac rehab programs, some believe that women, especially older women, may not be interested in exercise, and miss out on the chance to refer women to a program. Time can also be a factor. Most cardiac rehab programs are conducted during the day. A woman is more likely to have home responsibilities that can interfere with her attendance, or to work at a job from which she can't get the necessary time off. If this is true in your case, you may be able to persuade your employer that cardiac rehab is an important part of your recuperation by pointing to a 1989 study done at Coors Industries in Colorado, where workers who participated in cardiac rehab returned to work sooner, resulting in savings of over $10,000 in wages and disability expenses per participant.

WHO PAYS FOR CARDIAC REHAB?

If you have private health insurance or Medicare, you should be covered for cardiac rehabilitation if you have had a heart attack or unstable angina, or have had balloon angioplasty or coronary bypass surgery. If there's another reason for you to participate in cardiac rehab, such as repair of a congenital defect, your doctor should be able to convince the insurer it will benefit you.

If you don't have insurance, a good cardiac rehab program strives to keep its costs low, so the fee may be less than you think. If you want to continue going to cardiac rehab after your program ends, you'll probably have to pick up the cost yourself, but you may find that it costs less than joining a health club.

BE YOUR OWN CHEERLEADER

Lack of emotional support may be the most important factor of all in explaining why women take less advantage of cardiac rehab. Typically a male heart patient has a wife who can act as a cheerleader and encourage him to go. As a woman, you may be divorced, widowed, or otherwise living alone, with no one to give you the encouragement you need. If this is so, be your own cheerleader! Cardiac rehab may turn out to be the most important part of your recovery.

♥ Livesaving Tip: Even if you had your heart attack or surgery years ago, it's not too late to join a cardiac rehab program. Exercising will improve your health, increase your sense of well-being, add to your store of knowledge about your heart, and help you make new friends.

12
Open-Heart Surgery

I was sitting across the desk from the cardiologist, but his voice seemed to echo from a great distance. He was telling me I would need open-heart surgery. "Do you want to have it done in Hartford or New Haven? Just let me know and I'll find somebody good to do it," he was saying, casually.

Perhaps he was trying not to alarm me, but I didn't feel like being nonchalant. I'd met the cardiologist just that afternoon, and he was giving me news that stunned me. Up until a few weeks ago, I had not known anything was wrong with my heart. Now I was being presented with choices regarding open-heart surgery as casually as a waiter might ask what I wanted for lunch. It seemed unbelievable, but since then I've found that this approach is not unusual.

If you need heart surgery, you may find yourself being given the names of doctors and hospitals and being urged to choose quickly, without any consideration at all. Of course, if you suddenly find yourself faced with the need for emergency surgery, you may have little to say in the matter. That's true also if you belong to a managed health-care plan which limits your choice to one hospital. But most of the time, you'll have the opportunity to make a choice—which is what this section is all about.

Choices about the care of your heart can be among the most important you'll ever make. Dr. Bruce Lytle, a cardiovascular surgeon at the Cleveland Clinic, says, "When you have open-heart surgery, that is one of the most important events in your life. The outcome is very important. Whether you'll be alive, how long you will live, and how well you will do for the rest of your life are the types of things which are at stake."

If you're confronting a serious heart problem, that may seem enough in itself to cope with, and you may feel that making decisions about hospitals and surgeons is the last thing you need to worry about. But by becoming informed, you ensure that you'll get the best care.

♥ **Mindsaving Tip: If you're visiting a physician or cardiologist to investigate a significant medical problem, don't go alone. Learning that you have a serious heart problem or need surgery is a lot to deal with. Take along your spouse, a grown child, or a close friend to serve as your "listener" so that you can be certain what you've heard is accurate. Also, arrange to call the doctor back once you've absorbed the news and have formulated a list of questions to ask.**

CHOOSING A HOSPITAL

In these days of tough competition, hospitals are too often tempted to represent themselves as being all things to all people. Hospitals play up their strengths but are unwilling to reveal their weaknesses and risk losing patients. They eagerly recruit new patients with shiny brochures, impressive annual reports, and health fairs. But all hospitals are not alike.

SMALL HOSPITALS VS. LARGE

Most people feel more comfortable about being in a hospital close to home, even if it's small. There's no problem with that, as long as it can provide you with the care you need. The fundamental question in choosing a hospital, no matter what its size, should be "Is this where I'll receive the best care?"

> ♥ Lifesaving Tip: Many hospitals tout themselves as "heart centers," but have only a cardiovascular surgeon and a cardiologist or two on staff. This can spell danger for you. For your cardiac procedure, it's imperative that your hospital be a cardiac treatment center in reality, not just in name. At the bare minimum, your hospital should have two experienced cardiovascular teams. After all, members sometimes need to fill in for each other.

TEACHING VS. NONTEACHING HOSPITAL

Whether or not to select a teaching hospital is another often-debated question. At a teaching hospital, the doctors tend to be at the cutting edge of their profession and have access to the most advanced diagnostic technology and therapies. On the other hand, if you're in a teaching hospital, you may find that, while your care is supervised by an attending physician, you'll be attended by some doctors who are still in training. You may be attracted to the hospital because someone famous is on the staff, but you probably won't get a glimpse of the medical celebrity unless your case is quite exotic. You can also expect to be periodically visited by troops of student doctors. Such attention can be welcome, and a newly minted doctor can sometimes pick up a problem a veteran may miss. But such visits can also be exhausting.

HEART MEGA-CENTERS

Some hospitals are considered among the best of the best for heart care. They are named in articles such as the one in the June 15, 1992, issue of *U.S. News & World Report*. The magazine asked leading cardiologists to choose the best hospitals in the country. The selected dozen include the Cleveland Clinic, Massachusetts General Hospital in Boston, and the Mayo Clinic in Rochester, Minnesota.

Should you seek out such a center for your heart problem? If you're not considered to be at unusually high risk from heart surgery and your problem is relatively straightforward, probably not. But if you are considered high-risk, your problem is unusually complex, or you're undergoing open-heart surgery a second or third time (particularly if you did not do very well before), you should certainly consider seeking out such a facility.

ARE YOU A HIGH-RISK PATIENT?

Just by virtue of being female, you're at slightly higher risk from open-heart surgery. But if you're in otherwise good health, being female does not necessarily make you a high-risk patient. There are other factors to consider. If you fall into one of the categories below, you should choose your hospital and surgeon with extra care:

- You're undergoing surgery on an emergency basis.
- Your heart has been damaged by a heart attack or other cause.
- You have multiple heart problems. For example, you need a coronary bypass operation but you also have a leaky mitral valve which may require surgery.
- You underwent open-heart surgery before, most particularly if you did not do well.
- You already had a heart valve replacement, but now need to have that valve replaced a second or third time.
- You have other serious medical problems such as diabetes and/or high blood pressure.
- You're over sixty-five years of age. Open-heart surgery is now being done successfully on people in their seventies and even their eighties, but the risk is higher.

BUYER (AND PATIENT) BEWARE!

While it's reassuring to think of hospitals as benevolent institutions, that is not always the case. All hospitals are not created equal, and it pays to eye them critically. This is what Pat found out when she had her surgery. Her mother underwent the same procedure just two weeks after Pat did. In her small Connecticut hospital, Pat's every need was attended to, but for her sixty-five-year-old mother, who was in a large, inner-city hospital in another state, it was a different story.

"The accommodations were awful," Pat says. "Soap and towels were in demand. My sister had to bring them from home. She bartered for toilet paper. My mother had great doctors, but the hospital was a brutal introduction to inner-city life for her."

The growing competition among hospitals, coupled with the increasing tendency of patients to view themselves as consumers, has prompted hospitals to offer more publications. You can expect these materials to play up to the institution's strengths, but good ones offer valuable information as well. For example, the Cleveland Clinic now offers a free guide called "How to Choose a Doctor and Hospital If You Have Coronary Disease."

Some questions to ask when choosing a hospital:

· Is the hospital accredited by the Joint Commission on Accreditation of Healthcare Organizations (JCAHO)? While such accreditation is voluntary, it assures you that the hospital meets minimum standards of staffing, equipment, and safety regulations, note Charles B. Inlander and Ed Weiner in their 1991 book *Take This Book to the Hospital with You.*

· How many cardiac procedures are performed annually? The hospital you're considering should perform at least 200 to 300 open-heart operations annually, the majority being coronary bypass operations, according to joint guidelines published by the American College of Cardiology and the American Heart Association.

· What is the mortality rate? While most hospitals are more than happy to shower you with glossy annual reports and slick magazines, they're often less eager to show off their rates of death and surgical complications. That, however, is precisely the information you need. If the hospital won't tell you, that's a good reason to consider going elsewhere.

· The Health Standards and Quality Bureau of the Health Care Financing Administration publishes an annual report listing mortality rates of individual hospitals for Medicare patients who have undergone bypass surgery. The telephone number is 410–966–1133.

· What is the morbidity rate? While the mortality rate is the number of deaths which occur as a result of certain treatments or procedures, hospitals also keep track of their morbidity rate, the number of serious complications which occur. If you're a candidate for open-heart surgery, you want to know how often patients undergoing the procedure suffer strokes or heart attacks.

- Is the hospital in relatively good financial shape? Certainly a medical cost crisis exists across the country, but have newspaper articles been published in your community warning that the hospital is deeply in debt or about to go under? If so, staff and supply shortages could compromise your care.

- Is the hospital beset with labor problems? Although it's uncommon for hospital staff to go on strike, you don't want it to happen while you're a patient there. Watch newspapers in the hospital's area for articles about wage disputes or labor unrest. If the staff is underpaid and unhappy, you may not get the quality of care you need.

- How's the nursing staff? Ask former patients (your doctor's waiting room is a good place to find them) about the nursing care they received. Were the nurses well trained and caring? Distracted or unprofessional? Busy or hopelessly overworked? Were patients sent home with follow-up instructions?

- What percentage of the staff are temporary employees? As journalist Walt Bogdanich wrote in his investigative book about the nation's hospitals, *The Great White Lie*, some of the most dangerous slipups occur in hospitals which rely on temporary workers.

- What do your friends think of the hospital? Unless you're going to a medical center far from home, you probably have friends who have been treated at this hospital. If not, they may have friends or relatives who would be happy to share their experiences. Seek them out. Firsthand testimonials count!

CHOOSING A SURGEON

If you need surgery in an emergency, you won't have time to consider your choice. More likely, though, your decision to undergo surgery will be made after serious thought. The surgeon is the person to whom you're entrusting your life, so choosing someone you feel confident about is an important matter indeed.

In smaller institutions, a cardiovascular surgeon is a jack-of-all-trades. While such a surgeon generally performs all sorts of heart surgeries, the vast majority of them will be coronary bypass procedures. If you're to have another type of heart surgery, you want to be sure your surgeon does enough of these operations to be proficient. If your problem is unusual, such as a complicated congenital defect or an aortic valve repair, it's wise to seek a surgeon who specializes in this area. This may be a good reason to consider a larger hospital or medical center.

> ♥ Lifesaving Tip: If you are going to undergo valve or congenital heart surgery, inquire if intraoperative echocardiography is available. Echo imaging during such operations can now be used to guide the surgeon's progress and to assess the procedure's success. If the results aren't optimal, the surgeon can redo it before the heart is closed. The use of ultrasound technology during such open-heart surgery procedures has quickly become an important supportive service, and its use by your surgical team is an indicator of being up to date. If you ask about intraoperative echo and are told that it isn't available, or it's "not very important," think about having your surgery elsewhere.

It's important to remember that in choosing a surgeon you are, in essence, often choosing the hospital where the surgery will be performed. Most surgeons operate out of only one or two hospitals.

HOW IMPORTANT IS IT THAT YOU LIKE YOUR SURGEON?

"When I left my cardiologist's office, I went to see the surgeon he recommended," says Pat, who at the age of thirty-six had surgery to correct a congenital heart defect. "I liked my cardiologist, but, when it came to the surgeon, he seemed to feel the less the patient knew, the better. He gave me the impression he felt the patient should shut up, let him do his magic, and be appreciative." Still, even though Pat still bristles when she recalls her surgeon, she probably would not have chosen someone else. "This surgeon was presented to me as the best in his field. What should I have done, chosen second best?"

Ideally, the surgeon you choose will have both a fine personality and a high degree of skill. If it's not possible to have both, the nod should go to skill. But even if a surgeon is a star, that's no reason for a patient not to be treated with respect.

WHEN SHOULD YOU MEET THE SURGEON?

You should certainly meet the surgeon well in advance of the surgery. Dr. John Elefteriades, a cardiac surgeon at Yale–New Haven Hospital, meets with candidates for surgery in advance to discuss not only the procedures but any other options they may have. "Every patient deserves to know her condition, what's going on with her heart," Dr. Elefteriades says. "Patients also should know what their options are, both surgical and nonsurgical, and they should receive a description of the operation, the risks, the estimated length of their hospital stay and their recovery." If you're having emergency surgery, of course, this is not usually possible. Also, some hospitals keep their "star" surgeons so busy they simply don't have time to meet with patients.

My hospital roommate never laid eyes on her surgeon. I later learned he was legendary in this respect. In fact, the story goes, several of his former patients once turned up where he was giving a lecture, just to thank him! This surgeon may not have succeeded in the realm of patient relations, but his skill with a scalpel was such that his patients were willing to overlook it.

♥ **Mindsaving Tip: Your choice of a surgeon will probably come from your cardiologist. Ask for two or three names; this way, if you decide you don't want a particular surgeon, you can choose another more easily.**

THE SURGICAL TEAM

Having heart surgery is something like choosing a package-deal vacation: In choosing a surgeon, you're not only selecting the doctor who will perform the procedure, but the entire surgical team as well. While open-heart surgery has become quite common, it is still a very complex and precise operation which requires that every member of the surgical team, from the anesthesiologist to the scrub nurse, performs his or her job flawlessly. If you choose your surgeon wisely, you can have confidence that this will be so. No topflight heart surgeon would tolerate an inferior team.

Here are some questions to ask a surgeon:

· **What is your mortality rate when you do this type of proce-**

dure on a woman of my age and condition? Of course, mortality rates can vary; it's not surprising if a surgeon specializing in coronary bypass operations on patients with serious kidney failure has a higher death rate than others. But for open-heart surgery on a woman in otherwise good health, a surgeon should have an overall mortality rate no higher than 3 or 4 percent.

Many people feel uncomfortable asking such things. According to Dr. Bruce Lytle, a cardiac surgeon at the Cleveland Clinic, they shouldn't. "Your doctor is working for you, you are not working for your doctor, and you have the right to ask anything you want," Dr. Lytle says. He always volunteers the information about his mortality rate. Certainly you can phrase such questions diplomatically, or have a family member ask instead. But you should not be reluctant to press for this important information. A surgeon may not have precise figures but should be able to give you some idea. If a surgeon is very defensive, or refuses to discuss the topic, you might take that into consideration when deciding whether you want this surgeon to do the operation.

- **What is your morbidity rate for patients of my age and condition?** During open-heart surgery, the possibility of a stroke is among the most threatening complications for your future quality of life. But heart attack or serious lung or bleeding complications can also occur. These major complications are usually called morbidities. For open-heart procedures, they usually equal the mortality rate.

- **Do you offer alternative approaches to treating cardiac problems?** The field of medicine is ever-changing. To make sure you're getting the best care, your surgeon should be able to offer you the most up-to-date treatments. If your surgeon is not familiar with the latest techniques, such as valve repair instead of replacement, if possible, or an atherectomy instead of coronary bypass surgery, you won't receive the best in surgical care.

- **How many cardiac procedures do you perform?** Practice makes perfect. According to the American College of Cardiology and the American Heart Association, a cardiovascular surgeon should perform at least 100 to 150 open-heart operations annually. But while quantity counts, be wary of the surgeon whose procedures mount into the thousands. That surgeon may not have the time to give patients adequate before-and-after surgical care.

> ♥ **Mindsaving Tip: When quizzing your prospective surgeon, be tactful. You're entitled to this information, but that doesn't mean you have to come on like Attila the Hun.**

THE OPEN-HEART PROCEDURE

It was shortly after midnight on the day that I was to have open-heart surgery. I couldn't sleep. I was nervously leafing through a magazine for heart patients when I came across the statement that such operations had become "almost as routine as an appendectomy." "Hah! That's easy for you to say; it's not your heart," I thought. Open-heart surgery is the operation which evokes the most anxiety in us. As children we all learned that if your heart stops, you die. All the discussion in the world about the marvels of technology will not completely erase that fear. So if it's your heart for which surgery is being considered, you may not be able to consider it routine.

If you're about to undergo heart surgery, plenty of people will probably be eager to tell you how routine a procedure it has become. In a way, they're right: In 1989 alone, nearly 700,000 open-heart operations were performed in the United States, making it one of the most common surgical procedures in the country. If it is your surgery, however, there's no reason you should view it as routine. Open-heart surgery is very precise, delicate work which must be performed flawlessly. Over the years, surgeons' skill in performing this type of surgery has improved, and the rates of death and major complications have fallen dramatically.

BEFORE THE SURGERY: FINDING SUPPORT

If you are to undergo open-heart surgery, you'll probably discover that there is plenty of support and information available afterward, but not much before. My cardiologist's advice to "go home, have a cup of tea, and call me with any questions you have" was okay as far as it went. But what I really needed was to talk with someone who had gone through the surgery. Fortunately, I discovered that my friend Julia had a friend, Pat, who had undergone the same surgery I was to have. Thus began our friendship. We never met until after my surgery, but during those excruciating six weeks beforehand, Pat was often the last person I talked to by phone by night and the first person I called in the morning. In retrospect, I would never leave finding such support to chance. Neither should you.

Ask your doctor to suggest a patient to whom you can talk. Contact the hospital, too, and ask whether there are volunteers who meet with patients undergoing similar surgery. Often such meetings take place the day before surgery. Trust us, you'll want someone to talk to way before then. Ask to talk to another woman so that you can get as personal as you like. Or contact your local office of the American Heart Association, or Mended Hearts, a national organization listed in the "Recommended Reading and Resources" section.

> ♥ **Mindsaving Tip:** Many hospitals provide you with educational information about your surgery, but they usually give it to you afterward. Request such materials ahead of time to help you prepare.

ASK QUESTIONS   Back in 1979, when Cheri had open-heart surgery to correct a heart problem caused by Marfan's syndrome, a serious congenital condition, she fumed because "they told my husband everything, but they kept me totally in the dark." When she had cardiac surgery again in 1991, she was pleased to discover that that behavior had changed. Today, it's recognized that patients have the right to know what's going to happen to them.

> ♥ **Mindsaving Tip:** Be informed. What you're imagining the procedure is like is probably more frightening than the reality. If you're squeamish, feel free to decline information that's offered. But it should be your choice.

BANKING YOUR BLOOD   With the concern these days about AIDS, you're probably worried about your hospital's blood supply. Surprisingly, open-heart surgery in many hospitals does not currently require blood transfusions. However, complications can arise, and you might need a pint or two. As soon as you've decided to undergo the surgery, ask your doctor whether you can bank some of your own blood and check with the hospital to find how this is done. You can also ask your family and friends if they wish to donate blood, but remember their blood type *must* match yours. If you're not medically well enough to donate your own blood, or if you're having surgery out of state, find out what precautions the hospital takes to ensure that its blood supply is safe from such dangers as AIDS and hepatitis. This is an area where you can't be 100 percent sure, but the risk of failure to have needed surgery outweighs the risk of receiving contaminated blood.

OTHER PREPARATIONS Find out whether you require any additional tests such as a thorough dental check-up before the surgery, and whether you should discontinue any medications you're taking. Doctors may vary in their advice on this; for example, if you take birth-control pills, some surgeons suggest you switch to another method of contraception before surgery to avoid the danger of blood clots.

Things to do before surgery:

· Recruit emotional support.
· Obtain educational materials about your procedure.
· Plan your recuperation.
· Find out when you will enter the hospital, and any preparations or tests which need to be done beforehand.
· Inquire about banking your own blood.
· Find out whether you need to stop taking any of your medications.

♥ **Lifesaving Tip: If you haven't reached menopause and your surgery is not an emergency, ask your surgeon whether your operation should be scheduled when you're not menstruating. While you're on the heart-lung machine, your blood is infused with an anticlotting agent, which can sometimes result in bleeding problems.**

THE NIGHT BEFORE SURGERY When I had my surgery at the Cleveland Clinic, I was stunned to discover that the procedure was "TCI." In hospital parlance, that means "to come in." I was to arrive the morning of my surgery. Since I had always checked in the night before for less major procedures, I was amazed. "This is almost like walk-in open-heart surgery," I marveled.

While some large hospitals specializing in open-heart surgery use a TCI system, most require you to check in the night before. If you're hospitalized, you'll probably be visited by the anesthesiologist, whose job it is to put you to sleep the next day. You'll be asked questions about your health, allergies, and medications, and such lifestyle questions as whether or not you smoke. The anesthesiologist's job is to select the types of drugs which will be used during your surgery. Be honest in your answers; it's very important that you receive the right type of anesthesia.

> ♥ **Mindsaving Tip: Wherever you spend it, in the hospital or at home, the night before heart surgery is bound to be anxiety-provoking. Plan some pleasant distractions for yourself, such as inviting a good friend or relative to come see you. Or treat yourself to some long-distance phone calls.**

THE DAY OF YOUR SURGERY   The day of the surgery, you'll be given a sedative to relax you. Preparations vary from hospital to hospital. Sometimes they're done before you're put to sleep, or sometimes afterward. Your body will be scrubbed with an antiseptic. Part of your pubic area may be shaved in case your femoral artery (the one near the groin) needs to be accessed during surgery. If a leg vein is to be used for a coronary bypass, part of your leg will be shaved. Some of these preparations may be done the night before.

> ♥ **Mindsaving Tip: Sometimes surgery is delayed. You're probably the last person anyone will think to tell. Relax; the delay probably is caused by the surgical schedule, and has nothing to do with you medically at all.**

THE SURGERY ITSELF

Because of the sedative, some people don't recall being in the operating room, but others do. Before long, though, you'll be put to sleep. When you awaken, you'll be in the recovery room. The exact procedures for coronary bypass, valve surgery, and the correction of a congenital defect are discussed in Chapter 11. But these preliminary steps are the same no matter what type of open-heart surgery you're having.

During this preparation time, after you're unconscious, the

anesthesiologist places a breathing tube through your mouth, connecting you with a machine which will regulate your breathing during surgery. Various tubes and monitors are connected to you as well so that your body's functions can be monitored closely.

The heart-lung machine is the device which makes open-heart surgery possible. It temporarily takes over the function of the heart and lungs. It consists principally of a pump, which does the work of your heart, and an oxygenator, which does the work of your lungs. Your blood flows from your heart's main veins into the machine. There it is cleansed of carbon dioxide, filled with oxygen, and recirculated throughout your body.

For the surgery, your chest is opened and your heart exposed. This requires cutting through the breast bone. The surgeon places tubes in your heart which enable your blood to begin flowing through the circuitous tubing of the heart-lung machine. This recirculation of your own blood lowers the probability that you will need any blood transfusion. It also enables the surgeon access to a "bloodless field" and helps him or her see and work on your heart more easily.

An important part of open-heart surgery involves the lowering of your body temperature. This is done for two important reasons: First, lowering the temperature of your heart slows down its beat, and second, when your heart is cooled, it requires far less oxygenated blood. Once your chest is opened and preliminary steps complete, the surgeon stops the blood flow to your heart by clamping your aorta. A mixture of cold water and saline is applied to your heart to stop it from beating.

Again, the surgical procedures for a coronary bypass, valve repairs and replacements, and congenital defects are discussed in Chapter 11. Whatever the procedure, once it's completed, the surgeon directs the perfusionist (the technician who operates the heart-lung machine) to gradually begin allowing your heart and lungs to resume their normal functions. Your own rewarmed blood will begin flowing slowly back through your heart. This infusion of warm blood is enough to start your heart beating again. It's not unusual for a heart to begin beating erratically. If this happens, the surgeon applies an electric shock, which gets the heart beating in its own rhythm again. Once your heart is beating satisfactorily on its own, your chest will be sewn up and you're transferred to an intensive care ward.

♥ Mindsaving Tip: During the operation, you'll be given narcotics to make sure you'll remain asleep. Surveys have shown that many people fear waking up during the operation, but this virtually never occurs. You will be monitored and if it appears you're not sleeping deeply enough, you'll be given more drugs.

COMPLICATIONS OF OPEN-HEART SURGERY

Earlier in this chapter, we dealt with such complications of open-heart surgery as death and stroke. There are some other risks to this type of surgery as well.

The risk of stroke is higher if you're elderly, but no matter what your age, it's also slightly increased in procedures during which the cardiac chambers themselves must be opened. This is not done in coronary bypass surgery, which is performed on the surface of the heart, but in procedures to repair congenital heart defects or replace valves. When the heart chamber is opened, it increases the chance that a tiny air bubble could enter your bloodstream and travel to your brain.

One particular type of complication seems related to the use of the heart-lung machine: neurological problems. This is an area that doctors sometimes don't feel like discussing, but if you're not aware of the possibility and it does occur, you may be unnecessarily worried.

No matter how miraculous this man-made machine is, it cannot do its job as perfectly as your own heart and lungs in providing your brain with perfectly oxygenated blood. So sometimes being on the heart-lung machine can result in mental changes. On very rare occasions, there can be a permanent change, such as losing the ability to do calculations or analyze problems. Subtle mental alterations, such as memory loss, personality change, or cloudy thinking are more common. Such problems are most often temporary. Dr. John Elefteriades, a cardiac surgeon at Yale–New Haven Hospital, says, "I've operated on hundreds of patients, including people like doctors and professors, who need their intelligence for their work. With the exception of those rare patients who suffer a stroke during surgery, nobody has ever come back to me and said they were unable to carry out their job."

How will I feel when I come to? Once you awaken, you may feel groggy. Your first sensation, though, is likely to be the most unpleasant: You'll probably awaken fighting the breathing tube. If you're unprepared for this, you may be frightened. Try not to fight the machine, but to breathe with it. Most likely, a nurse will be nearby to assist you. The staff is aware that the breathing tube is uncomfortable, and it will be removed as soon as possible, but not before you are fully awake and able to breathe normally on your own. This usually means the morning after the surgery, but most people are only aware of the breathing tube for the last hour or two before it's removed because they're sleepy.

What will I feel like after surgery? After I came to (and got rid of that darn breathing tube!), I recall doing a mental inventory from my feet up to my head. I was surprised to find that I felt, basically, okay. The only annoyance I recall is that everything looked fuzzy. I soon realized that was because I wasn't wearing my glasses!

When you first regain consciousness, you probably won't feel too great. On the other hand, some women feel better than they expected to. How you feel can depend on how much anesthesia you were given, how long your procedure was, and its complexity. Despite all these factors, there is no simple formula; individuals simply differ in the way their bodies respond to surgery.

But times have changed, and open-heart surgery is not the long ordeal it used to be. Cheri was born with Marfan's syndrome and developed a life-threatening aneurysm at the age of twenty-one. It grew slowly until Cheri was twenty-nine, when it became so large there was no choice but to remove it. Still, the surgery was deemed so risky at the time that she was sent to Texas, where Denton Cooley, the world-famous heart surgeon, performed the operation. Cheri was hospitalized for a month and spent an additional three months recuperating. In 1991, she underwent open-heart surgery again, to correct another aneurysm. After her first experience, she was understandably terrified, but her recent surgery turned out not to be anything like what she'd expected. "There was a big difference. This time, I was home in several days and the recuperation period was much shorter. I felt pain, but not the kind of pain that I remember from 1979. Either I'm fooling myself or it's been fantastic. I have to slow down occasionally because I just get carried away, I feel so good."

TIPS ON SURVIVING (AND EVEN LOVING) YOUR HOSPITAL STAY

Here are our favorite tips for making a hospital stay not only survivable, but even sometimes fun:

- Appoint an advocate. During your hospital stay, there will be times when you won't be able to look out for yourself. Ask your partner, a relative, or a close friend to look out for your interests and question any tests, medications, or procedures ordered for you.
- Bring your underwear! Those drafty hospital gowns are a necessity right after surgery, but later on most hospitals won't mind your wearing underwear. Warm flannel or cotton underwear makes a big difference.
- Bring a few inexpensive mementos from home. This can be a few family pictures or a favorite souvenir. But don't bring anything you couldn't bear to lose if it were misplaced or even stolen.
- Be pleasant to the staff. It may be unfair, but it's true; nobody wants to be around a grouch. The old saying "You can catch more flies with honey than you can with vinegar" is as true on the hospital ward as anywhere else. If you're nice, the staff will do their best to brighten your stay.
- A bright piece of costume jewelry (perhaps something heart-shaped?) or a whimsical pin can brighten a hospital gown. For one woman, her son's gift of oversized "Snoopy" slippers kept up her spirits and provided her with a sense of identity as well. Padding up and down, she cheered up the whole floor!
- Tired of TV? Take along an inexpensive radio or cassette player with earphones. This way you can listen to your favorite music or enjoy that novel you always wanted to read, on tape.

♥ Mindsaving Tip: Heart surgery is serious business, but don't lose your sense of humor. If it will cheer you, bring along comedy tapes or humor books.

STARTING YOUR RECUPERATION

Soon you'll begin getting out of bed, at first with a nurse at your side. Before long, you'll be padding down the hall. Then you'll be complaining about the hospital food. Hallelujah, you've survived!

A WORD ABOUT THOSE BEEPS . . .

Although it looks as if you're on a regular hospital floor, you'll soon discover that all your fellow patients are heart patients. This is because you're in a "telemetry" unit, which refers to the constant monitoring of your heart. You're connected to devices which record your heartbeat even when you're walking down the hall. One reason for this is that after heart surgery your heart is prone to such problems as an irregular rhythm.

> ♥ **Mindsaving Tip: If you've had heart surgery, your heart's electrical patterns, while normal for you, may appear abnormal on an electrocardiogram. If this is true in your case, ask your cardiologist for a copy of your EKG to carry with you. This way, if an EKG is ever done on you in an emergency, it won't be erroneously assumed that what they're observing represents an undiagnosed heart problem.**

ONCE YOU'RE HOME

With costs rising, hospitals are under pressure to release you as soon as they possibly can. If there are no complications, you'll probably stay in the hospital a week or so. Just when you're beginning to feel able to get around, you'll find yourself being discharged.

YOUR RECUPERATION

Just as you plan for a successful vacation, you should plan for a successful recuperation. If you leave things to chance, they may not work out at all the way you want them to.

Despite the woman's movement, it remains largely true that men work outside the home while women work at a job, then come home to another day's worth of responsibilities. This alone creates extra pressure when you return from the hospital.

Your needs during recuperation will vary, depending on what stage of life you're in. When Pat returned from the hospital, she had three young children including a baby to care for. Eleanor, in her late forties, had teenagers who relied on her to chauffeur them to school activities. Hope, in her mid-sixties, lived alone, with no one to help out.

The best time to make arrangements for your after-care is before your surgery. Sue Dehner, a nurse at the Cleveland Clinic who provides postsurgical education, says, "We tell patients they can't lift anything greater than eight to ten pounds for six to eight weeks. That means no vacuuming or lifting of laundry baskets or small children. Often that poses problems for women. So we encourage them not to be shy about asking for outside help."

Janice Anderson, a nurse who heads the cardiac rehabilitation program at Norwalk Hospital in Connecticut, notes that some women face a special problem. Since women tend to develop coronary heart disease at an older age, they may have husbands who have heart problems as well. "Sometimes one spouse can become too protective of the other," Anderson notes. More often, though, the woman will be a widow. This can led to depression, because her own illness can bring up painful memories of the time when her husband was ill.

Here are the advantages of planning your recuperation in advance:

- You'll be faced with a minimum of pressure and disorganization when you can least cope with it—when you first get home.
- You'll be sending a message to your family that it won't be "business as usual" when you get home, that you'll need their help.
- You'll be thinking about your life after surgery, a subtle but strong message that you will survive. This can lessen everyone's anxiety.

♥ **Mindsaving Tip:** If your husband, a close friend, or a relative can take some time off from work, the best time to do it is your first week at home, rather than the week you're in the hospital. That's when you'll need the help more.

On your return home, you may find you still feel some pain. How much pain depends on the individual and the type of procedure. For example, women who have had bypass surgery done with mammary grafts appear to feel more postoperative chest pain. Many patients (and sometimes their doctors) erroneously believe they will become addicted to pain medication after surgery. Recently, though, the federal government urged doctors to give such painkillers more freely after surgery because their appropriate use actually speeds recovery.

As you recuperate, you'll discover that your energy ebbs and flows. It's normal to feel peppier on some days than others, or start the day with a burst of energy and start drooping around noon. Gradually, the time during which you feel like your old self should become longer and longer. This can take as little as a few weeks for some, up to a year or even longer for others. The important thing is to remember you're an individual, and not to compare yourself with others. "The one thing I resented was people telling me I'd be a new woman," said fifty-eight-year-old Ida. "They'd heard of others recuperating within a few weeks. I felt everyone was blaming me because it didn't happen that way for me."

♥ **Mindsaving Tip: Consider keeping a journal of your progress as you recuperate. You can note the day you walked one block, then two, then three. Before long, you'll discover that, overall, you're doing better than you realized.**

BACK TO WORK

Studies have shown that more men than women return to work after open-heart surgery. One difference is that most women patients tend to be older, so they're closer to retirement. Or they're homemakers.

After surgery, you can expect to return to your regular activities in about six weeks, although it may certainly take you longer to regain your customary stamina. Before you're allowed to return to work, your doctor may order an exercise stress test. This test not only provides medical information about your heart, but it reassures you that your heart is up to the rigors of your everyday life.

If you work, try to return part-time, at least for the first week or so. You may find yourself eager to go in the morning but spent by early afternoon. *I recall my own experience years ago after abdominal surgery. I'd returned to my reporting job at a small newspaper part-time, but I couldn't resist the lure of a night editing job at a larger paper. After two days, I discovered I was walking bent over! That was the last time I tried to convince my recuperating body that I knew better than it did.*

> ♥ Mindsaving Tip: When we talked to women in the course of researching this book, we were surprised to discover how many had only the vaguest idea what had been done to them. They were dismayed about this as well. After your surgery, ask your doctor for a copy of your "operative report" (made after every surgery) or a written description of your operation.

YOUR EMOTIONS

Any threat to your heart can knock your emotions topsy-turvy. Depression is sometimes a by-product of bypass surgery, and can pose a serious threat to your health. After heart surgery, you may also experience some reluctance when it comes to having sex. Women who suffer heart attacks experience similar problems, so these subjects are covered in Chapter 10.

YOUR INCISION

If you're having open-heart surgery, a permanent memento of your experience will be your incision. If you're undergoing bypass surgery, you don't have a choice: You'll be the recipient of the famous "zipper" incision which runs from the base of your neck down to the middle of your chest.

This surgical incision affects many women differently. But too often women get the impression that they shouldn't give their impending incision a thought or that they're only entitled to be concerned if they're young. Grace, a seventy-nine-year-old, impeccably groomed fashion designer, is eager to set the record straight on that misconception. Talking about her reaction after her bypass, she says, "I think the greatest shock was in the morning, when I awoke for the first time, and I saw this horrible scar that started at the pit of my neck and went all the way down to my navel." But not all women think that way. Barbara, a bypass patient in her fifties, doesn't mind her incision at all. "When I think of the incision, I look down and say to myself, 'That's why you're alive, kid.' So it's really not a problem."

THE HORIZONTAL OR SUBMAMMARY INCISION If you're having coronary bypass surgery, there's no alternative to the vertical scar. But if you have another type of heart surgery, there may be a more cosmetically pleasing alternative. This is the "submammary" or horizontal incision, which may be appropriate for such cases as simple congenital heart defect repair or certain types of valve surgery.

With this type of incision, you're opened across your middle, rather than cut vertically down your chest, and most of the incision is hidden in the crease under your breasts. The incision is low enough to be invisible beneath the most daring of swimsuits.

Don't necessarily expect to be offered this alternative. Most cardiovascular surgeons spend the majority of their time performing bypasses, and the submammary incision is not suitable for those cases. So they may be unfamiliar with it and therefore uninterested in performing it.

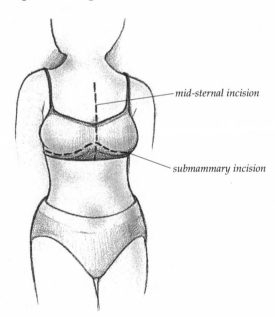

Submammary Incision. The vertical line shows the midsternal incision, generally used in most open-heart surgery. The submammary incision, shown by the horizontal dotted line, is made along the underside of the breastline and is mostly hidden by the overhanging breasts.

"When I asked if there was an option of having a submammary incision done as opposed to an incision down the middle, my surgeon treated me as if I was vain and somewhat simple-minded," says Pat. "He was very sarcastic about it also and implied that I thought cosmetics were more important to me than my life." Dr. Eliot Rosenkranz of the Cleveland Clinic, on the other hand, specializes in repairing congenital defects and uses a submammary incision when it does not compromise other requirements for a safe operation. This incision, he says, "provides the heart surgery patient with a cosmetically more acceptable scar while at the same time providing the surgeon safe, easy access to the heart." However, he adds, it should never be done if there are medical considerations which dictate a vertical incision, such as the possibility you may need to undergo surgery again. This is because the submammary incision does not lend itself to being redone. This is also a difficult incision to perform if a woman has very large breasts. Such an incision does require cutting some of the sensory nerves in the chest, which can result in a loss of sensation in the areas of the breasts. This should eventually return to normal, but sometimes it never does. So this is a factor you should consider.

If you think you may be a candidate for a submammary incision, but your surgeon resists the idea, you might consider seeking out a surgeon who is more receptive, possibly one who specializes in congenital heart defects. Remember, though, your first priority should always be the skill of the surgeon.

ABOUT YOUR INCISION, NO MATTER WHAT TYPE Whether you have a vertical or submammary incision, in time it should become less noticeable. Unfortunately, many incisions don't heal as nicely as we would like. Many times they form a noticeable scar. There are two types of abnormal scars: hypertrophic scars and keloids.

A hypertrophic scar is a thick covering which remains within the bounds of the incision. A keloid, on the other hand, exceeds these boundaries, and can even come to resemble a tumor on the skin. Although it's not known why, blacks and those of Southern European heritage develop keloids more often.

Should a plastic surgeon close my incision? "I don't think having a plastic surgeon close an incision guarantees you a better scar," says Dr. Randall Yetman, a plastic surgeon at the Cleveland Clinic. "I think heart surgeons close their wounds very carefully. Unfortunately, it's not who closes the wound, but where the wound is located and the individual patient and how he or she scars that are usually the determining factors."

According to Dr. Yetman, scarring can occur whether your incision is vertical or horizontal. When it does, it tends to be most visible in the area of the breast, possibly because of the weight of the breasts on the incision.

During the first weeks after surgery, some doctors recommend massaging the incision, or applying moisturizing oil, with or without vitamin E. While Dr. Yetman finds that both measures promote healing, he questions their usefulness in avoiding abnormal scarring. He says people who have a tendency to form abnormal scars generally do, no matter how they try to avoid it. If you're unhappy with the way your scar looks, or it's "symptomatic," that is, it still burns and itches after you should have adequately recuperated, you might consider a procedure called scar revision.

SCAR REVISION Sheila, who is in her mid-thirties, had surgery when she was only a child to correct a congenital defect. Although her incision has healed quite well, she's always hated it. "The scar made me feel different," she says. "It's always bothered me and affected my self-image and self-esteem." She recently made an appointment for a scar revision.

Scar revisions are done by plastic surgeons. During the procedure, you are awake but sedated; the doctor uses a local anesthetic. When Dr. Yetman does his scar revisions, for example, he uses a combination of methods. He cuts away the thickened part of the scar and applies cortisone, a synthetic corticosteroid drug, to promote better healing. Afterward, he has found it helpful to have his patients wear a special silicone covering over the incision for about a year. This sheetlike material covers the incision but must be washed and changed every few days. Dr. Yetman performs most of these scar revisions for patients who complain of burning and itching, but finds they're usually pleased by the improvement in their appearance as well.

♥ **Mindsaving Tip:** If you're considering scar revision, find a surgeon who has experience in the procedure. Don't believe it if you're told the scar will be eliminated. The appearance of scars can be improved, but they can't be made to completely disappear.

After heart surgery, the time you require to recuperate may vary, but before long, you'll probably be back to your routine. If you're returning to work, you may find you pick up your life much as it was before. If you're not returning to work, it doesn't mean you can't return to an active lifestyle. Boredom is the enemy of heart health. Several of the older women we spoke with enjoy an active schedule filled with hobbies and volunteer work. If you're interested in volunteer work, here's an idea: Who's more qualified to talk with other women facing heart surgery?

HEART TRANSPLANTS

It's very rare that a heart becomes so weakened as to require a heart transplant. Much less drastic measures are available to treat, and even correct, the majority of heart problems.

In the few cases in which the heart is so badly weakened and damaged that a heart transplant is the only hope, transplants have become much safer. In his 1971 book, *Hearts,* journalist Thomas Thompson chronicled several heart transplant cases performed between 1968 and 1971. These were the early, heady days of heart transplants, before doctors fully realized the daunting problems presented by the body's immune system. Many of these early heart transplants failed.

But doctors learned a great deal in this early, experimental period. Techniques have been refined and important drugs discovered which suppress the body's immune system. In 1990, 2,071 heart transplants were performed in the United States. The most recent statistics show that 72 percent of heart transplant patients are still alive after five years. Many of them have been able to return to active lives.

Careful selection has also contributed to the increased survival rate among transplant patients. Candidates for heart transplants are usually under sixty years of age. They're usually male, as women often develop heart disease later in life. There's no lower age limit for heart transplants: children with very severe congenital heart defects are now receiving them.

In adults, candidates usually have very little chance of survival without a transplant. They are usually in the final stages of congestive heart failure, caused either by coronary heart disease or a heart muscle disorder, such as a cardiomyopathy, usually from a virus that attacks the heart. They need to be in otherwise good health, free of such diseases as diabetes or cancer.

One of the biggest barriers to a heart transplant remains the shortage of donor organs. Often a candidate for a heart transplant is placed on a long waiting list or may have to travel to an area where donor hearts are more available. It's unfortunate but true that the odds of receiving a donor heart are better in larger cities, where higher accident rates contribute to the availability of organs for transplant. Health insurers are also increasingly assuming a major role in determining where a transplant patient will be treated.

Heart transplants are similar to other types of open-heart surgery, which is covered in Chapter 12. As in other open-heart procedures, the patient is placed on the heart-lung machine. Although it may sound from the term "heart transplant" as if the entire heart is removed, this is not accurate. In a heart transplant, the major portion of the heart which is diseased—the ventricles—is removed. The "back walls" of the heart and remnants of the atrium remain, and the new heart is put in place. The major blood vessels are then reconnected, and the procedure is complete.

Because of the risk that the donor heart may be rejected, patients who undergo heart transplants must remain on strong immunosuppressive drugs, such as cyclosporine, for the rest of their lives. (Such drugs suppress the body's immune system so that the transplanted organ is not rejected.) Transplant patients also must guard their new hearts against infection and return to the hospital frequently for tests.

Psychologically, a heart transplant can be a very difficult experience. Often the wait for a donor heart is an emotional roller coaster ride, with hopes raised, then dashed. All of our beliefs about our hearts, even the most primitive, rise to the surface when the topic is a heart transplant. Patients may wonder whether they will be somehow "different" with another person's heart beating within their chest. If you're a candidate for a heart transplant, patient organizations such as Mended Hearts (listed in the "Recommended Reading and Resources" section) can be of tremendous help.

Although heart transplants are relatively uncommon, they have become far safer over the years, and may offer the best chance for some patients to lead a normal life.

WHAT ABOUT ARTIFICIAL HEARTS?

During those early days, there was great hope that an artificial heart could be perfected that a person could live with indefinitely. In the early 1980s, the whole world followed the story of Barney Clark, the dentist who lived with an artificial heart for 112 days before he died. Researchers had underestimated how perfectly the heart performs, and they discovered that artificial hearts, at least up to now, cannot simulate the work of the heart precisely enough to keep many of the body's organs from eventually deteriorating. Today artificial hearts are used only as a temporary measure, keeping the patient alive for a few days or weeks until a human donor heart can be found and a heart transplant performed.

13

Hormone Replacement Therapy: The Big Question Mark

"The Dilemma of Estrogen Replacement"; "The Estrogen Question"; "Menopausal Hormone Therapy: A New Risk?" These are some titles of recent magazine articles which examine whether women should take hormones to replace those which naturally decline at menopause. Actually, "The Estrogen Question" was used twice. That shows that when the topic is hormone replacement therapy, a giant question mark invariably hangs over it.

Recently the size of the question mark has grown even larger, thanks to studies which show that women who took estrogen dramatically decreased their risk of cardiovascular disease.

"The data we have show that estrogen users have at least a fifty percent reduction in coronary disease as compared to non-users," says Dr. Trudy Bush of Johns Hopkins University. "No other therapeutic modality we have can even approach a fifty percent reduction." In fact, Dr. Bush believes this therapy may be medicine's strongest weapon in the fight against cardiovascular disease in women.

Whether or not older women should have hormone replacement therapy is the hottest issue in women's health today. Right now, 43 million American women are either approaching or experiencing menopause, and that number will mushroom during the coming decades, thanks to the baby boomers.

Supporters of hormone replacement therapy contend it's a health bonanza for women, bringing them younger-looking skin, stronger bones, healthier hearts, and even better spirits. Critics argue that women are being ill used by drug companies out to brainwash them, convincing them they need a drug to see them through a natural part of life. The studies on heart disease have further fueled the controversy. Before we get to that, here are some facts about menopause.

WHAT IS MENOPAUSE?

Menopause is the time in a woman's life when her reproductive life ceases. It's usually considered to occur between the ages of forty-one and fifty-five, with the average age fifty-one. The onset of menopause begins gradually with a period of subtle hormonal changes called the climacteric. This phase ends with estrogen levels falling so low that eventually the woman has her last menstrual period. This occurs over several years, sometimes beginning when the woman is in her mid-thirties. If you haven't yet reached menopause, you most likely will around the same age your mother did. Studies have found that women who smoke enter menopause a few years earlier than they would if they didn't smoke.

The changes that women undergo during menopause are primarily due to the decline in the production of estrogen, the so-called "female" sex hormone which governs the sexual and reproductive system. This reduction was once thought to primarily affect a woman's reproductive system. While this effect of estrogen is indeed enormous, researchers are only now coming to realize how the decline in this hormone affects the rest of the body as well.

Symptoms include hot flashes, night sweats, moodiness, cloudy thinking, vaginal dryness, loss of sexual desire, and such urinary problems as incontinence. Women can also develop thinning hair or baldness, or unwanted facial hair. Depression is cited by some as a symptom of menopause, but others argue that "feeling blue" during this time can be better explained by the fact that women reaching this stage in their lives may be grappling with other pressures, such as children leaving home, caring for an aging parent, or the problems of growing older in our youth-oriented society.

Every woman's experience of menopause varies. Some barely notice it; others develop debilitating symptoms. Experts estimate that 15 to 25 percent of women breeze through menopause. On the other end of the spectrum, an equal percentage of women suffer symptoms which can stretch on for years. The majority fall somewhere in between.

Generations ago, when a woman's life span was shorter, menopause was something to be dreaded, as it signaled the approach of old age. Today, nothing could be further from the truth. Currently a U.S. woman's life span is seventy-five years, and in the absence of disease, experts say, eighty-five years is a realistic expectation. By the time you reach menopause, your life may be barely half over.

It's no wonder that these days women wish to consider menopause nothing more than a minor pause in their busy lives. But the biological changes which come with menopause are far from minor. Just as momentous changes in your body heralded the start of your life as a female capable of reproduction, so do major changes within your body now herald the end of this phase of your life.

THE CHECKERED HISTORY OF ESTROGEN REPLACEMENT THERAPY

The controversy over hormone replacement therapy is not new. It's been around for half a century, ever since an oral form of estrogen was developed. The debate intensified in the 1970s, a decade when oral estrogen was trumpeted as the veritable fountain of youth for aging women. Then, it was found that giving estrogen alone to women increased their risk of developing uterine cancer, also known as endometrial cancer. This unwelcome discovery understandably dampened the enthusiasm for estrogen replacement therapy.

Since then, hormone replacement therapy has undergone a major change. In the mid-1970s scientists discovered that combining progesterone, the other hormone produced during a woman's menstrual cycle, with estrogen greatly reduced the risk of uterine cancer. Given together, these hormones more closely approximate a woman's natural reproductive cycle, with estrogen stimulating the growth of the uterine lining during the first part of the menstrual cycle and progesterone responsible for its sloughing off toward the end. This strategy proved quite successful: When the two hormones are used in combination, the risk of uterine cancer is not eliminated, but it falls to the level at which it would normally occur in women not on such therapy.

Nowadays, when replacement therapy is discussed, it generally refers to this combination of estrogen and progesterone, which we'll refer to as hormone replacement therapy, or HRT. Some women, mainly those who have had a hysterectomy, may still receive pure estrogen. This is because during a hysterectomy the uterus is removed, which eliminates the possibility of uterine cancer. The use of estrogen alone is usually referred to as estrogen replacement therapy, or ERT. To avoid being drowned in alphabet soup, we'll refer to it as estrogen therapy.

How can HRT benefit me? As of this writing, there are three FDA-approved indications for the use of estrogen in menopausal women. They are:

- **For the relief of hot flashes.** Although hot flashes are not life-threatening, HRT can seem like a lifesaver to women who suffer from them, as well as drenching night sweats, disrupted sleep patterns, and other symptoms of menopause.
- **To prevent vaginal atrophy.** As a result of declining estrogen levels, many women experience a thinning of their vaginal tissue, which becomes easily irritated and susceptible to vaginal infection. This can make sexual intercourse painful.
- **To prevent osteoporosis.** Nearly half of the 40 million women in the United States over the age of fifty have osteoporosis to some extent. This natural part of the aging process can result in loss of bone density, particularly in white women. Osteoporosis is blamed for 1.3 million fractures per year. Hip fractures in the elderly are particularly devastating, as they can lead to disability and even death.

Noticeably absent as of this writing is any mention of using HRT as a means of preventing heart disease. But prescribing HRT for that purpose (a practice which can be done now at a doctor's discretion and is referred to as off-label prescribing) could easily dwarf the current three FDA-sanctioned uses.

There are three common means of hormonal replacement therapy. The therapies may be combination preparations with progestin (the synthetic form of progesterone), or estrogen preparations alone. Which method you choose depends on your preference, your medical history, and the reasons for which you're taking replacement hormones.

Replacement hormones are administered in one of three ways:

- **Tablets.** In this form, pure estrogen, often made from the urine of pregnant mares, is taken orally. If you're taking progesterone as well, a typical regimen would be for you to take estrogen for most of the month, with progestin added during the latter part of the cycle. Since this usually results in menstruation-like bleeding at the end of the month, doctors now vary the schedule to avoid this unwanted side effect.
- **Estogen cream.** This preparation is inserted into the vagina with an applicator and absorbed directly through the vaginal lining. Estrogen cream works very well in rejuvenating the tissue in the vagina, but is not useful in protecting against osteoporosis or cardiovascular disease.
- **Transdermal patch.** In this method, estrogen is administered directly into the bloodstream via a skin patch which is changed about every three days. The patch is also considered preferable for smokers because of the way in which cigarette smoke affects metabolism. If you're taking combined replacement hormones (HRT) in this manner, the estrogen is delivered by way of the patch and you take the progesterone orally.

HRT AND HEART DISEASE

Although estrogen is primarily considered a sexual hormone, it's now being credited with affording the natural protection that women enjoy against heart disease. Since the early part of this century, it has been known that women begin catching up to men after menopause in the rate at which they develop coronary heart disease and suffer heart attacks.

In the 1950s, this sharp disparity led to some classic experiments which found that animals given estrogen were less likely to develop coronary heart disease. In recent years, studies involving not animals but women have led to a mounting body of evidence that estrogen is indeed effective in preventing coronary heart disease.

A 1991 follow-up of 48,470 menopausal women between the ages of thirty and sixty-five enrolled in the Harvard Nurses' Health Study found that the participants taking estrogen had about half as many heart attacks and cardiovascular deaths as women who did not take the hormone. This study came on the heels of several others which have shown similar results. Another example is the 1991 study of 8,881 postmenopausal women which found that the death rate from all causes in women who had been taking estrogen for more than fifteen years was reduced by 40 percent. Supporters of hormone replacement therapy point to several other studies with equally impressive numbers. Some studies also suggest that while replacement estrogen can benefit all older women, it's especially useful in preventing the progression of coronary heart disease in those who are already afflicted. Researchers have not only been seeking to learn whether hormone therapy lowers the risk of heart disease; they also need to find out why.

Coronary heart disease (known also as coronary atherosclerosis), the biggest killer of both women and men, is caused by the narrowing of the coronary arteries due to the formation of atherosclerotic plaques, or raised patches in the inner lining of the arteries. Playing an important role in the buildup of these deposits is the cholesterol contained in the blood. But not all cholesterol is "bad" cholesterol. Cholesterol is made up of different types, including a high-density component (HDL cholesterol) and a low-density component (LDL cholesterol). The LDL cholesterol, so-called "bad" cholesterol, helps form the deposits, while the HDL cholesterol, the so-called "good" cholesterol, helps whisk them away and keep the arteries clear.

At all ages, women have a higher proportion of HDL cholesterol than men, but after menopause the balance begins to shift. Although the mechanism of that shift is still not completely understood, the decline in estrogen level appears to play a pivotal role. Estrogen has been found to increase the level of HDL cholesterol and decrease the level of LDL cholesterol in a manner which researchers suggest should protect against heart disease. Indeed, studies are backing this up.

But cholesterol levels probably don't tell the whole story. Recent research suggests that estrogen has other positive effects on a woman's body as well. Such findings indicate that estrogen may favorably influence a woman's insulin levels, help lower her blood pressure, and prevent spasms of the coronary arteries. Elderly women are also at risk of strokes; although the evidence is inconsistent, some studies show that estrogen may reduce the incidence of strokes as well.

One problem is that these studies have mostly involved women taking oral estrogen. Questions arise when you consider the different methods of hormone replacement now available, as well as what may happen to estrogen's protective effect when progesterone is added to prevent uterine cancer. These are major questions only now under study, but they are of utmost importance if you're considering hormone replacement therapy to prevent coronary heart disease.

How does the method of administration affect estrogen as a protection against coronary heart disease?

Most of the cholesterol which is in our blood is manufactured in our liver. When estrogen is taken orally, it's metabolized in the liver. This is not the case when estrogen is administered through a skin patch or vaginal cream. This raises the concern that by taking estrogen other than orally, a woman will lose estrogen's positive effects on her cholesterol profile. However, since studies also suggest that estrogen's positive effects are more than just those on cholesterol level, some experts believe estrogen still offers significant cardiovascular benefits, no matter how it's administered.

But what happens when you add progesterone?

Although mounting evidence shows that estrogen given in its pure form helps prevent heart disease, very little research has been done to determine whether adding progesterone eliminates the benefits. Here's what is known so far: The hormone progesterone acts in a way which directly counteracts the bodily changes produced by estrogen. Some studies have found that adding progestin (the synthetic form of progesterone used in HRT) lessens the beneficial effect of estrogen on a woman's blood cholesterol level. This has led to the understandable concern that, by reducing a woman's risk of uterine cancer, the protective effects of estrogen on heart disease will be canceled out. However, some small studies suggest this is not the case, and that although progestin lessens the protective effect of estrogen replacement therapy, other cardiovascular benefits remain. Still, some experts, such as Dr. Nanette Wenger, professor of medicine at Emory University School of Medicine, says there is not enough research to show whether or not this is definitely true. "No randomized studies have been done with these drug combinations to know whether there are cardiovascular benefits, so the answer is not there," Dr. Wenger says.

Does adding progesterone negate estrogen's effect on osteoporosis?

Although not a lot of study has been done in this area, research suggests that estrogen used in combination with progesterone still protects against bone loss caused by osteoporosis, according to Dr. J. Christopher Gallagher of the Creighton University School of Medicine in Omaha, Nebraska. In fact, Dr. Gallagher says, there is some indication that adding progesterone "might possibly produce an additional effect above that seen with estrogen only. More research is needed to determine whether this is so," he said.

When should I go on HRT?

Some doctors prefer to wait for a year after a woman has had her last period, but others say this unfairly deprives women of the hormone. If you're experiencing menopause-like symptoms, your doctor can perform a blood test to measure your estrogen levels and determine whether your estrogen level is indeed declining.

What are the side effects of HRT?

No matter how "natural" replacement hormones are viewed, they're still medication. As can any drug, they can make you feel better or worse. Many women dislike the side effects of replacement hormones, such as bloating and breast tenderness, so much that they stop taking them. Switching to a different type of hormone formula or reducing the dosage may help.

What if I went through menopause early because I had a hysterectomy?

A hysterectomy does not always include removal of the ovaries. However, if your ovaries have been removed and your body no longer produces estrogen, you should definitely consider estrogen replacement therapy as a means of securing protection against heart disease and osteoporosis. "If a woman has her ovarian function removed ten years prematurely, she's going to have her hip fracture ten years sooner or her heart attack ten years sooner," says Dr. Delbert L. Booher, director of the Cleveland Clinic's Program for Mature Women. "These are women who are at particularly higher risk of experiencing problems related to a lack of estrogen because it began earlier in their lives."

If you have undergone a hysterectomy, which by definition is removal of the uterus, your choice of hormonal replacement is somewhat easier. Since your uterus has been removed, you have no possibility of developing uterine cancer. You're a candidate for estrogen alone. On the other hand, just because you're no longer at risk for one type of cancer doesn't mean that you're immune from other types, including breast cancer. Weigh the information on HRT and breast cancer set forth below.

Is it ever too late to go on HRT?

Doctors who are enthusiastic about HRT contend that women can enjoy such benefits as relief from menopausal symptoms and a decreased risk of cardiovascular disease even if they went through natural or surgically induced menopause years ago. Traditionally the age of seventy has been viewed as an unofficial cutoff, but some doctors are now prescribing HRT for women over seventy if they are experiencing such postmenopausal problems as urinary incontinence, or to decrease the risk of cardiovascular disease.

HORMONE REPLACEMENT THERAPY AND BREAST CANCER

By using progestin in combination with estrogen, scientists have succeeded in eliminating much of the concern over uterine can-

cer. However, the question whether hormone replacement therapy increases a woman's risk of breast cancer, and if so by just
how much, has proved more difficult to answer.

Over the years, numerous studies have been done to try to
learn whether there is a link between HRT and cancer. Some have
found an association, but some have not. This has understandably led to confusion. Fears about a possible link between estrogen replacement therapy and breast cancer were fueled by a 1989
Swedish study which found a significant increase in the risk of
breast cancer for 23,244 women taking estrogen. However, results
of the Harvard Nurses' Study published in 1991, which found
that estrogen replacement therapy significantly reduced heart disease, also found that women who had used estrogen in the past
but had since stopped had the same risk of breast cancer as
women who had never used the therapy. The study also found,
however, that a woman currently on the therapy had about a 35
percent higher risk than one who was not on it, no matter how
long she had used it or what dosage she was taking. And yet another major study done at the Vanderbilt University School of
Medicine found no increased risk at all.

To sort out some of these inconsistencies, researchers have
turned to carefully analyzing the several hundred other studies
done on the topic. Even here there are conflicting results. In a
1991 analysis of thirty-one major studies on the topic done over
the past eighteen years, it was concluded that hormone replacement therapy given at the current suggested dosage for less than
fifteen years did not increase a woman's chance of getting breast
cancer at all. Women taking such therapy for more than fifteen
years, and at a higher dosage, did experience an increased risk,
although it was marginal.

What does all this add up to? Most experts agree that hormone replacement may increase the risk of breast cancer, but at
worst the added risk would not be major. Doctors who favor hormonal replacement also contend that while concern over breast
cancer is valid, it's overshadowed by the paralyzing dread
women have of this disease. While breast cancer is a deadly disease that should not be minimized, the simple fact remains that
a woman is much more likely to develop heart disease than she
is to develop breast cancer.

An editorial published in 1991 in the *New England Journal of
Medicine* noted that most women between the ages of fifty and

ninety-four have a 31 percent risk of dying of coronary disease, compared to only 2.8 percent for breast cancer. "If estrogen's effects are applicable over this longer interval," the authors noted, "even a small relative benefit for heart disease would dwarf all the other effects."

This fear of breast cancer and the extent to which it has discouraged women from taking replacement hormones are not surprising when you consider the results of polls in which interviewers ask women about their biggest health concerns. These polls show that, even though women have a one in nine chance of developing breast cancer, it is their number-one fear. Cardiovascular disease, the number-one killer of American women, often doesn't even make the list.

THE PEPI TRIALS

The great hormonal replacement debate is bound to continue for a while. The good news is that more definitive information should be on the horizon. Researchers involved in the HRT controversy have long acknowledged that one problem with the studies is that they are all done retrospectively, which means they attempt to draw conclusions by studying women who happen to be on hormone replacement therapy. Such women usually tend to be white, better off economically, and more concerned with their health than other women, all factors which would contribute to a lower rate of heart disease anyway.

This problem points to the need for a large-scale, tightly controlled "prospective" study to evaluate the effects of HRT. Such a study ideally would be a "double blind," meaning that women would be given either HRT or a placebo, and that neither the woman nor her doctor would know which she was taking.

The good news is that such a study is now under way. The $10-million study is being conducted by the National Heart, Lung and Blood Institute, which is part of the federal government's National Institutes of Health. Called the PEPI Trials (the Post-Menopausal Estrogen/Progestin Intervention Trials), this is a continuing nationwide study of 800 women between the ages of forty-five and sixty-four. The study is designed to measure the effects of estrogen, the method of administration, and the effect of adding progesterone, and weigh the benefits and risks of these therapies related to heart disease, cancer, osteoporosis, and quality of life. This is an important study and long overdue.

The earliest results of the PEPI Trials are not expected until 1995. Even then, some of the questions surrounding the long-term use of hormonal replacement may not be answered. But at least there will be more information to help women judge the benefits and risks.

If you've been skeptical about the relevance of scientific research, the PEPI Trials provide an excellent example of research which will make a real difference in all our lives. Funding for the PEPI Trials is guaranteed for only the initial three-year phase and is expected to come up for renewal at about the same time this book is published. Consider urging your representatives in Congress to support the continuation of this research project, as well as other studies which benefit women.

MAKING YOUR OWN DECISION ABOUT HRT

No one likes to think that she makes decisions regarding her health by taking an educated gamble, but we do it every day. We swallow cold capsules in hopes that they'll cure our cold (they won't). We weigh the odds when we decide to undergo surgery. If we decide not to have an operation, we weigh the risks of that decision as well. Keeping this in mind should help you make a decision about HRT.

Your doctor can help you decide whether, based on your medical history, you should use HRT. Several books currently on the market address this question, including *The Complete Guide to Women's Health,* which is listed in the "Recommended Reading and Resources" section.

If there's no medical reason that you should not take HRT, you have a decision to make. One logical way of thinking about it is to consider what benefits HRT can bring to you. Then weigh in your personal risk factors, including those for breast cancer, heart disease, and osteoporosis. By approaching this subject with a cool head, you can decide what's right for you.

To determine whether you're at high risk for developing coronary heart disease, see Chapter 3.

The major risk factors which increase your chances of developing breast cancer include:

- A family history of breast cancer. The strongest risk factor for breast cancer is having a mother who had breast cancer; this doubles your risk.
- Never having had children.
- Having had your first child after the age of thirty.

The major risk factors which increase your chances of developing osteoporosis include:

- Being Caucasian or Asian.
- Being slender.
- Leading a sedentary lifestyle.
- Smoking.
- Eating a diet low in calcium.
- Having entered menopause early.
- Drinking alcohol or caffeinated beverages excessively.

IF YOU OPT FOR HRT . . .

No one can guarantee that if you go on replacement hormones, you won't develop breast cancer—or any other health problem, for that matter. But here are some livesaving and mindsaving suggestions which may minimize your risk:

1. If you decide you want to go on hormonal replacement, consider doing so for a short term so that you can reevaluate your decision as more information becomes available on long-term effects. Within a few more years, additional data should be available.
2. Make sure you're on the lowest possible dosage of estrogen considered sufficient to relieve menopausal symptoms and provide protection against osteoporosis and heart disease.
3. Follow the American Cancer Society's Recommendations for Mammograms and Breast Examinations. The society's current recommendations for women who do not have symptoms of breast cancer are:

- All women should have a "baseline" mammogram by the age of forty, and every one to two years after that until the age of forty-nine.

- At the age of fifty, and every year after that, a woman should have a yearly mammogram.
- Women between the ages of twenty and forty should have a clinical examination of their breasts done every three years, and every year after they turn forty.
- Women age twenty and older should make monthly breast self-examinations a habit.

ALTERNATIVES TO HRT IN PREVENTING CORONARY HEART DISEASE

There are lifestyle changes you can make to improve your cardio-vascular risk without turning to such artificial treatments as re-placement hormones (see Chapter 4). Here are some extra points to remember if you're approaching menopause.

- Studies have shown that menopausal and postmenopausal women who exercise can benefit in three ways:
  1. Middle-aged women who participate in aerobic exercise can increase their level of cardiovascular fitness.
  2. Performing weight-bearing exercises, such as walking and weight-lifting, helps prevent osteoporosis.
  3. Exercise can improve your ratio of HDL, or so-called "good" cholesterol, as compared to LDL, or "bad" choles-terol.
- A calcium-rich diet can prevent osteoporosis. See Chapter 16 for a woman's calcium requirements. If you're lactose-intolerent, ask your doctor about calcium supplements.
- Cigarettes increase your risk of coronary heart disease and osteo-porosis. Give quitting another try. You will eventually succeed!

To sum up: Deciding whether hormone replacement therapy is for you requires careful consideration. If your doctor is abrupt with you, you may want to see another doctor, perhaps one who specializes in treating the health problems of older women. Going through menopause is a delicate and sensitive process, just as reaching womanhood was. Menopause should be the start of an-other vibrant and exciting chapter in your life.

14

A Woman's Stress

Nancy loved her teaching job, but was being pressured by her superiors to switch to a new technique. She was convinced her students couldn't learn as well under the new system, but she had no choice. To keep her job, she had to change her methods. Shortly after the start of the new school year, she suffered a heart attack. "The doctors don't know why I had a heart attack," says Nancy, now forty-two. "They can't explain it. In my opinion, though, my heart attack was caused by stress from my job. The stress built up until I short-circuited."

Veronica attributes her heart attack at the age of thirty-seven to her hard-driving ambition and the unrealistic expectations she put on herself, both on and off the job. "I'm a very intense individual. I was a perfectionist," she says. "I never felt like I was accomplishing anything. That's what led to my heart attack."

Roberta, the fifty-eight-year-old psychiatric nurse, says there's no mystery as to why she suffered a heart attack: Her abnormal cholesterol levels resulted in coronary disease. "My high cholesterol level led to my heart attack, I'm sure. But my job had been getting more and more difficult. The last night I worked was particularly hectic. Two days later, I had my heart attack. I really think it was the stress of my job that pushed me over the edge."

Did stress really cause these women's heart attacks? They believe it did. But what does the research show?

Scientists have long pondered why some of us develop heart disease and others don't. Why does someone like Carol, who leads a heart-healthy lifestyle, suffer a heart attack while her neighbor, Penny, a sixty-two-year-old chain-smoking, exercise-hating pizza-chomper, remains in apparently robust health?

In their search for other causes of heart disease, scientists have turned to issues known as "psychosocial" or behavioral factors. Such factors include stress, poverty, lack of education, social isolation, and discrimination.

But just as there is a lack of studies on women and the diagnosis and treatment of heart disease, there is a dearth of information on how these other factors may affect a woman's heart. Proving links can be difficult. Some studies have shown that the behavioral factors of hostility and anger are linked to atherosclerosis, but other studies have found no such connection. We agree with the experts who contend that although stress is probably not linked to the development of heart disease in the same major way as are risks such as smoking, an early family history of heart disease, high blood pressure, or diabetes, it should be considered a contributing factor. In other words, if you smoke and favor a diet high in fatty foods, blaming your health problems on stress alone may be wishful thinking. But being under continual stress can certainly contribute to such unhealthy behaviors, such as smoking and eating too much, and may damage your health in other subtle ways as well.

WHAT IS STRESS?

The dictionary defines stress as "any interference that disturbs a person's healthy mental and physical well-being." Dr. Hans Selye, a leading stress researcher, differentiated in the 1930s between the emotional feelings engendered by two different types of stress. Positive stress, he noted, is associated with joy, exhilaration, and a feeling of a job well done, while negative stress engenders anger, frustration, anxiety, fatigue, and a general sense that something is amiss.

In our daily lives, it's impossible to escape from all forms of stress. Nor would we necessarily wish to. What is draining stress for one person can be energizing for another. "Stress itself is not necessarily a negative force. When a deadline or a major project gets the adrenaline flowing and the spirits in high gear, stress can be positive. Call it good stress," says Rita E. Watson, coauthor of the 1991 book *Sisterhood Betrayed*, which discusses psychological pressures faced by women in the workplace. But Watson adds, "When there's no letup, when the adrenaline doesn't stop flowing, the stress overwhelms the body's ability to handle it. Then we're talking bad stress."

HOW STRESS AFFECTS YOUR HEART

Although stress is something that you usually "feel" consciously, your response to it activates mechanisms within your body of which you may not be aware. Bodily responses are controlled by the autonomic nervous system, which gathers information about the environment and enables the body to respond without our awareness. When faced with a stressful situation, the autonomic nervous system responds by increasing production of such hormones as cortisol and epinephrine, which increases the heart rate, raises the blood pressure, and speeds up the metabolism.

This response to stress dates to prehistoric times, say scientists, who call this the "fight or flight" response. This physiological response still governs our bodily functions, even though the dangers we face have changed, such as the need to jam on the brakes and avoid a car accident. Most of the time, though, our physiological "fight or flight" responses are mobilized to deal with the ups and downs of daily life. When we respond in such a major way to situations which are chronically stressful, we may be damaging our cardiovascular system.

Researchers believe that the release of the hormones governing the "fight or flight" response can affect your heart in two ways. One is by affecting your cholesterol profile. In your bloodstream flow HDL, or so-called "good" cholesterol, and the sticky, "bad" LDL cholesterol, which increases the likelihood of blockage in your coronary arteries. Some researchers theorize that the hormonal increase you experience under stress keeps the LDL cholesterol circulating in your bloodstream longer, which can eventually result in the development of atherosclerosis, leading to coronary artery disease.

The second way in which stress can cause heart problems, researchers hypothesize, has to do with people with a high degree of "emotional arousability"—people who are easily angered or made impatient. These people may be vulnerable to hormone surges. In rare cases, it is believed, these surges can trigger a malfunction of the heart's electrical system, resulting in a heart attack or even death.

Among theories on ways in which stress may affect women's hearts in particular is one which focuses on estrogen level. Since women usually develop heart disease after menopause, it's very likely that estrogen, the "female" sex hormone, plays a key role in protecting the female heart. So some researchers are looking at how stress may affect a woman's estrogen level. Some of this research is coming from the animal kingdom.

Dr. Carol A. Shively, an assistant professor of comparative medicine at Bowman Gray School of Medicine in Wake Forest University, Winston-Salem, North Carolina, studies cynomolgus monkeys, a species which has many similarities to humans, including the way in which they develop heart disease. Female cynomolgus monkeys have menstrual cycles very similar to women's, and it's believed that the estrogen they produce may protect their hearts, much like what apparently occurs in human females. Dr. Shively studies how behavioral factors affect the hormonal cycles of these monkeys.

Dr. Shively and her colleagues found that female monkeys who are subordinate to the dominant females produce less estrogen and tend to have more heart disease. In another study, they looked at social isolation, which has also been connected with a higher rate of heart disease. They also found that monkeys who were socially isolated tended to develop heart disease at a significantly higher rate than the monkeys who were allowed to live together, as they normally would in the wild. "You have to be really careful not to think of the monkeys as little people, but to the extent that they function like we do in certain areas, we can study them and determine what type of research to focus on in humans," says Dr. Shively. Perhaps these monkey studies will turn out to be a "missing link" in showing how stress and other behavioral factors influence our female hearts.

IS THERE A TYPE A PERSONALITY, AND DO WOMEN HAVE IT, TOO?

In 1959, two Californian cardiologists, Dr. Ray H. Rosenman and Dr. Meyer Friedman, first described the "Type A personality," which has dominated most of modern thinking about stress. These doctors wondered whether the then-accepted risk factors of smoking, diet, and exercise really explained why people got heart disease, or whether there were other dynamics at work as well. By studying heart patients, they were able to categorize the personality of those more likely to get heart disease. This was dubbed "Type A," the "coronary-prone" personality. According to this theory, someone who was a Type A personality embodied a certain set of characteristics, including impatience, anger, hostility, competitiveness, high job involvement, and desire for achievement. The Type A person was also assumed to be a white, middle-aged male. Indeed, the Type A personality was seen as the possible explanation for what appeared at the time to be an epidemic of middle-aged, white men keeling over at their desks with heart attacks. There was a second personality type, Type B. Those who fit its characteristics were said to be less driven and competitive and more easygoing. Although both personality types were equally likely to achieve success, it was the Type A's who most often went on to develop heart disease.

Whether a woman can have a Type A personality, and what, if anything, this means for her heart, are much more difficult to determine. Researchers have noted that it's difficult to come to conclusions regarding women because most such studies have been done on men. Some researchers still subscribe to the theory of the Type A personality; others disagree, contending that it's not the Type A personality as a whole which is harmful, but that some components may be damaging. Among these researchers is Dr. Lynda Powell, an epidemiologist at the Yale School of Medicine.

"What we are starting to realize now is that components such as job involvement, achievement orientation, and perhaps even competitiveness really have very little to do with heart disease," says Dr. Powell. "What seems to be important are the characteristics such as anger or hostility and time urgency."

Dr. Powell has found that being a woman certainly does not exclude you from feeling simmering hostility, no matter what your age or whether or not you work outside the home. She and her researchers are involved in a study which is trying to determine what women and men who have suffered heart attacks find stressful.

"In these interviews, a lot of the men are the Archie Bunker types," says Dr. Powell. "They are always doing the traditional Type A behaviors, like pounding their fists, flailing their arms, talking fast, and so forth. The women, or at least the women who are fifty-five and older, don't have these characteristics at all. They have characteristics which are more consistent with resentment. They may be angry inside, but instead of pounding their fists, what they tend to do is say things quietly like, 'I don't expect my husband to pick me up at the airport. He never did anything like that for me in his life. Why should he start now?' So you don't get those overt manifestations of anger, but you know there is a lot of anger inside."

Younger women also exhibit characteristics of stress, but such feelings seem to be triggered by different factors than those for older women," notes Dr. Powell. "I have this videotape of a woman with coronary disease who is about sixty years old. She feels abandoned by her husband and kids. The kids are all grown up and they've moved away. Her husband appears only to be interested in his golf game, and she's resentful of that. Since her kids are grown, she's been stripped of her role as a mother. Her husband has a life of his own and doesn't need her to take care of him. Now she doesn't know what to do with herself, and even if she did, she doesn't have the self-confidence to do it."

The stresses felt by older women may be different than their younger counterparts who came of age during the women's movement, she has found. "The women in the younger group were trained to have a lot of skills associated with the traditional woman's role. On the other hand, they've been told they don't have to be just mothers, that they can really have it all. So what you see now is women involved in demanding occupations, managing houses, raising children, caring for husbands and other family members, and eventually being overloaded with responsibilities. It will be interesting to see if this overload has an adverse effect on the heart as these women begin to pass through the menopause and come of heart attack age," Dr. Powell said.

TYPES OF STRESS WOMEN FACE

Here's a look at some of the stresses women face which we believe can affect a woman's heart. This is not to say that these factors can inflict the same type of damage as smoking or diabetes, but they may contribute to the probability of a woman's developing heart disease.

THE STRESS OF WORK

If you bring up the topic of women and heart disease at a dinner party, it probably won't be long before someone declares, "Well, the reason women are getting heart attacks now is that they're out in the work force, competing with men, and trying to climb the corporate ladder."

Actually, so far as we know, women have always gotten heart attacks. But is there any truth to the notion that a woman is more at risk of heart disease because she's taking her place in the boardroom instead of staying home, scrubbing the bathroom? Again, the role work plays in contributing to heart disease is exceedingly difficult to evaluate, especially because of the lack of research on the effect of the workplace on women. Some studies have found that working can make a woman more prone to developing heart disease, while others have shown just the opposite.

Dr. Ellen Hall, an assistant professor of behavioral science and health education at Johns Hopkins University, studies women and occupational stress. In discussing her work Dr. Hall chooses her words with care. Too often, she says, research which finds negative aspects in women's working has been used to exclude women from certain occupations or to justify their being paid less or given less responsibility. But she is concerned that the myth that "women can have it all, women can do it all" can be damaging to a woman's heart.

On the whole, most large-scale studies have shown that working, in and of itself, is not detrimental to a woman's health. On the other hand, Dr. Hall believes that the type of work that a woman is called on to perform can have either a positive or negative effect, depending on whether the woman is enjoying a middle- or upper-class lifestyle or belongs to a lower economic class. "The women you see portrayed in movies like *Working Girl* or on the television show *L.A. Law* find it life-enhancing to be in the workplace," she says, noting that the reality for the majority of working women is much different. They can be found in less glamorous and more physically punishing situations, such as factory work or low-paying service jobs.

Dr. Hall is also concerned that most studies fall far short of accurately portraying a woman's workday because they use methods adapted from studies of working men. When it comes to measuring the effect of work on women, she says, there are other factors which must be taken into account. Unlike men, who usually work straight through their adult years, from their twenties until they are sixty-five, women tend to rotate in and out of the workplace, so it's more difficult to measure their reaction to their time on the job. Another aspect which Dr. Hall says should be considered is that studies show not only that women usually have less control over the work tasks they perform, but that they don't have the same choice of type of job they take in the first place. The vast majority are still employed in traditionally female occupations, as opposed to men, who have a huge variety of careers open to them, which may have enormous psychological implications.

Yet another factor often not measured by labor studies is the amount and importance of the social support some women gain from their jobs. Studies have shown that social isolation is much more stressful for women than for men. So a woman who is allowed to interact with her coworkers can find her job a much different place than a night cleaning woman who works alone, says Dr. Hall.

Special stresses are faced by women who try to cross over into nontraditional occupations. A woman entering a male white-collar profession may not face the same problems as a woman who becomes a plumber, for example. Often, women entering male blue-collar professions face a great deal of harassment, a factor which Dr. Hall notes is not usually included in labor studies. Until studies are designed which take all these factors into consideration, it will be difficult to evaluate the true effect of outside jobs on women, says Dr. Hall.

THE STRESS SANDWICH

Since the research doesn't show that working is necessarily bad for a woman's heart (and, under some circumstances, could actually be good for it), let's look at some types of stress which may take a toll.

Consider Shirley, a fifty-eight-year-old woman who has worked on a factory production line for some twenty years. Last year she was promoted to line supervisor. The move freed her from monotony. But she has a new problem. Before, she was just "one of the girls," faced with the same workload as her friends along the line. Now Shirley is responsible for keeping the production line moving. She isn't supposed to care that her friend Eleanor's arthritis is so painful it keeps her hands from moving fast enough, or that Diane came in late because one of her kids is in trouble with the police. None of that is supposed to matter. Shirley is no longer "one of the girls." The boss pressures her, her former friends distrust her, and Shirley is miserable. As a result, she's eating more, smoking more, and is a prime candidate for a heart attack.

Shirley is caught in a "stress sandwich," an emotionally wrenching pressure-cooker of a situation from which she has no way out. In our society women are particularly vulnerable to being caught in such a situation. Women are socialized to be "pleasers," trying to make everyone they encounter happy. As a result, they're too often torn between loyalties, divided among husband, children, their coworkers, and boss.

A WOMAN'S MULTIPLE ROLES

Today, the vast majority of women work outside the home, either out of choice or from economic necessity. Whatever the reason, women must cope with multiple roles.

In the old days, these roles were spread out across a woman's life span. If a woman wanted to work outside the home, she could afford to wait until her youngest child entered school. But the number of working women with children less than one year old has grown from 23 percent in 1970 to 48 percent in 1988, says Dr. Margaret Chesney, a professor in the Department of Epidemiology and Biostatistics at the University of California at San Francisco. "The numbers of women who have to leave their ba-

bies every day to work outside the home has grown unbeliev-
ably," she says. "You used to be able to stay home until your children were in grade school and then go back to work. Now
women can't afford to do that."

Baby boomers are also in the "sandwich generation," caught
between the demands of children and the needs of aging parents.
Studies have shown that it's most often the woman who is called
on to minister to these needs. "A woman who has to care for her
children or parents is also likely to be working as a teacher or a
nurse, or as a secretary where she is also taking care of her boss's
needs," says Dr. Hall. "So there is a double burden that falls upon
women."

Because of these multiple roles, the woman's workday, unlike
the man's, doesn't end when she goes home. Indeed, another part
of her workday may just be beginning. Dr. Chesney cites a 1989
Swedish study which looked at male and female managers at a
Volvo plant. The study found that, throughout the workday, most
female and male managers experienced signs of cardiovascular
arousal, including an increase in norepinephrine, one of the so-
called "stress" hormones, in their blood. But at the end of the workday, when the men returned home, their norepinephrine levels
declined. Not the women's, though. Their "stress" hormone levels
continued to climb into the evening. This indicated that unlike the
men, the women were unable to "wind down," but instead had to
gear up to meet the demands of homemaking.

Studies show that the pressure on working women is growing even worse, with more women being forced to take up second jobs. "When I see a woman literally killing herself at two
jobs, I want to scream, 'Stop! Why are you doing this to yourself?' " says author Rita Watson. "But the statistics show that
women are working two jobs because they need the money."

UNREALISTIC EXPECTATIONS

It's not only getting squeezed in "stress sandwiches" and juggling
multiple roles that may engender stress in women. Women also
are socialized to take too much responsibility on themselves.
"Women have very unrealistic expectations," says Dr. Chesney.
"We take responsibility for everything, even the weather. If we in-
vite people to a picnic and it rains, we apologize for it."

Women also place unrealistic demands on themselves. In our

society, men tend to compete with one another, but studies show that women tend to compete against unrealistically high expectations they hold for themselves—and naturally to come up short.

WHAT ABOUT DISCRIMINATION?

It's indisputable that some differences in health are found among people of different races and ethnic groups. Still, the relationship between race and health factors remains a sensitive subject. It's known, for example, that black women face a higher risk of developing heart disease, which is likely due to their being more prone to high blood pressure. But what accounts for this higher rate of blood pressure among African-Americans? Some researchers are looking at heredity. Others are looking at possible biological adaptations to slavery. Dr. Nancy Krieger, a researcher at the Kaiser Foundation Research Institute in Oakland, California, is trying to learn whether black women may have high blood pressure in response to the type of discrimination they endure daily. She asked black women how they responded to what they perceived as unfair treatment. The black women who said they usually accepted unfair treatment with little or no outward response were also more likely to also report high blood pressure.

ARE YOU UNDER STRESS?

Some people say they can't change their response to stress. "Personality-wise, you are who you are," declares Helen, the forty-five-year-old school-bus driver who suffered a heart attack. Even though she was told to try and cut down on her stress, she's found that advice difficult to follow. "Some people can go through life and not have anything floor them, and for some people, everything floors them," she says. "I'm in that category. I let everything bother me."

But experts believe there are ways we can learn to make stress more manageable.

STRATEGIES FOR REDUCING STRESS

Leslie, who is forty-seven, suffered a heart attack about a year after her promotion to supervisor of a word-processing department. She'd enjoyed her previous job, but now she found herself squeezed in a "stress sandwich" between her demanding boss and her former coworkers. Before returning to work, Leslie voiced her concerns to her boss. He offered her the opportunity to keep her supervisory position but transfer to a new department. Leslie was lucky. The receptiveness she found is rare. Usually we must learn to change our reactions to stress.

According to Dr. Lynda Powell, those of us who find it difficult to reduce stress have a high degree of "emotional arousability." An event that would mildly annoy another, like having someone cut in front of her in a grocery store check-out line, infuriates such a person. When she works with these sorts of people, Dr. Powell tries to get them to see that they have a choice whether to respond or not. She tells them to think of such incidents as "hooks."

"Each morning when you wake up, you are like a fish swimming downstream in clear water," she says. "All of a sudden, a baited hook drops." If you rise to the bait and snap at the first hook by becoming upset, the chances are high you'll snap at the next one and the next, and spend the whole day feeling upset, angry, and simmering with harmful hostility. On the other hand, if you think about these unexpected hooks as predictable parts of everyday life and let that first hook pass, it makes it easier to let the next ones glide by as well. "If you can learn to say to yourself that one word to yourself, 'Hook!' at the time the hook drops, you'll find your anger, irritation, aggravation, and impatience will decrease."

Ways to avoid snapping at "hooks" and channel your stress can be learned in stress management courses, which are offered by local hospitals, community centers, and adult education programs. Techniques used in such courses may include biofeedback, in which you learn to control your unconscious bodily responses; relaxation techniques; role-playing, in which you rehearse your responses to stressful situations, and "self-talk," in which you learn to replace negative thoughts with positive ones.

♥ **Mindsaving Tip: Learning to manage your stress can have other benefits as well. Researchers have found that** when they manage stress, women who want to lose weight are more likely to stick to their diets and women who want to stop smoking are more likely to succeed.

Here are some short-term ways to relieve tension:

- **Exercise.** Even if it's only going out for a walk, exercise has been shown to be an excellent way to reduce stress.
- **Pamper yourself.** Take a hot bath, get a massage, lose yourself in a novel (or try to write one), or find other ways to add enjoyment to your life.
- **Get a hobby.** Did you once paint, sing, or dance? Try it again. Creative hobbies can be a great stress reliever—don't worry, you don't have to be a Picasso. For some people, oil painting is relaxing; others find rug hooking or knitting does the trick.
- **Play with your pet.** Studies have shown that stroking a dog or cat is so relaxing it even lowers blood pressure.
- **Work for change.** For those who are easily emotionally aroused, becoming involved in a political campaign, a company union, or a community group may just be inviting more stress. Others, though, may find it personally empowering and stress-reducing. Even stuffing envelopes for a candidate you support can be relaxing and can have a positive long-term result.

15
Paying for Your Heart's Care

As she talked, Laurie busily arranged a display of potpourri jars on some shelves at the gift shop she owns. "I have this jumping and fluttering in my chest. My doctor doesn't think it's anything serious, but she wants to do some tests to be sure. The trouble is, the only health insurance I could afford comes with a thousand-dollar deductible. If I have these cardiac tests done, I won't have enough money to buy inventory for the Christmas shopping season."

Nora, a thirty-five-year-old free-lance writer, has health care coverage for her children through her ex-husband's policy. She decided against continuing her own health coverage when the choice came down to paying for that or car insurance. "I live in the country," she says. "Without my car, I can't work, so I basically didn't have any choice."

Denise, fifty-three, started her own business after she was laid off, earns a good living, but can't find a health insurer who will cover her because of the cardiac valve replacement she had a few years ago. "They say it's a preexisting condition, so they won't cover me," she says. "I'm so worried about it I can't sleep at night."

Hope, a long-divorced artist, developed coronary disease at the age of sixty-two. "Thank God for Medicare," she says. "I had my other hospital stays before I turned sixty-five, so whatever the insurance didn't pay, I had to pay. I used to break out in a rash trying to figure out what I was supposed to pay, what I wasn't, and how to find the money for it."

What's a section on health insurance doing in a book which tells you how to take care of your heart? Frankly, we're tired of seeing health-care books which celebrate the latest in medical technology but make no mention of who pays for it. What good is it to know what an echocardiogram does if you don't have insurance to cover its cost? Why spend time locating the best medical center for your heart problem if your insurer won't pay for your treatment there? As noted by Cheryl Jensen, coauthor of *The Complete Guide to Health Insurance* (1988), "The death or severe illness of a loved one is a tragedy, but it may not be a catastrophe. The catastrophe comes when you cannot pay for it."

As of this writing, policy-makers are debating several plans for ending our nation's health-care crisis. If the problem has been resolved by the time this book is published, just skip this chapter. Unfortunately, we think the chances of that happening are slim.

WOMEN AND THE HEALTH-CARE CRISIS

Increasingly the spotlight has been shining on how America's system of health insurance works, and doesn't work. Being unable to afford health-care coverage used to be a hardship which only affected the poor, but a 1992 Gallup Poll showed that the cost of health care has become one of the top concerns of all Americans. We're all discovering, much to our dismay, that health insurance coverage no longer provides the worry-free guarantee it once did.

Although this problem touches both sexes, women are most likely to be affected. Of the estimated 35 million Americans who don't have health insurance, it's estimated that 20 million are women and children. In a report released on Mother's Day in 1992, the Older Women's League reported that 3.7 million Americans over the age of forty-five have no health insurance. In addition, nearly 1.5 million women aged forty-five to sixty-four are considered "underinsured." This includes those whose health insurance policies exclude such expensive preexisting conditions as heart disease or cancer.

"We hear from so many women who say they are listed as 'insured' in the statistics, but they tell us they might as well be among the uninsured because their health coverage covers so little," says Dr. Anne S. Kasper, a sociologist who coordinates the Campaign for Women's Health, a project of the Older Women's League, which is made up of more than seventy women's organizations working for health-care reform. "There are millions of American women with breast cancer or heart disease who cannot get insurance. So they tell us they might as well not have any insurance at all."

According to the Older Women's League many built-in societal factors account for women's disadvantage when it comes to health-care coverage. An estimated 30 percent of American women (compared to 8 percent of men) are listed as dependents on their spouses' health insurance plans, making them vulnerable to losing their coverage if their husbands lose their jobs or they divorce or become widowed. Women are also more likely to hold low-paying jobs or work part-time for small businesses, making it less likely they will get health-care coverage.

The report also showed that women are more likely than men to have to turn to private insurance instead of group insurance. Private insurance often costs more, is harder to get if you've had health problems, and often covers fewer preventive services, such as mammograms, Pap smears, and blood cholesterol profiles.

You may think that if you're older, Medicare will cover your costs. But this doesn't give the total picture. According to the report, people age sixty-five and older spend an average of $2,135 annually for acute health-care costs. This represents 28 percent of the annual median income of older women, compared to 15 percent for men.

Until changes are made, the health insurance crisis will probably get worse, not better. The rising cost of insurance has resulted in fewer businesses covering their employees. According to the report by the Older Women's League, in 1980 72 percent of employers offered full coverage as a workers' benefit, but by 1988 that number had fallen to 51 percent.

WHAT YOU CAN DO ABOUT HEALTH INSURANCE

Some of the problems of health insurance are built into the system and will not be remedied until it's changed. We don't have a solution to this complex problem, but we do have some ideas on how you can become a smarter consumer and increase the possibility that if you do have to undergo medical treatment, you'll be able to pay for it. That's why, in addition to the **Lifesaving** and **Mindsaving Tips** in the other chapters, we've added some **Moneysaving Tips** in this chapter as well.

♥ Moneysaving Tip: It's not enough to be a smart patient when it comes to taking care of your heart: You also need to be a smart consumer when it comes to shopping for and using health-care coverage. It's no longer enough to sit back and assume that your health insurance will cover you if you get sick. You need to know for certain beforehand. If you develop a heart problem, the costs of cardiac tests and treatments can mount up very fast.

This section is not intended to be a full-scale discussion of how to shop for health insurance; we've listed books in the "Recommended Reading and Resources" section to help you with that. But here are some of the things you should be thinking about.

THE ABC'S OF HEALTH INSURANCE

It used to be that health insurance came in one basic type; now there are a multitude of choices. These include traditional health insurance, where you (or your employer) pay a monthly premium and the insurer reviews and pays any medical bills after they come in. There are also HMO's, or health maintenance organizations, in which one fee covers treatments and services by primary care physicians and a variety of specialists. And there are variations on these two models as well. If you're starting a new job, or are already employed, at some point you may be asked to choose among a mind-boggling variety of plans.

If you have traditional health insurance, here are tips for getting the most out of your coverage:

1. **Know your health insurance plan.** In the past, a health-care policy was too often stuck in a drawer. Today you need to know what your health-care plan covers. Are the benefits adequate? What is your maximum out-of-pocket cost? Is your health insurance renewable, or can it be canceled if you become ill?

2. **Face facts. No matter what type of health insurance you have, these days it probably won't cover 100 percent of your bills.** First of all, insurance has gotten so expensive that few people can afford a policy without any deductibles; indeed, many insurers no longer offer such a luxury. Second, although your insurer may imply that you have 100 percent coverage, that's often not the case. Most insurers use a payment schedule that includes a loophole known as "reasonable and customary charges." Often this amounts to something like 80 percent of what the insurers consider the prevailing fees for the area where you live. For example, say your cardiologist charges $110 for a physical, but your insurer considers $80 the reasonable and customary charge for that procedure. Unless your doctor participates in that particular insurance plan, you'll have to convince him or her to accept the lesser figure or pay the difference yourself.

3. **Know your company's policy on "preexisting conditions" and waiting periods.** If you have a heart problem, or any other health problem, sometimes insurers can use it as a reason to raise your rate, exclude you from coverage for a given period, or even refuse to cover your problem at all for a certain time. Know the ins and outs of your heart problem; if it's relatively minor, you may be able to use that information to convince your insurer that the company's practice is unfair. If you take this route, send a copy of your letter to the agency in your state which regulates insurance companies. If your insurance company is not on firm medical ground, it may change its stand.

♥ **Mindsaving Tip:** Some states have taken steps to ensure that health coverage is denied to no one with the means to pay for it. For example, Connecticut has created a "high-risk pool," similar to a high-risk pool for car insurance. If you have a preexisting condition, an insurer may assign you to such a pool. You may need to pay higher premiums, but at least you can get the coverage you need. Find out whether your state has such a system or consider lobbying your legislators to create one.

4. **Know your insurer's appeal process—and use it.** *When I had my heart surgery, I spent my entire recuperation period checking and double-checking medical bills. This meant reading and re-reading my insurance policy, learning to decipher the code numbers used instead of names for treatment, making numerous calls to both hospital and insurer (finding out their toll-free numbers when they had them), and availing myself of the appeals procedure. I appealed almost every charge that was denied. This was time-consuming and frustrating, but it turned out well. First, I was able to whittle down the more than $1,500 my insurer wanted me to pay to about $165 (I'm not sure what that was for; I finally gave up out of exhaustion and sent in the check), and I used my experience to write a news-paper column detailing all the errors I found and the contradictory information I was given. An example? The day before my surgery, I underwent several tests that were required for my heart operation. The costs of these tests amounted to several hundred dollars. My in-surance company later told me my policy covered only the first test when multiple procedures were done on the same day. This sounded bizarre. Sure enough, I checked my policy and found no such stip-ulation. I called back, saying that if this was indeed the case, I would like it in writing. "No problem," I was told. I received a call the very next day and was told there had been a change (just the day before; what a coincidence!). The tests were covered and an amended statement to that effect was already in the mail.*

5. **Know whether your health insurer is financially sound.** After the booming 1980s, not only banks went bust; some health insurance companies did as well. We've heard heartbreaking stories of people who paid their insurance premiums only to find out later, when they needed coverage, that it wasn't there. Some went into bankruptcy or lost their homes. There's no surefire way to make certain this won't happen to you, but experts suggest a couple of steps:

   · **Check to make sure the insurer is licensed to sell insur-**

ance in your state. This assures you that the company has met certain financial guidelines. In addition, if a licensed insurer fails, your state's insurance guaranty fund can help cover your unpaid claims.

· **Check the insurance company's financial rating.** Insurance companies are rated by such independent rating companies as Standard & Poor's Corporation and Moody's Investors Service, both of New York. You can find such ratings directories in your library. Consider buying from companies with only an "A" rating or better, but keep in mind such a guarantee today is still not ironclad tomorrow. Some agencies offer telephone call-in services for a more up-to-date rating.

7. **Think about options for group coverage.** If you're self-employed, you may find it difficult or too expensive to get individual coverage. However, group insurance may be available through your labor union, a professional organization, or such groups as the National Organization for Women. You also may be able to obtain group coverage by joining a professional organization or your local Chamber of Commerce or Council of Small Businesses.

6. **Plan ahead if there is a possibility you may lose your group insurance benefits.** There are non-health-related reasons for losing your group insurance coverage, such as leaving your job, getting divorced, or becoming widowed. Whatever the reason, you may be able to continue that insurance by participating in a federally sponsored plan established under CO-BRA (the Consolidated Omnibus Budget Reconciliation Act). COBRA requires employers with twenty or more workers to provide them and their families with the option of continuing health insurance (eighteen to thirty-six months, depending on the circumstances). The Older Women's League points out that in 1990, 27.7 percent of all those who elected COBRA coverage were spouses and dependents.

THE ABC'S OF HMO'S

One of the movements which has changed the landscape of health care in our country has been the growth of HMO's and other managed health-care plans. This movement, which began many years ago in California, has now spread throughout the country.

WHAT IS AN HMO?   An HMO (health maintenance organization) provides comprehensive health-care services to its enrolled members for a prepaid, fixed monthly fee. It differs from traditional health insurance in not charging for each service provided. There are limitations, however. Most plans allow you to use only the doctors who are on the HMO's staff, and you may be limited in your choice of clinics or hospitals as well.

Over the years, variations on the HMO have also sprung up. For example, there is also the PPO, or preferred provider organization. This is a network of physicians who supply care. These doctors are contracted by a third party, usually a self-insured employer, union trust, or insurance carrier. The participating physicians provide care at a discount to the third-party payer, resulting in lower costs. Another variation is the independent practice association, or IPA, in which a group of doctors in private practice contract with an HMO to provide care for subscribers.

WHAT IS MANAGED HEALTH CARE?   As health-care costs have risen, more stipulations have been clamped down on consumers by private as well as group insurers. Currently, insurers throughout the country are adopting a system called "managed health care," which comes into play in two ways. If you're a managed health-care policy-holder, you're usually required to get second opinions for some procedures, and also must notify the insurer ahead of time for permission to enter the hospital. If you don't follow these procedures, you may be penalized when it comes time to receive your benefits. From the insurer's perspective, this plan is designed to minimize unnecessary hospital stays, eliminate unnecessary surgery, and get you home as soon as possible. For you, managed health care usually means restrictions to which you're unaccustomed.

"One of the biggest issues today is what type of health insurance people have," says Dr. Bruce W. Lytle, a heart surgeon at the Cleveland Clinic. "I can't tell you how many times someone has called me up and said they want me to operate on them, and I'll say, 'Fine.' Then they'll say, 'Well, my insurance says I have to go to such-and-such a hospital.' So I can't do it. People need to understand what their health insurance covers and what it doesn't."

If you have a managed health-care plan, your insurer may allow you to go elsewhere if you pick up part of the tab yourself. If you're used to thinking you have 100 percent coverage, you may find this unfair. But if you're a high-risk patient with a serious heart problem, you may be better off in the long run seeking out the most expert care you can find, even if you do have to pay part of the cost yourself.

WHAT ELSE CAN YOU DO?

If you want health care which truly answers your needs, become involved in the debate. Study the pros and cons of various plans and decide what type of health care you'd like to see. Beware of proposals with hidden factors which may discriminate against certain groups, such as women. For example, Dr. Nancy Jecker, an assistant professor at the University of Washington School of Medicine in Seattle, notes that some proposals support keeping health costs down by promoting the concept of health-care rationing based on age. While this might seem to make sense, it actually discriminates against women.

"The expense of caring for growing numbers of older individuals can create strong incentives to ration health care based on age," Dr. Jecker wrote in the *Journal of the American Medical Association* in 1991. "While not directed explicitly at women, this form of rationing would affect women disproportionately because more women than men occupy the ranks of older Americans." Moreover, older women are more likely to rely on public health funds, which would be cut under such a proposal, Dr. Jecker added. They also are less likely than men to have private health insurance, and they have fewer personal financial resources to make up the gap.

The outcome of the health-care debate is terribly important for the well-being of everyone in our country. The solution, of course, is a plan which would provide care to everyone but maintain the standard of medical care that has been justifiably called the best in the world. There is no easy answer, but it's important for everyone to take part in the debate. The decisions made in the next few years may well shape the future of Americans' health care—including the care of women's hearts.

16

How to Keep
a Healthy
Heart

EVERY WOMAN'S EATING PLAN FOR LIFE

When it comes to your heart, there are some excellent reasons for eating right. If you eat right, you reduce your risk of heart disease. You're less likely to be overweight; excess weight has been clearly linked to an increased risk of heart disease by the Framingham Heart Study and the Nurses' Health Study, a study of 121,700 women compiled by Harvard Medical School and Boston's Brigham and Women's Hospital.

Studies have also found that eating "wrong," that is, eating a diet high in fat and cholesterol, can increase your chances of developing coronary artery disease. On the other hand, eating right can improve your blood cholesterol profile, thus lessening the risk. But while it's easy to agree that maintaining your desirable weight is a positive thing, for some of us that means going on a diet.

Men and women react very differently to the idea of going

on a diet. Imagine this scenario. It's been a long winter for the co-authors of this book. Neither of us has been as active as we'd like. We haven't been paying attention to what we eat, and we've each gained ten pounds. Here are our reactions:

Dr. Pashkow: "I've put on ten pounds. I'd better start watching what I eat more closely and cut out snacks. It won't take long to lose that weight."

Charlotte Libov: "Oh, my God! I've gained ten pounds! This is horrible! I hate myself! How could I have let myself get out of control that way? I should go out into the garden and eat worms. No, that's too fattening; I should go out into the garden and eat lettuce!"

Are we exaggerating? Not much. Women in general have so well absorbed our society's obsession with thinness that many can no longer think about eating rationally. More and more American women are dieting, and at younger and younger ages. Eating disorders, formerly rare, are becoming quite common. The desire to lose weight has fueled a multibillion-dollar diet industry. But most of that money just goes to waste, as studies show that diets don't last. In fact, an estimated 75 to 90 percent of women diet only to gain back the weight they've lost, and often more pounds besides.

This is not to build a case for being fat; that is neither healthy nor desirable. Obesity is a risk factor for heart disease as well as other ailments. But obesity is generally defined as being 20 to 30 percent above ideal weight. Many women far more slender than this are obsessed with losing weight.

Studies have shown that women more than men tend to have unrealistic images of their body, invariably for the worse. It's not unusual for a slender woman to look in the mirror and see fat that simply is not there. As a result, women often follow such stringent diets that it's not surprising they become obsessed with food. If they eat anything at all, they feel guilty. For these women, the very word "diet" can trigger an eating binge. For this reason, we've banished the word "diet" from this book as it is used to denote the limiting of food. (We do use it occasionally as a synonym for "eating plan.")

Reasons we abolished the "D" word:

1. This chapter is not just for women who want to lose weight. Its suggestions are aimed at women who want to create a healthier way of eating.

2. Diets don't work. The word "diet" implies a regimen you're adopting for a limited period. People go "on" diets and "off" diets with alarming frequency. Unless you permanently change the way you eat, it's highly unlikely you will succeed in losing weight and keeping it off.

3. For many women, the word "diet" is so emotionally loaded it may send them right to the pastry shelf. Both of your coauthors love food. We were raised in families where a table laden with food was seen as a symbol of love. Also, neither one of us is naturally svelte. By adopting the strategies we've outlined in this chapter, we've been able to maintain healthy bodies and eat our cake (on occasion) as well.

It's always amusing to see the latest diet product advertised on television. Hidden somewhere in the dazzling claims is the fine print, which says something like, "to lose weight, follow the enclosed diet plan." Following *any* diet plan in which you ingest less calories than your body burns will result in your losing weight, no matter what the gimmick.

ARE YOU A COMPULSIVE EATER (OR DIETER)?

As we've noted, for many women eating has become a compulsion, often manifested in "yo-yo" dieting. Often this pattern begins quite early. A young girl who is slightly overweight decides to lose the weight. That's all well and good. But she may starve herself to get the last few pounds off. More often than not, it's difficult to lose because she's dipping below her realistic weight. To keep it off, she starves herself. Since she's starving herself, she becomes obsessed with food. Before long, a "starve and binge" cycle can set in.

Are you a compulsive eater? Ask yourself these questions:

· Do words associated with food conjure up feelings of guilt and shame?
· Can you keep anything "good" in the house without devouring it immediately?
· Do you constantly go on diets only to go off them just as quickly?

· Do you hate your body?
· Do your thoughts constantly revolve around food?

Some women are addicted to compulsive eating; others fall prey to the addiction of dieting. While some women find the idea of "going on" a diet threatening, others find the idea of "going off" a diet equally scary. For them, dieting is a way of life. Before you consider embarking on any eating plan, you must get this diet monkey off your back. Some people find this easier than others. There are books on the market that may help.

THE IMPORTANCE OF EXERCISE

To maintain your desirable weight, or lose weight and keep it off, you must step up your level of physical activity. Being active not only helps you burn more calories, but also improves your self-esteem and lessens depression. For many women, poor self-esteem and depression can lead to eating. To get the most out of our eating plan, use it with its companion section, "Every Woman's Exercise Guide for Life." These two guides together will give you our best advice to create a healthier lifestyle.

STRATEGIES FOR EATING RIGHT

Here is our basic strategy for eating right (drumroll, please): **The eating plan you're most likely to stick with is the one closest to the way you normally eat.** Perhaps it seems as if the foods you eat daily are mostly chosen at random, i.e., "There's a muffin shop across from my office, so I start the day with a muffin." Such choices may actually not be random at all; your food preferences are probably far more deep-seated. After all, when you go "off" a diet, you automatically revert to your old eating habits. It follows that if your eating plan is similar to the one you would normally follow, it's harder to "go off it."

This is one reason we believe that following a "diet" of someone else's creation doesn't work in the long term. Such a plan does not admit your preferences or fulfill your needs. This is why we can't create an "eating plan" for you: You must create such a plan for yourself, based on the foods you usually prefer. If you're a hard-core dieter, you may have suppressed your own food preferences for so long you don't even remember the foods you used to enjoy eating.

CREATING YOUR PERSONAL EATING PLAN

We suggest you compare the way you eat with the U.S. Department of Agriculture's recommendations for a healthy diet. Your taxpayer dollars paid for it. If you look closely, you'll see it resembles the kinds of plans you have to pay lots of money for when you join diet clubs. Since you've already paid big bucks for this one, take advantage of it. The USDA will send you lots of information on how to use this eating plan, create menus, bag lunches—all kinds of good stuff, free or at very low cost. For information on ordering, see the "Recommended Reading and Resources" section.

The following menu comes from the USDA's dietary guidelines for both men and women. Since most women require less food than men, you should use the lower number of suggested servings—especially if you want to lose weight.

Type of Food	Suggested Daily Servings
Vegetables	3–5 servings (raw, leafy vegetables, 1 cup, other types, ½ cup)
Fruits	2–4 servings (1 medium apple, orange, or banana counts as 1 fruit, as does ½ cup diced fruit or ¾ cup of fruit juice)
Breads, cereals, rice, and pasta	6–11 servings (1 serving equals 1 slice bread; ½ bun, bagel, or English muffin; 1 ounce of dry cereal; ½ cup of cooked cereal, rice, or pasta)
Milk, yogurt, and cheese	2–3 servings (1 serving equals 1 cup of milk or yogurt or ½ ounce of cheese)

Meats, poultry, fish, dry beans and peas, eggs, and nuts	2–3 servings (Your daily total should be about 6 ounces. Beef should be lean and chicken cooked without skin. A 3-ounce portion is about the size of a deck of cards.)

What's a serving size? If you're trying to maintain your ideal weight or reduce your weight, the size of your servings counts. It's natural to think that if you start carefully monitoring your portions, you'll end up eating less. Interestingly, though, some people who are obsessed with gaining weight and dieting may tend to *overestimate* the size of a serving, and actually shortchange themselves.

To measure your portions, you'll need a set of measuring cups, measuring spoons, and a small food scale. Measure all your food until you get an idea of the size of the portions; then you can stop. But do check frequently to be certain "portion inflation" hasn't crept in. (If you're a veteran dieter who has portion size indelibly etched into your brain, you can skip this step. But be honest and test yourself first.)

How should I determine what my eating plan should be? Two types of women will read this chapter: those who are close to their ideal weight and want to make sure their diet is as healthy for their hearts and their entire bodies as possible, and those who want to shake the "diet" habit once and for all, lose weight in a healthy fashion, and maintain their weight. For both groups, many of our recommendations are the same. Much of what we suggest revolves around limiting the amount of fat you ingest each day.

According to research, the best way to reduce your risk of heart disease is to reduce the amount of fat in your diet. Happily, studies also show that limiting fat is a great way to lose weight. Since this is the strategy your coauthors both follow, we can attest to the fact that limiting fat intake is the best way to lose weight and not feel hungry.

Depending on which statistics you read, Americans derive from 37 percent to 50 percent of their daily calories from fat, far higher than the current level of 30 percent recommended by the American Heart Association. Now, you may have learned that "a calorie is a calorie is a calorie." Technically, that's true. But the great thing about cutting out fat is that you can feel as if you're eating more even while consuming fewer calories. One gram of fat contains nine calories, but a gram of carbohydrate or protein each contains only four calories. So every time you choose protein or carbohydrates instead of fat, you're saving five calories per gram consumed.

♥ **Lifesaving Tip:** Lowering the fat in your diet reduces your risk of developing not only coronary artery disease, but also breast cancer and diabetes.

So if you're eating less fat, what are you eating? You'll probably be consuming more protein and carbohydrates. You'll probably also be consuming more fiber. This is great for your heart: There's evidence that eating such insoluble fiber as oat bran lowers your cholesterol level. You're also more likely to eat more fruits and vegetables, which are rich in "antioxidants," such as vitamin E and vitamin C (ascorbic acid), and are believed also to help protect you from coronary artery disease. In addition, as you learn to choose foods lower in fat, you'll probably eat less beef and more fish. This increases your intake of the Omega-3 fatty acids in fish oil, which seem to have a positive effect on the blood fats and perhaps a blood-thinning effect.

As a woman, it's important that you not overlook the need for calcium in your diet. Calcium can help prevent osteoporosis, the "brittle bone" disease that can come with aging. According to the USDA, women ages nineteen to twenty-four should ingest 1,200 milligrams of calcium a day, 800 milligrams for women ages twenty-five to fifty. According to their surveys, women actually eat less than that, taking in about 565 to 665 milligrams a day. Although dairy products are the best source of calcium, other choices include bread and grain products, such vegetables as broccoli and spinach; meats, fish, and tofu.

♥ **Moneysaving Tip:** The USDA offers a low-cost guide to the nutrients you need every day. This seventeen-page set of fact sheets lists the recommended amounts of everything from vitamin A to zinc. Information on ordering it appears in the "Recommended Reading and Resources" section.

What if I want to lose weight? Considering our society's obsession with thinness, we suspect that many of you reading this chapter for information on how to lose weight are actually at or close to your true desirable weight. If so, you should relax, follow the guidelines on cutting fat in your diet, and exercise. If you are overweight, however, reducing your weight is an admirable goal.

There is only one way to lose weight: You have to ingest 3,500 fewer calories for each pound of weight you wish to lose. To calculate how many fewer calories you need to eat, you have to know how many calories you are eating each day in the first place. Then, you need to calculate how many fewer calories you need to eat in order to lose your desired amount of weight. Here's how to do it:

Step 1. Figure out how many calories you are now eating by keeping a food diary.

For at least one day, but preferably two or three, write down everything you eat. Using a calorie counter, figure out the exact number of calories you are eating. Figure out the fat grams as well. (We'll tell you how to do this below). Knowing what you normally eat is necessary before you can begin to figure out the dietary modifications you'll need to make. Also write down when you eat and why. Were you hungry? Tired? Depressed? Anxious? Most of us eat not only when we are hungry but for psychological reasons as well. You can use this information to choose alternative activities to eating when you are actually not hungry.

Keeping a food diary is easy to do, but it will only work if you are not on a constant diet already or if just keeping such a diary makes you unbearably anxious. If this is the case, it may indicate you need to change your attitude towards food before you consider losing weight.

Step 2. Calculate how many calories you need to maintain your ideal weight.

Take your desirable weight (and make sure that is a realistic weight, which is not necessarily what you weighed in high school), and multiply every pound times 15 calories. If you do not use a realistic weight, the resulting calorie count will be too low, dooming your reducing plan to failure.

According to these calculations, a moderately active woman whose ideal weight is 125 pounds would need to eat 1,875 calories per day. Since women (especially those who are less active) generally need slightly fewer calories than men, some experts advise using a figure of 12 or 13 calories instead. If you use both the upper and lower figures, this can give you a range of, say, 1,500 to 1,875. This gives you the number of calories you need to eat to maintain your ideal weight.

Step 3.   Calculate the number of calories you need to eat to lose weight.

To lose a pound of weight, you need to burn 3,500 more calories. How do you apply this to yourself? If your ideal weight is 125, consuming 1,500 to 1,875 calories a day would maintain your normal weight. If you want to be certain to lose weight, it's probably better to take the lower figure. So, take 1,500 calories each day and multiply that by seven days, to get a figure of 10,500 calories. Then, subtract the 3,500 calories you want to lose and divide by 7 for 1,000 calories a day. If you find yourself too hungry, use the "15-calories-a-pound" figure. This would give you 1,375 calories. If you find yourself not losing weight, you can always pick a figure somewhere in between 1,000 and 1,375.

Step 4.   Subtract the number of calories you need to lose from the number of calories you are currently eating, and you should be left with the number of calories you need to eat in order to lose weight.

♥ Mindsaving Tip: In calculating your ideal caloric intake, make certain you use your *ideal* weight, not some unrealistically low weight our Barbie-doll-conscious society may have instilled in you. If you start off with an unrealistically low calorie goal, it becomes virtually impossible for you to lose pounds and maintain the lower weight.

HOW TO USE THIS PLAN   *"Only one pound a week! That's too slow!"*
On the contrary, many nutritional experts would say it's too fast. They contend it should be a half pound a week, but most of us would find that excruciatingly slow. Still, losing weight gradually is the only way to accomplish a permanent weight loss. Unfortunately, it's human nature to want to lose lots of weight fast. So if you adopt this strategy, there's one pitfall you need to be aware of.

Let's say you've followed our plan; you've changed your eating habits and have lost about half the weight you want to lose.

Invariably, you run into a friend. She's lost a lot of weight and looks terrific. "I went on so-and-so's plan and lost fifteen pounds in three weeks!" she exclaims. How depressing! You've been diligently following our eating plan for two months and you've only lost half the weight she lost in two weeks. Here's where the *real* test of your willpower comes in. What you must do is smile graciously and congratulate your friend, realizing that by the next time you see her again, you may well have lost all your weight, but the chances are great that she'll have regained hers.

> ♥ Mindsaving Tip: You've been very good all day, but now you're starving. You could eat an apple, but that would put you about 135 calories over the higher daily number of calories you've allocated yourself. Eat the apple, we say. In the long run, it won't make a difference in your weight, and you'll be more likely to stick with your plan.

EATING A HEART-HEALTHY DIET AND MAINTAINING YOUR CURRENT WEIGHT

If you want to maintain your current weight and eat a healthier diet, you should limit your daily fat intake to 25 or 30 grams. If you want to lose weight, you need to watch both your fat grams and your calories. Part of the problem here is that while the food industry has lately worked to reduce the fat content of many foods, there are a lot of so-called "low-fat" and "fat-free" foods which are in reality quite high in sugar and calories. So just counting fat grams probably won't do it, unless you also make a conscious effort to eat as little sugar as possible. Counting both fat grams and calories is the most accurate way of determining whether you're eating the right amount of food to reduce your weight.

COUNTING FAT GRAMS

Determining your caloric intake is fairly simple, as there are many guides to counting calories and many foods list calorie counts on their labels. Evaluating the fat content of your food is not so easy, as fat is expressed in *grams*.

If you want to maintain your current weight, take the

number of calories a day you need to do that and multiply it by the percentage of fat you should be consuming daily. The American Heart Association recommends 30 percent, although many experts now use 25 percent. Let's take the woman we were using as an example. If she wants to eat less fat, say 25 percent, she should take the ideal number of calories she needs to maintain her ideal weight (1,875) and multiply that by 25 percent. That comes out to about 47 grams of fat a day. So if she's following a 1,125-calorie-a-day plan, she should be limiting herself to 28 grams of fat a day. You can eat a wide variety of foods, including a moderate amount of meat, as well as carbohydrate and protein, on such a plan. To make fat gram counting easier, pick up one of the fat gram counters on the market.

> ♥ Mindsaving Tip: If you're counting fat grams, here's a tip from Dr. Victoria Clyne, a primary care physician from Cleveland, Ohio. When her patients read food labels, she tells them that for every 100 calories of food, there should be no more than 2 grams of fat. That ensures that under 20 percent of that food's calories come from fat.

CALORIE AND FAT GRAM "BANKING"

Now that you've figured out what you're eating, decide what modifications to make. Often people find that the best way to cut down on eating is to eliminate snacks. If that's not enough, limit your desserts to one serving a day, or substitute fruit. Again, eating is a very individual thing. You may find it impossible to cut snacks out but relatively painless to substitute, say, sugar-free cocoa and four vanilla wafers for the doughnut and hot chocolate you normally have.

Let's face it: One of the reasons diets don't work is that we tend to go off them. You might go on a cruise where you're surrounded by food, or travel to an exotic locale and not want to miss out on the culinary delights. Perhaps you're at a wedding and can't bear to pass up the cake. Perhaps you've been avoiding desserts all week and are now dreaming of a chocolate bar. You can work these treats into your eating plan.

The best way to get into a healthy eating plan for life is to learn the principles of calorie and fat "banking." This is the feature which will make your eating plan adaptable so that you can really learn to live with it. Picture your calorie and fat allotments as the balances in your checking account. You can draw on these amounts just as you would a real bank account. Say you go to that wedding and are faced with what you estimate is a 400-calorie wedge of wedding cake. Using the checkbook analogy, it's like going into a store and falling in love with a $400 dress. You can deal with this dilemma in one of two ways. If you know ahead of time that you're going to want to spend the 400 calories, you can decrease your calorie count by 100 calories a day the week before. That gives you 700 calories. You can have the cake and a glass of champagne to go with it and feel virtuous at the same time. You've saved these calories and they're yours to enjoy without an iota of guilt, just as if you'd spent a month saving to buy that dress.

Here's the second way to handle the dilemma. Say you planned to go to the wedding but believed you'd have enough willpower to pass up the cake. But now it's just too tempting. Go ahead! You may be "overdrawing" on your calorie balance today, but it's only a temporary measure. For the next five days, simply trim an extra 100 calories off your calorie allocation. Voilà! You've got a balanced metabolic checkbook again.

Once you've lost the weight you want to lose, the best way to keep from regaining it is to gradually add back the calories until you've reached the level you need to maintain your ideal weight. If you gain more than a few pounds (allowing for your normal weight fluctuations), go back on the plan for a few weeks. Using this system, you can keep your weight under control forever, and not feel deprived.

ABOUT "FAT-FREE" FOODS

During the 1960s, about the only "diet" foods available were low-calorie soft drinks. Since then, there has been an explosion of low-calorie, low-fat foods. Some of these can be a real boon to us food-lovers. There are absolutely delicious low-fat, and even no-fat, frozen yogurt, puddings, and even cakes. But watch out—a lot of these foods have loopholes. Some may be low in fat but high in sugar. Others get their low calorie counts by virtue of minuscule portions. By the time this book is published, new government labeling regulations will, we hope, have cleared up much of the confusion. But there may still be loopholes. Become a wary label-reader to avoid being tricked.

♥ **Mindsaving Tip:** Skipping breakfast to lose weight is not a good idea. Eating breakfast "wakes up" your metabolism, and you burn calories more efficiently throughout the day.

WHY WE EAT

Remember that food diary? It had two parts. It listed what you ate and also when and why you ate it. Eating can be a complex activity. If you're hungry, eating satisfies you. But eating also has emotional causes. Many of us eat not only when we're hungry, but often when we're depressed, bored or lonely, or even happy or excited.

If food has become your way of dealing with your emotions, you're probably misinterpreting your bodily and emotional clues. You leap from your desk to the candy machine without giving a second thought to what your body is really trying to tell you. Maybe you need a good stretch or a walk around the office. Maybe you're tired and need to go to bed earlier. Or maybe you're lonely and really long to chat with a friend. Keeping track of why and when you eat can help you get a handle on these needs and provide you with alternate ways to fulfill them. So instead of automatically heading into the kitchen for something to eat, ask yourself what it is you really need. Maybe it's not a candy bar at all, but a hug!

EVERY WOMAN'S EXERCISE PLAN FOR LIFE

For too many of us, our only exercise is trotting around the aisles of the supermarket, dashing from one corporate suite to the other, or helping our husband or boyfriend search for the TV remote control. That's not good for our hearts. In fact, the American Heart Association in 1992 made it official: A lack of exercise is now considered a risk factor for heart disease.

Want some proof? Here you go. In the Healthy Women Study results published in 1992, Dr. Jane F. Owens of the University of Pittsburgh found that women who exercised regularly experienced less of a decrease in HDL cholesterol, the so-called "good" cholesterol that declines with aging. Studies also show that exercise improves your heart's capacity for work. In addition, new research shows that aerobic exercise affects your body's metabolism, resulting in changes which can slow or even halt the development of atherosclerosis, the process which narrows your coronary arteries.

Thus the heart association takes exercise very seriously. So do we, and so should you. But the best exercise is exercise that's fun, a factor we kept in mind when writing this chapter.

This chapter was created with the invaluable assistance of Peg Pashkow. A licensed physical therapist and exercise physiologist, Peg (with her husband, this book's coauthor) founded HeartWatchers in 1977, an international expert resource group for cardiac professionals. Most importantly, Peg truly exemplifies the benefits of exercise. Vibrant and enthusiastic, she begins nearly every day with a vigorous exercise program. She's also an avid jogger, swimmer, and bicyclist. For Peg, exercising is as necessary and natural as breathing. As a special bonus in this section, along with our usual **Lifesaving** and **Mindsaving Tips**, there are lots of **Moneysaving Tips** and special exercise advice from Peg called **Peg's Tips**.

This chapter really contains recommendations for every woman's heart. No matter what your age or physical condition, whether you're young or old, athletic or sedentary, there's information here that you can use to design your own exercise plan. This is generally also true if you have a heart problem. If that's the case, though, you should definitely check with your doctor before beginning new physical activities.

Before we get down to basics, here are the answers to some questions you may have.

Exercise: What's in it for me? Quite a lot. Exercise is a small investment that reaps big benefits. Exercise can:

- Help you lose weight and keep it off.
- Help you quit smoking and stay off cigarettes.
- Strengthen your heart and improve your circulation.
- Tone your muscles.
- Help you sleep.
- Reduce stress.

· Enhance your self-esteem.
· Help reduce high blood pressure.
· Help control diabetes.

EXERCISE AND DIABETES

If you have diabetes, or a family history of the disease, exercise can be very important. Regular physical exercise can help control diabetes, possibly helping a diabetic who is not insulin-dependent to stay off insulin. Exercise helps prevent overweight, which can contribute to the development of diabetes. Some promising research also indicates that exercise itself may help prevent diabetes from developing.

EXERCISE AND OSTEOPOROSIS

Exercise builds muscle mass, a major way of warding off osteoporosis. However, you must choose carefully the type of exercise you do. We'll tell you how in this chapter.

EXERCISE AND STRESS

Being physically active has been shown to be a great stress-reducer. As Peg notes, "By exercising, you get a sense of stretching your mind as well as your body. Exercising makes you feel very free."

IF YOU'RE OLDER . . .

Studies show that exercise can benefit older women tremendously. Of course, you should consult your doctor before starting an exercise program. Your doctor should be delighted to know that you want to, but if he or she is not encouraging and there's no medical reason that you shouldn't exercise, it may be that the doctor believes old myths about the appropriateness of exercise for older people. You can educate your doctor or find a new one. Point out that studies show that by exercising, older people can become more fit than younger sedentary people. If you have kids, you'll probably enjoy telling that to them as well.

Here are some commonly asked questions and answers about exercise.

I spend a lot of time on my feet just doing my daily activities at work and at home. Isn't that enough? No. To get the most out of exercise, your activity should not be related to the type of work you normally do. If you're doing housework, chasing after the kids, or trotting from one office to another, your mind is on the task at hand, not on exercising your body. Exercise is something you do for *you*, not for anyone else.

Most books on exercise include six- or eight-week plans. Where's one of those nifty charts which tells me exactly what I should do? We could have included a chart here and it might even pay off for you in the short run, but just as most diets don't work in the long run, neither do most exercise plans. When you talk about a "plan," you're summing up the whole problem. To many people, a plan suggests that you're going to do something only for a specific period, then quit. That's how people usually view exercise, as a quick fix. Formulating a plan is fine if it's one you can follow for life. For example, you can plan to go cross-country skiing in the winter and swimming in the summer. Or, as this chapter suggests, you can plan to build more activity into your daily life.

But if there's no set plan, how do I know what my goal should be? We live in a very goal-oriented society. We set goals all the time; we'll lose weight in two months, stop smoking in three, and transform ourselves into Jane Fonda in four. Such goals are unrealistic, and unrealistic goals are self-defeating.

Since no one knows you better than you know yourself, you should set realistic goals for yourself. Maybe your goal will be to get into condition so that you can walk briskly to work without huffing and puffing or go dancing without feeling winded. If you'd like a goal suggestion from us, here's one: **"My goal is to become more active than I currently am."**

Now that you have a realistic goal in mind, we'll give you some information on exercise so that you can choose the types of activities which are best for your body—including, of course, your heart. We'll also present the principles of our "Every Woman's Exercise Philosophy," which is designed to transform even couch potatoes into exercise-lovers—or at least exercise-likers.

♥ **Peg's Tip: Being "physically fit" doesn't mean being an Amazon. Being physically fit means you can accom-**

plish such everyday activities as raking leaves, taking brisk walks, or playing with your kids (or your grandkids). You can maintain this level of conditioning throughout your life.

THE BASICS OF HEART-HEALTHY EXERCISE

Here is the basic tenet of our exercise philosophy: Whatever you do is better than doing nothing at all. But you need to understand the three types of exercise which will strengthen your body in different ways:

- Aerobic exercise (for endurance)
- Weight-bearing exercise (to retard osteoporosis)
- Anaerobic exercise (for strength)

You must do all three types if you want to fully condition and strengthen your body.

AEROBIC EXERCISE   This type of activity is vital if you want to improve the functioning of your cardiovascular system, which includes your heart. Aerobic exercise also improves your endurance and strengthens your musculoskeletal system, the bony skeleton of your body and the muscles attached to it. Aerobic exercise makes use of rhythmic, repetitive movements which use your large muscle groups. It's a sustained form of exercise during which your heartbeat must remain in an elevated range, also called your "target heart range." How to find your target heart range is discussed later in this chapter.

It was once thought that to be beneficial, aerobic exercise must be performed for at least a twenty-minute period three times a week. Some studies have shown, however, that you can also derive benefit from doing aerobic exercises for shorter periods, say for ten minutes at the start and end of each day.

Aerobic activities include brisk walking, jogging, race walking, swimming, water aerobics, bicycling (either stationary or on a real bicycle), aerobic dancing, folk dancing, using rowing and skiing machines, calisthenics, and using free weights and pulleys.

♥ **Peg's Tip: Playing softball or volleyball is fun, but it doesn't qualify as an aerobic workout. Some teams solve** that problem by doing aerobic workouts before the game. Square dancing, too, is fun but may not be vigorous enough to qualify as an aerobic workout. For a more intense workout, widen the dance circle. For an easier workout, walk, don't skip, around the circle.

WEIGHT-BEARING EXERCISE   As a woman, you especially need to incorporate weight-bearing exercise into your daily life. Aerobic exercise is marvelous for the cardiovascular system, but alone does not help prevent the loss of bone mineral which, as you age, can result in osteoporosis. Weight-bearing exercises are those which provide impact on the joints and, in doing so, stimulate the ends of your bones.

There are two ways to build weight-bearing exercise into your activities. One is by choosing aerobic activities which apply some force to the bones. Swimming provides aerobic exercise, but because your body is suspended in water, no force is applied to your bones. Walking, jogging, aerobic dancing, and racquet sports all qualify as both aerobic and weight-bearing exercise.

ANAEROBIC EXERCISE (STRENGTH-RESISTANCE TRAINING)   Women especially should be aware of the need to keep up the strength in their upper arms. "Women tend to focus on their hips and thighs, but as we age, we need to build up our arms," says Peg Pashkow. "This enables us to carry packages more easily, for example, and keeps the skin on our arms firm."

A good way to strengthen your upper body is to work out with weights. A simple exercise using dumbbells or other weights will accomplish your goal. Most sporting goods stores carry a variety of inexpensive weights and exercise books or videotapes. A gym or health club can also provide you with a good program.

♥ Moneysaving Tip: If you don't want to buy weights, use cans of food instead. Or buy some detergent in plastic bottles with grip handles. Not only is this inexpensive, but you can lighten the weight, if necessary, by using some of the detergent.

♥ Peg's Tip: Some women find the kind of muscles they can build by "pumping iron" quite attractive, but many do not. Should you decide to work with weights, don't worry about becoming muscle-bound. Working with weights will give you a stronger, firmer body, but unless you perform daily, lengthy workouts, you won't end up looking like Linda Hamilton in the movie *Terminator 2.*

Here are some basics for getting started:

1. **Before beginning to exercise, you must take the following guidelines from the American College of Sports Medicine into consideration:** If you are in *good general health,* and are fifty years of age or younger, and you plan to increase your activity very gradually (the best way to do it), you probably do not need to see your doctor before beginning an exercise program. If, however, you know you have a heart problem; if you're at risk for coronary heart disease; if you have another medical problem (such as asthma or diabetes), or you have *any* reason to doubt your physical condition, you should check with your doctor before starting.

    For example, if you have two or more major coronary risk factors (which include smoking, diabetes, high blood pressure, abnormally high blood-cholesterol levels, or a family history of early coronary heart disease) but are experiencing no symptoms, you should see your doctor if you are planning to start a vigorous exercise program. If, on the other hand, you are suffering from chest pains or palpitations, you should have a physical examination and exercise stress test before beginning even a moderate exercise program. This holds true whether or not you are at risk for coronary heart disease.

    These guidelines are not intended to discourage you from exercising (nor are they an excuse for not exercising!) We just want you to take care.

    ♥ Lifesaving Tip: If you have heart disease, you must consult with your doctor before starting an exercise program. As you start to increase your level of activity, if you experience any symptoms such as chest pain, shortness of breath, dizziness, or undue fatigue, consult your doctor.

♥ Peg's Tip: Before beginning an activity, take a medical inventory of yourself. Recall any injuries or problems with your back, ankles, arms, or legs. Make certain that the activities you choose will not damage, but instead will strengthen these problem areas. Research shows that higher rates of injury are associated with weight-bearing activities like jogging and running. Those most likely to injure themselves are people who run for long distances, have a personal history of injury, or suddenly step up their exercise schedule.

2. **Whenever you exercise, start with a warm-up and end with a cool-down period. Never overlook the importance of warming up and cooling down.** Immediately throwing yourself into vigorous activity is too demanding for your body. You need to warm up your muscles and stretch your joints slowly to avoid strains and cramps. A ten-minute warm-up also gradually increases the circulation to your heart and muscles in preparation for more vigorous exercise. A ten-minute cool-down period is needed to gradually slow your heartbeat to its normal rate. If you've been exercising vigorously, cooling down will prevent dizziness, lightheadedness, nausea, and muscle cramps. If you exercise in a class or with an exercise tape, make certain that warm-up and cool-down periods are included. Even if you're only starting with a brisk ten-minute walk, build in a warm-up and cool-down period. Increasing your flexibility is an important benefit of warming up and exercising in general. Stretching is a great way to warm up, but you need to stretch slowly to avoid the "rubber-band" effect. "If you pick up a new rubber band and stretch it, you'll think you've really stretched it out," explains Peg. "But if you put it around a vise and hold it there for five minutes, when you let it go, it's more likely it will be stretched out. The same is true of your muscles."

3. **Drink plenty of fluids.** Be *sure* to drink plenty of fluids before, after, and during exercise. Those water bottles which look so chic in exercise class actually serve a purpose. But don't drink a solution with sugar in it—your stomach will demand priority circulation to digest the sugar instead of sending blood to the muscles you're exercising.

♥ Peg's Tip: Too often women tend to believe that if they don't drink water, they'll lose weight more quickly. This is a dangerous fallacy—your body needs water.

4. **Monitor your heart rate.** Whether your vigorous activity is walking, running, or doing calisthenics, if you want to be certain you're benefiting aerobically you need to monitor your heart, making sure it stays at its target rate. By monitoring your heartbeat at various points during your exercise, you can make sure the exercise is neither too mild nor too intense. Some people mistakenly think that if pushing your heart rate to its target rate is good, pushing it higher is even better. This is definitely not true. If your heart rate goes too high, you're no longer exercising aerobically; you're exercising anaerobically, which has no cardiovascular benefits.

When you exercise aerobically, your body is meeting your muscles' increased need for oxygen. "Aerobic" means "requiring air to live." Oxygen serves to release energy from your body's store of fat, glycogen (starchy stored material), and sugars. If you exercise too vigorously and exceed your heart's target rate, your body begins exercising anaerobically—not using oxygen. Short bouts of anaerobic exercise are also called isometric exercise. But while this type of exercise can be useful for building strength, it does not build endurance and can result in muscle fatigue and exhaustion.

To find your target heart range, subtract your age from 220. Multiply that figure by 0.6 and 0.80. That figure will give you your heart rate if you're working at 60 to 80 percent, which is considered a good level for cardiac conditioning. For example, if you're forty years old, your maximum heart rate is about 180 beats per minute. Your 60 to 80 percent target range is 108 to 144. Often in an aerobics class, the instructor will have you take a ten-second measurement, feeling your pulse at wrist or neck. Dividing by 6, this means your target heart rate should fall between 18 and 24 for a ten-second count. If it's higher than that, don't stop abruptly, but slow down. In an exercise class, an easy way to do this is to march in place. If your pulse rate is too low, put a little more intensity into your activities.

♥ Peg's Tip: If you've been tested for exercise capacity, on a treadmill or stationary bicycle, for example, and you were given a target heart rate, use it instead of the above calculations, since the rate is specific to *your* body.

There's another easy way to test the intensity of your activity, especially if you and a friend are walking or using a treadmill or stationary bike. This is called "the talk test." If you can talk to your partner easily, your level of activity is probably appropriate.

♥ Peg's Tip: Individuals vary. Regardless of your heart rate, if the exercise feels too strenuous, slow down or stop. If you're still winded ten minutes after you stop exercising, or still tired after an hour, you're overdoing it. Contact your doctor if exercising brings on difficulty in breathing, faintness, dizziness, nausea, confusion, chest pain, extreme fatigue, or leg pain.

Following are some tips for two of the most popular types of exercise.

WALKING　 Studies find that a brisk walk three times a week can afford the type of cardiovascular benefits once associated with more strenuous activities like running and jogging. Walking is a great exercise, and all you really need is a pair of well-fitting walking shoes. You can get earphones and enjoy tape-recorded music while you walk; you can walk with a friend or alone. If you live in a climate where it's sometimes too cold, rainy, or snowy, consider walking in a shopping mall. Many have organized walking clubs.

♥ Peg's Tip: Browsing doesn't count! If you pick a mall for walking, but also love to shop, go before the stores open. *Briefly* window-shop and then take your walk. Afterward, you can return.

Eventually you may want to increase your walking speed to an easy jog, or even a run. Be sure to increase gradually. To go from walking to running, you might start out by alternating between them. For example, if you walk on a track, try running past the bleachers, then resume your walking pace. If you're walking in a city or town, alternate a block of walking with a block of running. Increase very gradually, and before you know it you may be out jogging or running instead of walking.

If you're a beginning runner, here are a couple of tips:
- **Beware of hard surfaces.** Running on grass can be easier on your ankles and legs and help you avoid injury. Once you're accustomed to running, try doing it on an uneven surface. This forces you to lift your legs higher, improves your balance, and strengthens your ankles.
- **Put your money where your feet are.** Once upon a time, sneakers were the only "athletic shoes" available. But the sneaker has grown up, and proper shoes can help you exercise better and prevent injuries. Check magazines such as *Consumer Reports*, which in its May 1992 issue ranked the most popular running shoes and included tips on shopping for them, such as shopping at the end of the day, when your feet have swollen to their largest, wearing the socks you'll run in, and trying on both left and right shoes, as most people have slightly different-sized feet. *Consumer Reports* often ranks exercise equipment as well; it's a great guide for those who are money-savvy, or want to be.

SWIMMING AND WATER EXERCISES   Swimming and water exercises are a refreshing way to condition yourself if you've been sedentary or if you're elderly, disabled, or have previously injured yourself. Working out in the water provides overall fitness and conditioning and can also strengthen your body. If you swim, doing laps is a terrific way to get into good condition. But even if you don't swim, check with health clubs or community pools to find out about water aerobics classes. Sometimes these classes are surprisingly intense, so be certain to find one at the right level for you.

One of Peg's favorite pool exercises is water walking. It's harder to do than you think. Stand in waist- to chest-deep water and try to walk as you would on land, swinging your arms as you go. Belts available in mail-order catalogs can help maintain buoyancy.

♥ **Peg's Tip: Don't do water exercises on your toes. Your body may naturally want to do this, but it's important to keep your heels down—otherwise, you may** get leg cramps. If you have to stand on tiptoe, the water is too deep.

As with other exercise, warming up and cooling down are important. Lap swimmers always start off with some stretching. Do a slow lap at the end, or some slow exercises, to cool down before you leave the water.

♥ Peg's Tip: Take care, particularly if you have joint problems, not to overdo your water exercise. You may be tempted because using your limbs in the water feels so good.

EXERCISING AT HOME

Some people enjoy exercising alone at home. That's great. Others prefer to exercise in a group. Consider getting a few friends together to form your own class, with the help of a videotape. The advent of cable television and VCR's have made it easier to exercise at home than ever before. There are a wide variety of exercise videos designed for women of all ages, exercise ability, and musical tastes. You can order them at video stores or through mail-order catalogs. Some tapes, such as Richard Simmons's more recent videos, are particularly good because they incorporate not only aerobics but some simple strength-building exercises as well.

♥ Moneysaving Tip: Your library or local video store probably has many different exercise tapes which you can borrow or rent. Try them out and find the one that's right for you.

CHOOSING A HEALTH CLUB

A health club can be a terrific place to exercise or an expensive rip-off. Too often people sign up for an expensive health club contract, go a lot during the first few weeks, and then stop because they're bored, they've overdone it, or their needs are not being met. Before joining a club, ask yourself these questions:

·   How convenient is the facility to you?
·   Do the exercise times fit in to your schedule?

- What is the facility itself like?
- Are the exercise classes too crowded?
- Is there a long wait to use equipment?
- Does the facility offer a variety of equipment?

The answers to these questions can indicate whether you'll use the club for years, or whether it will be just a passing fancy.

A main reason that many people join health clubs is to take advantage of the exercise classes offered. The class, though, is only as good as its leader. Ask to meet the staff and participate in a trial workout. You should be able to tell whether the exercise leaders are sincerely interested. Does the leader use the class for his or her own exercise? The answer should be no. The leader should exercise along with you, but concentrate on your needs.

If an instructor is a certified exercise fitness instructor, so much the better. But skill and enthusiasm are very important; some instructors may not have credentials, but still lead excellent exercise groups. Also, while the fitness instructor doesn't necessarily have to look like Jane Fonda or Arnold Schwarzenegger, she or he should appear to be in good shape. It's easier to be inspired by someone who lives by what he or she teaches. But watch out for the instructor who looks too good and is just there on an extended ego trip.

The right music can make exercise seem effortless; the wrong music, torturous. If you enjoy working out to Motown, make sure the leader doesn't favor heavy metal. If it's a dance-oriented class, check out the routines. You may be unfamiliar with the steps at first, but it should be easy to catch on. If you always feel lost, you won't be getting the kind of workout you need.

Most of us like to feel that we fit in. Peek into the class ahead of time, or ask the instructor what clothes people usually wear. If a great-looking leotard makes you feel more like exercising, buy one by all means. If you don't look great in a leotard (and most of us don't), opt for a colorful oversized T-shirt. Some women won't step into an exercise class without full makeup, while others wouldn't give it a second thought. Do what's comfortable for you.

♥ **Peg's Tip: Don't feel embarrassed to leave a class if you don't feel well, it's too intense, or you don't like it. You're there for you.**

♥ Moneysaving Tip: Joining a health club can be a substantial monetary investment. Be sure to read any contract very carefully before you sign. In many states, there is a "cooling-off" period during which you can cancel a contract without penalty. Also, although many health clubs are on firm financial footing, some have been known to go out of business. Check with your local Better Business Bureau and state consumer protection division to find out whether any complaints have been filed against the club you're considering and what monetary protections you might have.

♥ Moneysaving Tip: Many colleges and hotels have excellent physical fitness facilities which they allow the public to use; the fee may be less than a health club membership. If you live near your alma mater, your alumni status may enable you to use its facilities free or at a reduced rate.

TEN PRINCIPLES OF BECOMING ACTIVE

Some of our principles may sound a little unconventional. Probably no one had ever suggested that you not worry about starting an exercise "plan," that you underdo it, or that you lower your standards. But especially if you're unaccustomed to exercising, we believe these are the keys to becoming more active. If you go easy on yourself, you'll find that exercise can be fun. Eventually you'll be surprised at how much you're actually doing, and you'll be having fun, too.

1. **No matter how little activity you do, it's better than no activity at all.** For example, a brisk twenty-minute walk three times a week is a good form of exercise, but if you're very sedentary, this may be too ambitious. Even a ten-minute walk is far better than no walk at all.
2. **Safety first!** As a woman, it's especially important that you keep safety in mind. If you're going to walk, bicycle, jog, or do other outdoor activities, make sure you pick a park or other place which is safe. Go with a friend and steer clear of high-crime areas. If you're choosing a health club, particularly if you're going to use it at night, make certain the parking lot is

well lit and that the club is in an area where you feel safe. If you ride a bike, wear an approved helmet.

3. **Underdo, don't overdo.** By far the biggest mistake people make when they begin exercising is to overdo it. You sign up for a bunch of exercise classes, or you decide to swim five days a week, or walk everywhere instead of taking the car. What happens? You exhaust yourself, become waterlogged, or get drenched in the rain. Before you know it, you're back on the couch again. If you're busy, instead of trying to squeeze in an exercise class three times a week, find one that meets twice a week. You'll be more apt to stick with it, and that's what counts in the long run.

4. **Choose the activities you enjoy.** You're an individual; why should you tailor yourself to someone else's idea of exercise? There are many ways you can build activity into your day— don't waste your time doing things you hate.

5. **Build in variety.** Pursue different activities; drop the ones you don't like, keep the ones you do, and always be ready to try new ones. Besides staving off boredom, different types of activities use different parts of your body. Professional athletes call this cross-training. For example, a runner training for a marathon may run five days and take a leisurely bike ride on the sixth day.

6. **Always have a backup plan.** You should be able to switch to another activity if the need arises—if your exercise class takes a break, your walking companion gets sick, or you mildly twist your ankle. In each of these cases, if you've planned ahead, you can switch to swimming, or some other activity, without skipping a beat.

7. **Lower your standards.** Often people new to athletic activities compare themselves to the pros and become discouraged. We could compare ourselves only to ourselves, but we usually have unrealistic expectations of ourselves as well. So relax your standards! If your prowess at tennis consists mainly of running around the court chasing balls, but you enjoy it, that's fine. On the other hand, if feeling perennially klutzy is making you uncomfortable, consider finding an activity to which you're better suited, or take a few lessons. But remember, you don't have to be perfect!

8. **Increase your activity level gradually.** If you're doing a mile on a treadmill, don't add another mile; start with a quarter

of a mile for, say, a week, then continue for a few weeks at one and a quarter miles, then add another quarter of a mile, and so on. The same holds for other activities.

9. **If you stop exercising, when you resume, cut back significantly on your activities.** It is sad but true that it doesn't take long at all for your body to begin getting out of condition again. If you have to stop for a while because you're ill, or even after a vacation, you'll have to start slowly again.

10. **Give yourself permission to quit (occasionally).** Far too often, we decide we're going to exercise for a certain period. Then we go on vacation, get sick, or just get bored, and miss a time or two. "That's it," we say to ourselves. "It's no use! Back to the couch!" You can't stay on the couch forever. At some point, pick yourself up and go back to the health club or try another type of activity. The most difficult part of getting back into an exercise routine is returning for the first time. But almost everyone has been through a similar experience, and before you know it, you'll be happily exercising again.

Glossary

ACE inhibitor—A type of drug that blocks a specific enzyme (angiotensin converting enzyme); used to treat high blood pressure and heart failure.

Aerobic activity—Exercise in which the body is able continuously to meet the muscles' increased demand for oxygen. Aerobic exercise conditions the cardiovascular system.

Anaerobic activity—Strenuous activity in which oxygen is used faster than the blood circulation can supply it.

Aneurysm—A ballooning out of the wall of a blood vessel or the heart muscle due to a weakening caused by disease, injury, or an abnormality present at birth.

Angina pectoris—Discomfort or pressure, usually in the chest, caused by a temporarily inadequate blood supply to the heart muscle due to coronary heart disease. Discomfort may also be felt in the neck, jaw, or arms.

Aorta—The large artery which leaves the heart's left ventricle and branches into other arteries to carry oxygen-rich blood to the body.

Aortic stenosis—A malformation of the aortic valve or a stiffening which comes with age and prevents the valve from opening normally.

Aortic valve—The heart valve between the left ventricle and the aorta.

Arrhythmia—An irregular heartbeat.

Arteriography—A testing procedure in which dye is injected into the bloodstream and then X-ray pictures are taken and studied to see the condition of the arteries.

Artery—A blood vessel which carries blood away from the heart to various parts of the body.

Artificial heart—A mechanical version of the heart used as a temporary measure to keep a patient alive until a heart transplant can be performed.

Atherectomy—A procedure designed to dilate (widen) a blood vessel; atherectomy is similar to angioplasty but uses an instrument other than a balloon.

Atherosclerosis—A buildup of fatty material in the artery wall which causes it to become thick and irregular. This buildup is sometimes called plaque. The condition it causes is known as coronary heart disease or coronary artery disease.

Atrial fibrillation—An arrhythmia caused by impulses coming from the atria that are disorganized, irregular, and rapid.

Atrial septal defect (ASD)—A congenital defect, a so-called "hole" dividing the upper chambers of the heart.

Atrium—An upper chamber of the heart; the plural is "atria."

Bacterial endocarditis—see Endocarditis.

Balloon angioplasty—A procedure used to dilate (widen) narrowed arteries. Known also simply as angioplasty, this procedure calls for a catheter with a deflated balloon on its tip to be passed into the segment of artery which is narrowed; the balloon is then inflated and the artery dilated. Also known as percutaneous transluminal coronary angioplasty (PTCA).

Balloon valvuloplasty—A procedure in which a balloon is inserted into the opening of a narrowed heart valve. The inflating of the balloon dilates (widens) the valve.

Beta blocker—A type of drug that reduces stimulation of the heart; related to the production of adrenaline, slows heart rate, lowers blood pressure, and reduces angina.

Biological valve—An artificial valve made from animal (usually pig) tissue, used to replace a malfunctioning heart valve.

Blood clot—Blood tissue that has turned from liquid to solid by clotting factors in the blood. Blood clots can form inside an artery whose lining is damaged by atherosclerosis, causing a heart attack or stroke.

Blood pressure—The force or pressure exerted in the arteries by blood as it is pumped around the body by the heart.

Bradycardia—A heart rate of less than sixty beats per minute. "Brady" means slow and "cardia" means heart.

Calcium channel blocker—A type of drug which blocks spasm of the blood vessels, lowers blood pressure, and reduces angina.

Capillaries—Tiny blood vessels which allow oxygen-carrying red cells to pass through and nourish the tissue cells.

Cardiac—Pertaining to the heart.

Cardiac arrest—The stopping of the heartbeat, usually because of interference with the heart's electrical system.

Cardiac catheterization—A procedure in which a tube is inserted into an artery in the arm or leg and guided to the heart; contrast dye is injected and X-ray movies are taken of the coronary arteries, heart chambers, and valves.

Cardiac rehabilitation—A program of exercise, education, and psychological and social support designed to return people to normal health or better after a heart attack or other cardiac crisis.

Cardiac spasm—A potentially dangerous constriction of the heart's blood vessels.

Cardiology—The study of the heart and its functions.

Cardiomyopathy—A serious disease involving deterioration of the heart muscle which results in decreased cardiac function.

Cardiovascular—Pertaining to the heart and blood vessels, "cardio," meaning of the heart, and "vascular," meaning of the blood vessels. The cardiovascular system is the circulatory system of the heart and blood vessels.

Cardiovascular drugs—Medications which control blood pressure, stabilize the heartbeat, and ease the symptoms of heart disease.

Cerebral embolism—A blood clot formed in one part of the body and then carried by the bloodstream to an artery of the brain, where it may cause a stroke.

Cerebral hemorrhage—Bleeding within the brain resulting from a ruptured aneurysm or a head injury.

Cerebral thrombosis—Formation of a blood clot in an artery that supplies blood to part of the brain.

Cholesterol—A pearly, fatlike substance which is an essential component of the body's cells. Also found in some foods.

Circulatory system—Refers to the heart, blood vessels, and the circulation of the blood.

Coarctation of the aorta—A congenital defect in which the aorta is pinched or constricted.

Congenital heart defect—A malformation of the heart or of its major blood vessels at birth. Also known as congenital heart disease.

Congestive heart failure—The condition created when the heart is not able to circulate adequate amounts of blood; the accumulation of fluids in the lungs, hands, ankles, or other parts of the body that results from inadequate circulation.

Coronary arteries—The heart's major arteries, arising from the aorta. They arch down over the top of the heart, branch, and provide blood to the working heart muscle.

Coronary bypass surgery—A procedure in which a graft (a "conduit") is sewn around an area of blockage in the coronary artery. Blood flow is then rerouted to allow blood to flow to the heart. Referred to also as coronary artery bypass grafting.

Coronary care unit—A hospital area designed specifically for the treatment of heart patients.

Coronary thrombosis—Formation of a clot in one of the arteries that carries blood to the heart muscle.

Costochondritis—Inflammation of the rib joints which may cause chest pain that can be misinterpreted as a symptom of heart disease.

Cyanosis—Blueness of the skin caused by insufficient oxygen in the blood.

Diabetes—A disease in which the body doesn't produce or properly use insulin, the substance which converts sugar and starch into energy. There are three forms: Type 1, which is inherited and occurs before age forty; Type 2, which occurs in adults after that age; and gestational diabetes, which occurs during pregnancy and disappears afterward.

Diastolic blood pressure—Pressure in the arteries when the heart is relaxed between heartbeats. In a blood pressure reading, this is reported as the lower of the two numbers.

Diuretic—A type of drug that enables the kidneys to rid the body of excess salt and water. May be referred to as a water pill.

Dyspnea—A medical term for shortness of breath.

Ebstein's anomaly—A congenital defect in which the tricuspid valve of the heart is malformed.

Echocardiography—A diagnostic method used to detect structural and some functional abnormalities of the heart; uses ultrasound, in which pulses of high-frequency sounds are transmitted into the body and the echoes returning to the surfaces of the heart and other structures are electronically recorded. See also Transesophageal echocardiogram.

Edema—Bodily swelling caused by an excess accumulation of fluid.

Eisenmenger syndrome—An irreversible condition in which the small blood vessels of the lungs are damaged by prolonged high blood pressure within the heart and the lungs, related to an abnormal flow of blood between the ventricles of the heart.

Electrocardiogram (EKG or ECG)—A diagnostic test which consists of a picture on graph paper of the electrical impulses traveling through the heart muscle. The picture is drawn by a computer from information supplied by electrodes attached to the chest.

Electrophysiological study (EP study or EPS)—A diagnostic test in which wires are threaded into the heart and stimulated in hopes of simulating an irregular heartbeat.

Endocarditis—A serious infection, usually bacterial, of the heart lining or valves. People with abnormal or replaced heart valves or congenital heart defects are among those at risk for developing this disease.

Esophageal dysfunction—A malfunction of the esophagus which can manifest symptoms that can be misinterpreted by the body as chest pain caused by heart disease. Also known as esophageal spasms or reflux esophagitis.

Esophagus—The muscular tube which carries food from the back of the mouth to the stomach.

Estrogen—A group of hormones essential for normal female sexual development and the healthy functioning of the reproductive system.

Estrogen replacement therapy (ERT)—Estrogen given to women to counteract the decline of their natural estrogen caused by menopause or surgical removal of the ovaries.

Exercise echocardiogram—A diagnostic test which combines an exercise stress test with an echocardiogram.

Exercise stress test—A diagnostic test in which an activity such as walking on a treadmill or riding a stationary bicycle is used to evaluate the effect of physical exertion on the heart.

Fainting—A temporary loss of consciousness caused by insufficient oxygen reaching the brain.

Fibrillation—Rapid, uncoordinated contraction of individual heart muscle fibers which results in the heart's being unable to efficiently pump blood.

Finger-prick test—A simple blood test which involves only a finger prick and which is used to measure total cholesterol level.

Genes—Units of inherited material contained in our body's cells.

Genetics—The study of how traits are passed down from one generation to another through genes.

Heart—The four-chambered, muscular organ which is responsible for pumping blood through the body.

Heart attack—Permanent damage to the heart muscle caused by a lack of blood supply to the heart for an extended period. Known also as a myocardial infarction or MI.

Heart block—A disorder of the heartbeat caused by an interruption in the passage of impulses through the heart's electrical network; the heart beats irregularly and usually more slowly.

Heart-lung machine—A machine that temporarily takes over the function of the heart and lungs and makes possible certain types of operations, including open-heart surgery.

Heart murmur—A clinical finding which refers to an abnormal sound made by the heart. Heart murmurs which do not signify a heart problem are known as innocent murmurs.

Heart transplant—Replacement of a damaged or diseased heart with a healthy heart taken from a donor.

High blood pressure—An unstable or persistent elevation of blood pressure above the normal range.

High-density lipoprotein (HDL)—A substance believed to reverse the accumulation of low-density lipoproteins (LDL) by transferring it away from the artery; the so-called "good" cholesterol.

Holter monitor—A small, portable recorder, connected by electrodes to the chest, that records the heartbeat over an extended period of time.

Hormone replacement therapy (HRT)—The use of synthetic or natural hormones to treat a hormone deficiency. In the context of this book, the combined use of estrogen and progestin, the synthetic form of progesterone, to counteract the symptoms and effects of menopause.

Hormones—A group of chemicals, each released into the bloodstream by a particular gland or tissue and specifically affecting tissues elsewhere in the body.

Hyperlipidemia—An inherited metabolic condition which results in an abnormal cholesterol pattern that is a risk factor for coronary artery disease.

Hypertension—The medical term for high blood pressure. There are two types. Essential hypertension, the most common, occurs for no apparent reason. Secondary hypertension is caused by an underlying disorder, such as with the kidneys, the adrenal glands, or a congenital disorder.

Hypertensive cardiovascular disease—A type of heart disease caused by untreated high blood pressure.

Hysterectomy—The surgical removal of the uterus. Sometimes the ovaries are removed as well.

Implantable cardioverter defibrillator (ICD)—A device implanted under the skin which can deliver an electric shock to reset the heart.

Ischemia—A condition in which not enough oxygen-rich blood is supplied to the heart muscle. Silent ischemia has no symptoms.

Kawasaki disease—An acute illness of children characterized by fever, rash, swelling, and inflammation of various parts of the body. In 20 percent of cases, the coronary arteries or other parts of the heart are affected.

Keloid—The outgrowth of a scar. Another type of scarring abnormality is known as a hypertrophic scar.

Lipid—A fatty substance insoluble in blood.

Lipid profile—A blood test which measures the different amounts of lipids in the blood.

Lipoprotein—The combination of lipid surrounded by a protein; the protein makes it soluble in blood.

Low-density lipoprotein (LDL)—The main carrier of harmful cholesterol in the blood; the so-called "bad" cholesterol.

Magnetic resonance imaging (MRI)—A diagnostic test which uses superconductive magnets and radio waves to obtain high-quality, detailed images of the body's internal organs.

Mammary artery—Also called the internal thoracic artery; located in the chest wall, it can be used as a bypass graft for coronary artery bypass surgery.

Marfan's syndrome—A rare inherited congenital disorder of the connective tissues, affecting especially the cardiovascular system, eyes, and musculoskeletal system.

Mechanical valve—An artificial valve made from materials such as titanium and ceramic, used to replace a malfunctioning heart valve.

Menopause—The term commonly used to describe the stage in a woman's life at which physiological and psychological changes occur as a result of reduced production of estrogen hormones by the ovaries.

Microvascular angina—A type of chest pain not caused by coronary artery disease or spasm. Known also as Syndrome X.

Mitral regurgitation—see Regurgitation.

Mitral stenosis—Stiffening and thickening caused by calcification of the heart's mitral valve.

Mitral valve—The heart valve between the left atrium and the left ventricle.

Mitral valve prolapse—An anomaly in which the leaflets of the mitral valve move out of normal position during the heart cycles. Most of the time this is not serious, but it can rarely cause serious mitral valve leakage.

Multiple-gated acquisition test (MUGA)—A diagnostic test which evaluates the strength of the heart.

Myocardial infarction—See Heart attack.

Nitroglycerin—A drug which causes dilation (opening) of blood vessels and is often used to treat angina pectoris, the chest pain from coronary heart disease. Known also as nitrates.

Obesity—A body weight 20 percent or more above the accepted standard for a person's age, sex, and body type.

Open-heart surgery—Surgery performed on the heart while the blood is diverted through a heart-lung machine.

Osteoarthritis—A degenerative type of arthritis which occurs in various joints of the body. When it occurs in the neck, the body may misinterpret the pain signals as coming from heart disease.

Osteoporosis—A disease of aging which primarily afflicts women and results in a loss of bone density that causes brittleness, fractures, and posture distortion.

Ovary—An almond-shaped gland situated on either side of the uterus which produces the so-called "sex" hormones, estrogen and progesterone.

Pacemaker—The heart's "natural pacemaker" is the sinus node, a small cluster of specialized cells in the top of the heart's right atrium that produces the electrical signals that cause the heart to contract or beat. An artificial pacemaker is an electrical device that can be substituted for a defective natural pacemaker. The artificial pacemaker controls the beating of the heart by emitting a series of rhythmic electrical discharges.

Palpitation—A heart rhythm disturbance, also described as a "pounding" or "flopping" heartbeat.

Patent ductus arteriosus—A congenital defect in which the passageway between the heart's two major blood vessels fails to close shortly after birth.

Pericarditis—Inflammation of the membranous sac which surrounds the heart.

Pericardium—The translucent outer sac that surrounds both the heart and the roots of the major blood vessels emerging from it.

Peripartum cardiomyopathy—A type of heart failure that may occur late in pregnancy or shortly after delivery.

Peripheral vascular disease—Narrowing of the blood vessels carrying blood to the legs and brain; a condition often found in people with heart disease.

Plaque—Hard, fatty matter embedded in the artery wall that develops with atherosclerosis.

Positron emission tomography (PET)—A diagnostic test which uses a radioactive isotope to create three-dimensional images of the heart.

Postural hypotension—A type of fainting caused by sudden changes in body position.

Pregnancy-induced hypertension—A general term referring to high blood pressure disorders occurring during pregnancy.

Premature atrial contraction (PAC)—An irregular heartbeat in which the upper chambers of the heart (atria) beat before they are expected to.

Premature ventricular complex (PVC)—An irregular heartbeat in which the lower chambers of the heart (the ventricles) beat before they are supposed to.

Pulmonary artery—The large artery that receives blood pumped from the right ventricle and channels it to the lungs.

Pulmonary hypertension—A type of high blood pressure which develops within the blood vessels of the lungs.

Pulmonary stenosis—A malformation of the pulmonary valve

which prevents it from opening normally. Also called valvular pulmonary stenosis.

Pulmonary valve—The heart valve between the right ventricle and the pulmonary artery.

Radio wave ablation—The use of low-frequency radio waves to destroy heart tissue transmitting an abnormal heartbeat.

Regurgitation—The abnormal backward flowing of blood through a valve in the heart. When this occurs in the mitral valve, it is known as mitral regurgitation.

Restenosis—The recurrent narrowing of a blood vessel after angioplasty or a similar procedure.

Rheumatic heart disease—Damage done to the heart, particularly the heart valves, by rheumatic fever.

Risk factor—A behavior or trait that has been proved to contribute independently to the development and progression of a disease.

Sedentary lifestyle—A way of life characterized by lack of exercise.

Septum—The muscular wall which divides the heart into the right and left sides.

Shingles—Known also as herpes zoster, an infection of the nerves which causes symptoms that the body may misinterpret as chest pain from heart disease.

Silent heart attack—A heart attack which is not recognized because of the body's misinterpretation of pain signals.

Stenosis—The narrowing or constriction of an opening, such as can occur with a heart valve.

Sternum—The breastbone.

Stress—Any interference that disturbs a person's mental and physical well-being.

Stroke—A sudden and often severe attack caused by a loss of blood to part of the brain. Known also as a cerebral vascular accident.

Sudden death—Death that occurs unexpectedly and instantaneously, usually for a cardiac cause. If a person is successfully revived after a heart stoppage, this is known as having undergone an episode of sudden death.

Syncope—The medical term for fainting.

Syndrome X—see Microvascular angina.

Systolic blood pressure—The pressure in the arteries during the heart's contraction. In a blood pressure reading, this is reported as the higher of the two numbers.

Tachycardia—A fast heartbeat; technically, a rate above 100 beats per minute.

Telemetry—A term referring to electronic monitoring devices for the heart.

Tetralogy of Fallot—A quartet of separate heart defects occurring together.

Thallium stress testing—A diagnostic test which combines an exercise stress test with a special nuclear study to create images of the heart.

Thrombolytic therapy—The administration of drugs called clot busters, used to minimize damage to the heart from a heart attack.

Tilt study—A diagnostic test in which the body is tilted at certain angles; useful in diagnosing causes of fainting. Also called a tilt table test.

Transesophageal echocardiogram—A type of echocardiogram used to obtain images of harder-to-visualize structures of the heart; the sound probe is swallowed and positioned behind the heart.

Transient ischemic attack (TIA)—A temporary strokelike event caused by a blocked blood vessel.

Tricuspid valve—The heart valve between the right atrium and the right ventricle.

Triglycerides—Fatty compounds found in combination with chylomicrons and very-low-density lipoproteins (VLDL); large amounts of triglycerides are implicated in the development of atherosclerosis.

Valve—A structure which controls blood flow between two chambers of the heart or between a chamber of the heart and a blood vessel.

Valvular pulmonary stenosis—see Pulmonary stenosis.

Vasospastic angina—Discomfort or pressure, usually in the chest, resulting from a blockage of blood flow to the heart caused by a spasm of the coronary artery.

Vasovagal syncope—A type of fainting caused by overstimulation of the vagus nerve, the major nerve running from the brain to the upper gastrointestinal tract.

Veins—Blood vessels which return blood back to the heart.

Vena cava—Either of two large veins which deliver oxygen-depleted blood back to the heart.

Ventricle—One of the two main chambers of the heart.

Ventricular septal defect (VSD)—A congenital defect in which there is a so-called "hole" between the heart's lower chambers.

White coat hypertension—A form of high blood pressure caused by anxiety, such as a visit to the doctor.

Wolff-Parkinson-White syndrome—A cardiac syndrome caused by abnormal conduction of electrical signals to the heart, resulting in episodes of rapid heartbeats, from 120 to 200 per minute.

Selected Bibliography

BOOKS AND PAMPHLETS

American College of Cardiology/American Heart Association Task Force, "ACC/AHA Guidelines and Indications for Coronary Artery Bypass Surgery," 1990.

American College of Cardiology/American Heart Association Task Force, "Guidelines for Percutaneous Transluminal Coronary Angioplasty," 1988.

American College of Sports Medicine, "Guidelines for Exercise Testing and Prescription," 4th Ed. Philadelphia: Lea & Febiger, 1991.

American Heart Association, *1993 Heart and Stroke Facts*. Dallas, 1992.

CANOBBIO, MARY M., R.N., M.N., *Cardiovascular Disorders.* St. Louis, Missouri: C. V. Mosby Company, 1990.

CLAYMAN, CHARLES B., M.D., *American Medical Association's Encyclopedia of Medicine.* New York: Random House, 1989.

DAVIS, GOODE P. JR., EDWARDS PARK, AND THE EDITORS OF U.S. NEWS BOOKS, *The Heart: The Living Pump.* Washington, D.C.: U.S. News Books, 1981.

DOUGLAS, PAMELA S., M.D., *Heart Disease in Women, Cardiovascular Clinics.* Philadelphia: F. A. Davis Company, 1989.

EAKER, ELAINE D., S.CD., BARBARA PACKARD, M.D., PH.D., NANETTE KASS WENGER, M.D., THOMAS B. CLARKSON, D.V.M., AND H. A. TYROLER, M.D., *Coronary Heart Disease in Women.* New York: Haymarket Doyma Inc., 1987.

PASHKOW, FREDRIC, M.D., PEG PASHKOW, M.S., R.P.T., AND MARJORIE SCHAFER, B.S.N., M.N.A., WITH CHRISTINE FERGUSON, *Successful Cardiac Rehabilitation.* Loveland, CO: HeartWatchers Press, 1988.

U.S. Department of Agriculture, "Nutrition and Your Heart: Dietary Guidelines for Americans," 3rd Ed., 1990.

U.S. Department of Health and Human Services, *The Healthy Heart Handbook for Women.* Washington, D.C.: U.S. Government Printing Office, 1989.

JOURNAL ARTICLES

ANASTOS, KATHRYN, M.D., PAMELA CHARNEY, M.D., RITA A. CHARON, M.D., ELLEN COHEN, M.D., CLARA Y. JONES, M.D., ET AL., "Hypertension in Women: What Is Really Known?" *Annals of Internal Medicine,* Vol. 115, No. 4 (August 15, 1991), 287–93.

AYANIAN, JOHN Z., M.D., M.P.P., AND ARNOLD M. EPSTEIN, M.D., M.A., "Differences in the Use of Procedures Between Women and Men Hospitalized for Coronary Heart Disease," *New England Journal of Medicine,* Vol. 325, No. 4 (July 25, 1991), 221–30.

BARRETT-O'CONNOR, ELIZABETH L., M.D., AND TRUDY L. BUSH, PH.D., M.H.S., "Estrogen and Coronary Heart Disease in Women," *Journal of the American Medical Association*, Vol. 265, No. 14 (April 10, 1991), 1861–8.

BARRETT-O'CONNOR, ELIZABETH L., M.D., BARBARA A. COHN, PH.D., DEBORAH L. WINGARD, PH.D., AND SHARON L. EDELSTEIN, M.SC., "Why Is Diabetes Mellitus a Stronger Risk Factor for Fatal Ischemic Heart Disease in Women Than in Men?" *Journal of the American Medical Association*, Vol. 265, No. 5 (February 6, 1991), 627–31.

BLYSKAL, JEFF. "Staking a Claim." *American Health* (March 1992), 48–50.

BOOTH, DAVID C., M.D., ROBERT H. DEUPREE, PH.D., HERBERT N. HULTGREN, M.D., ANTHONY N. DEMARIA, M.D., STEWART M. SCOTT, M.D., ET AL., AND THE INVESTIGATORS OF VETERANS AFFAIRS COOPERATIVE STUDY NO. 28, "Quality of Life After Bypass Surgery for Unstable Angina, *Circulation*, Vol. 83, No. 1 (January 1991), 87–95.

BROWN, GREG B., M.D., PH.D., "Coronary Vasospasm: Observations Linking the Clinical Spectrum of Ischemic Heart Disease to the Dynamic Pathology of Coronary Atherosclerosis," *Archives of Internal Medicine*, Vol. 141 (May 1981), 716–22.

CANNON, RICHARD O. III, M.D., "Microvascular Angina: Pathophysiology, Diagnostic Techniques and Interventions," *Heart Disease Update*. Philadelphia: W. B. Saunders Company, 1991.

CARALIS, DENNIS G., M.D., M.P.H., UBEYDULLAH DELIGONUL, M.D., MORTON J. KERN, M.D., AND JEROME D. COHEN, M.D., "Smoking Is a Risk Factor for Coronary Spasm in Young Women," *Circulation*, Vol. 85, No. 3 (March 1992), 905–9.

COLDITZ, GRAHAM A., M.D., ERIC B. RIMM, B.S., EDWARD GIOVANNUCCI, M.D., MEIR J. STAMPFER, M.D., BERNARD ROSNER, PH.D., ET AL., "A Prospective Study of Parental History of Myocardial Infarction and Coronary Artery Disease in Men," *American Journal of Cardiology*, Vol. 67 (May 1, 1991), 933–8.

DUNCAN, JOHN J., PH.D., NEIL F. GORDON, M.B.B. CH, PH.D., AND CHRIS B. SCOTT, M.S., "Women Walking for Health and Fitness: How Much Is

Enough?" *Journal of the American Medical Association,* Vol. 266, No. 23 (December 18, 1991), 3295–9.

DUPONT, WILLIAM D., PH.D., AND DAVID L. PAGE, M.D., "Menopausal Estrogen Replacement Therapy and Breast Cancer," *Archives of Internal Medicine,* Vol. 151 (January 1991), 67–72.

FELDMAN, TED, M.D., AND KENNETH M. BOROW, M.D., "Atrial Septal Defects in Adults: Diagnosis and Management," *Cardiovascular Medicine* (March 1986), 19–24.

FLETCHER, GERALD F., M.D., STEVEN N. BLAIR, P.E.D., JAMES BLUMEN-THAL, PH.D., CARL CAPERSEN, PH.D., BERNARD CHAITMAN, M.D., ET AL., "Statement on Exercise: Benefits and Recommendations for Physical Activity for All Americans, *Circulation,* Vol. 86, No. 1 (July 1992), 340–43.

FRANK, ERICA, M.D., M.P.H., MARILYN A. WINKLEBY, PH.D., DAVID G. ALTMAN, PH.D., BEVERLY ROCKHILL, M.A., AND STEPHEN P. FORTMANN, M.D., "Predictors of Physicians' Smoking Cessation Advice," *Journal of the American Medical Association,* Vol. 266, No. 22 (December 11, 1991), 3139–44.

GLASSER, STEPHEN P., M.D., AND PAMELA CLARK, R.N., B.S.N., "Interpretation of Exercise Test Results in Women," *Practical Cardiology,* Vol. 14, No. 8 (July 1988), 85–90.

GREENLAND, PHILIP, M.D., HENRIETTA REICHER-REISS, M.D., URI GOLDBOURT, PH.D., SOLOMON BEHAR, M.D., AND THE ISRAELI SPRINT IN-VESTIGATORS, "In-Hospital and 1-Year Mortality in 1,524 Women After Myocardial Infarction," *Circulation,* Vol. 83, No. 2 (February 1991), 484–91.

HALL, ELLEN M., "Gender, Work Control, and Stress: A Theoretical Discussion and an Empirical Test," *International Journal of Health Services,* Vol. 19, No. 4 (1989), 725–45.

HELMER, DIANNE C., DAVID R. RAGLAND, AND S. LEONARD SYME, "Hostility and Coronary Artery Disease," *American Journal of Epidemiology,* Vol. 133, No. 2 (January 1, 1991), 112–22.

HELMRICH, SUSAN P., PH.D., DAVID R. RAGLAND, PH.D., M.P.H., RITA W. LEUNG, A.B., AND RALPH S. PAFFENBARGER, JR., M.D., D.P.H., "Physical Activity and Reduced Occurrence of Non-Insulin Dependent Diabetes Mellitus," *New England Journal of Medicine*, Vol. 325, No. 3 (July 18, 1991), 147–52.

HUBERT, HELEN B., M.P.H., PH.D., MANNING FEINLEIB, M.D., D.P.H., PATRICIA M. MCNAMARA, D.P.H., AND WILLIAM P. CASTELLI, M.D., "Obesity as an Independent Risk Factor for Cardiovascular Disease: A 26-Year Follow-up of Participants in the Framingham Heart Study," *Circulation*, Vol. 67, No. 5 (May 1983), 968–76.

HUNG, JOSEPH, M.B., BERNARD R. CHAITMAN, M.D., JULES LAM, M.D., JACQUES LESPERANCE, M.D., GEORGE DUPRAS, M.D., ET AL., "Noninvasive Diagnostic Test Choices for the Evaluation of Coronary Artery Disease in Women: A Multivariate Comparison of Cardiac Fluroscopy, Exercise Electrocardiography and Exercise Thallium Myocardial Perfusion Scintigraphy, *Journal of the American College of Cardiology*, Vol. 4, No. 1 (July 1984), 8–16.

HUNT, STEVEN C., PH.D., KURT BLICKENSTAFF, M.D., PAUL N. HOPKINS, M.D., M.S.P.H., AND ROGER R. WILLIAMS, M.D., "Coronary Disease and Risk Factors in Close Relatives of Utah Women with Early Coronary Death," *Western Journal of Medicine*, September 1986, 329–34.

JECKER, NANCY S., PH.D., "Age-Based Rationing and Women," *Journal of the American Medical Assiciation*, Vol. 266, No. 21 (December 4, 1991), 3012–15.

JERESATY, ROBERT M., M.D., "Drug Therapy of Mitral Valve Prolapse," *Drug Therapy*, March 1991, 57.

KHAN, STEVEN S., M.D., SHARON NESSIM, D.P.H., RICHARD GRAY, M.D., LAWRENCE S. CZER, M.D., AURELIO CHAUX, M.D., ET AL., "Increased Mortality of Women in Coronary Artery Bypass Surgery: Evidence for Referral Bias," *Annals of Internal Medicine*, Vol. 112, No. 8 (April 15, 1990), 561–7.

KENYON, LORI W., PH.D., MARK W. KETTERER, PH.D., MIHAI GHEORGHIADE, M.D., AND SIDNEY GOLDSTEIN, M.D., "Psychological Factors Related to

Prehospital Delay During Acute Myocardial Infarction," *Circulation,* Vol 84, No. 5 (November 1991), 1969–76.

KRUMHOLTZ, HARLAN M., M.D., PAMELA S. DOUGLAS, M.D., MICHAEL S. LAUER, M.D., AND RICHARD C. PASTERNAK, M.D., "Selection of Patients for Coronary Angiography and Coronary Revascularization: Is There Evidence for a Gender Bias?," *Annals of Internal Medicine,* Vol. 116, No. 10 (May 15, 1992), 785–90.

KUMANYIKA, SHIRIKI, PH.D., "Obesity in Black Women," *Epidemiologic Reviews,* Vol. 9 (1987), 31–50.

LANGER, ROBERT D., M.D., M.P.H., AND ELIZABETH BARRETT-O'CONNOR, M.D., "Coronary Heart Disease Prevention in Women," *Practical Cardiology,* Vol. 17, No. 3 (March 1991), 45–62.

LONG, PATRICIA, "The Great Weight Debate," *Health,* February/ March 1992, 42–7.

LOOP, FLOYD D., M.D., F.A.C.C., LEONARD R. GOLDING, M.D., F.A.C.C., JULIE P. MACMILLAN, M.P.H., DELOS M. COSGROVE, M.D., F.A.C.C., BRUCE W. LYTLE, M.D., F.A.C.C., ET AL., "Coronary Artery Surgery in Women Compared with Men: Analysis of Risks and Long-Term Results," *Journal of the American College of Cardiology,* Vol. 1, No. 2 (February 1983), 383–90.

MANSON, JOANNE E., M.D., GRAHAM A. COLDITZ, M.B., B.S., MEIR J. STAMPFER, M.D., WALTER C. WILLETT, M.D., BERNARD ROSNER, PH.D., ET AL., "A Prospective Study of Obesity and Risk of Coronary Heart Disease in Women," *New England Journal of Medicine,* Vol. 322, No. 13 (March 29, 1990), 882–9.

MANSON, JOANNE E., M.D., MEIR J. STAMPFER, M.D., GRAHAM A. COLDITZ, M.B., B.S., WALTER C. WILLETT, M.D., BERNARD ROSNER, PH.D., ET AL., "A Prospective Study of Aspirin Use and Primary Prevention of Cardiovascular Disease in Women," *Journal of the American Medical Association,* Vol. 266, No. 4 (July 1991), 521–7.

MARKELL, MARY, "Women's Puzzling Outcomes after MI and CABG," *Cardiology World News,* April 1991, 23.

MAYNARD, CHARLES, PH.D., LLOYD D. FISHER, PH.D., EUGENE R. PASSAMANI, M.D., AND THOMAS PULLUM, PH.D., "Blacks in the Coronary Artery Surgery Study: Risk Factors and Coronary Artery Disease," *Circulation,* Vol. 74, No. 1 (July 1986), 64–71.

MAYNARD, CHARLES, PH.D., PAUL E. LITWIN, M.S., JENNY S. MARTIN, R.N., AND DOUGLAS W. WEAVER, M.D., "Gender Differences in the Treatment and Outcome of Acute Myocardial Infarction," *Archives of Internal Medicine,* Vol. 152 (May 1992), 972–6.

MCENIERY, PAUL T., M.D., JAY HOLLMAN, M.D., VALERIE KNEZINEK, KHOSROW DOROSTI, M.D., IRVING FRANCO, M.D., ET AL., "Comparative Safety and Efficacy of Percutaneous Transluminal Coronary Angioplasty in Men and Women," *Catheterization and Cardiovascular Diagnosis,* 1987, 364–71.

MEIER, BARRY, "Maker of Heart Valve Balks Over Some Warnings," *New York Times,* April 26, 1992, 30.

MURPHY, JOSEPH G., M.B., M.R.C.P.I., BERNARD J. GERSH, M.B., CH.B., PH.D., MICHAEL MCGOON, M.D., DOUGLAS D. MAIR, M.C., CO-BURN J. PORTER, M.D., ET AL., "Long-Term Outcome After Surgical Repair of Isolated Atrial Septal Defect," *New England Journal of Medicine,* Vol. 323, No. 24 (December 13, 1990), 1645–50.

NATIONAL INSTITUTES OF HEALTH CONSENSUS DEVELOPMENT PANEL ON THE HEALTH IMPLICATIONS OF OBESITY, "Health Implications of Obesity," *Annals of Internal Medicine,* Vol. 103 (December 1985), 1073–7.

OWENS, JANE F., D.P.H., KAREN A. MATTHEWS, PH.D., RENA R. WING, PH.D., AND LEWIS H. KULLER, M.D., D.P.H., "Can Physical Activity Mitigate the Effects of Aging in Middle-Aged Women?" *Circulation,* Vol. 85, No. 4 (April 1992), 1265–70.

ROBERT, ANNIE R., M.S., JACQUES A. MELIN, M.D., AND JEAN-MARIE R. DETRY, M.D., "Logistic Discriminant Analysis Improves Diagnostic Accuracy of Exercise Testing for Coronary Artery Disease in Women," *Circulation,* Vol. 83, No. 4 (April 1991), 1202–9.

ROBINSON, MATTHEW, B.S., JAMES A. BLUMENTHAL, PH.D., EILEEN J. BURKER, M.S., MARK HLATKY, M.D., AND J. G. REEVES, M.D., "Coronary

Artery Bypass Grafting and Cognitive Function: A Review," *Journal of Cardiopulmonary Rehabilitation,* Vol. 10, No. 5 (May 20, 1990), 180–9.

RODIN, JUDITH, AND JEANNETTE R. ICKOVICS, "Women's Health: Review and Research Agenda as We Approach the 21st Century," *American Psychologist,* Vol. 45, No. 9 (September 1990), 1018–34.

SALONEN, JUKKA T., M.D., PH.D., M.P.H., KRISTIINA NYYSSÖNEN, M.P.H., HEIKKI KORPELA, M.D., PH.D., JAAKKO TUOMILEHTO, M.D., PH.D., RITVA SEPPÄNEN, D.SC., ET AL., "High Stored Iron Levels Are Associated with Excess Risk of Myocardial Infarction in Eastern Finnish Men," *Circulation,* Vol. 86, No. 3 (September 1992), 803–11.

SAWADA, STEPHEN G., M.D., THOMAS RYAN, M.D., NAOMI S. FINEBERG, PH.D., WILLIAM F. ARMSTRONG, M.D., F.A.C.C., WALTER E. JUDSON, M.S., ET AL., "Exercise Echocardiographic Detection of Coronary Artery Disease in Women," *Journal of the American College of Cardiology,* Vol. 14, No. 6 (November 15, 1989), 1440–7.

SHAMAN, DIANA, "It Might Have Been a Beautiful Baby," *American Lung Association Bulletin,* 1982.

SHANGOLD, MONA M., M.D., "Advising Older Women About Exercise," *Journal of Musculoskeletal Medicine,* October 1991, 45–50.

STAMPFER, MEIR J., M.D., GRAHAM A. COLDITZ, M.B., B.S., WALTER C. WILLETT, M.D., JOANNE E. MANSON, M.D., BERNARD ROSNER, PH.D., ET AL., "Postmenopausal Estrogen Therapy and Cardiovascular Disease: Ten-Year Follow-up From the Nurses' Health Study," *New England Journal of Medicine,* Vol. 325, No. 11 (September 12, 1991), 756–62.

STEINBERG, KAREN K., PH.D., M.SC., STEPHEN B. THACKER, M.D., M.SC., JAY S. SMITH, M.S., M.I.S., DONNA F. STROUP, PH.D., M.SC., MATTHEW M. ZACK, M.D., ET AL., "A Meta-analysis of the Effect of Estrogen Replacement Therapy on the Risk of Breast Cancer," *Journal of the American Medical Association,* Vol. 265, No. 15 (April 17, 1991), 1985–90.

"Syndrome X," *Harvard Heart Letter,* Harvard Medical School, Vol. 1, No. 9 (May 1991), 1–4.

TOBIN, JONATHAN N., M.A., M. PHIL., SYLVIA WASSERTHIEL-SMOLLER, PH.D., JOHN P. WEXLER, M.D., PH.D., RICHARD M. STEINGART, M.D., NANCY BUDNER, M.P.H., ET AL., "Sex Bias in Considering Coronary Bypass Surgery," *Annals of Internal Medicine,* Vol. 107, No. 1 (July 1987), 19–25.

Transdermal Nicotine Study Group, "Transdermal Nicotine for Smoking Cessation," *Journal of the American Medical Association,* Vol. 266, No. 22 (December 11, 1991), 3133–8.

"Uncertainty About Postmenopausal Estrogen" (Editorial), *New England Journal of Medicine,* Vol. 325, No. 11 (September 12, 1991), 800–2.

WARNER, KENNETH E., PH.D., "Cigarette Advertising and Media Coverage of Smoking and Health," *New England Journal of Medicine* (February 7, 1985), 384–8.

WILLETT, WALTER C., M.D., ADELE GREEN, M.D., MEIR J. STAMPFER, M.D., FRANK E. SPEIZER, M.D., GRAHAM A. COLDITZ, M.D., ET AL., "Relative and Absolute Excess Risks of Coronary Heart Disease Among Women Who Smoke Cigarettes," *New England Journal of Medicine,* Vol. 317, No. 21 (November 19, 1987), 1303–9.

WOODMAN, SUE, "Target," *Mirabella,* April 1990, 80–84.

Recommended Reading
and Resources

Here are some books, support groups, and other resources which you may find useful in learning more about your heart.

BOOKS

THE HEART

ZARET, BARRY L., M.D., MARVIN MOSER, M.D., AND LAWRENCE S. COHEN, M.D., *Yale University School of Medicine Heart Book.* New York: Hearst Books, 1992.

CORONARY ARTERY DISEASE

BUDNICK, HERBERT N., PH.D., WITH SCOTT ROBERT HAYS, *Heart to Heart: A Guide to the Psychological Aspects of Heart Disease.* Santa Fe: HealthPress, 1991.

COHAN, CAROL, M.A., JUNE B. PIMM, PH.D., AND JAMES R. JUDE, M.D., *A Patient's Guide to Heart Surgery: Understanding the Practical and Emotional Aspects of Heart Surgery.* New York: HarperCollins, 1991.

HELLERSTEIN, HERMAN, M.D., WITH PAUL PERRY, *Healing Your Heart.* New York: Simon & Schuster, 1991.

KOWALSKI, ROBERT E., *Eight Steps to a Healthy Heart: The Complete Guide to Heart Disease Prevention and Recovery from Heart Attack and Bypass Surgery.* New York: Warner Books, Inc., 1992.

LEVIN, RHODA F., *Heartmates: A Survival Guide for the Cardiac Spouse.* Englewood Cliffs, N.J.: Prentice Hall Press, 1987.

OCKENE, IRA S., M.D., AND JUDITH K. OCKENE, PH.D., *Prevention of Coronary Heart Disease.* Boston: Little, Brown & Co., 1992.

CARDIOVASCULAR DRUGS

Pocket Guide to Cardiac Drugs, A Heartline Publication. The Coronary Club, 1991. (For information, see the Coronary Club under "Newsletters.")

EATING AND EXERCISE

The federal government offers useful information on diet, nutrition, and exercise free or at very low cost. For a free catalog, write Consumer Information Catalog, Pueblo, CO 81109. The publications available include "Dietary Guidelines and Your Diet," "Nutritive Value of Foods," and "Good Sources of Nutrients."

KWITEROVICH, PETER, *Beyond Cholesterol.* Los Angeles: Knightsbridge Publishers, 1991.

LAWRENCE, RONALD M., AND SANDRA ROSENZWEIG, *Going the Distance: The Right Way to Exercise for People Over 40.* Los Angeles: Jeremy P. Tarcher, Inc., 1987.

ORBACH, SUSIE, *Fat Is a Feminist Issue.* New York: Berkley Books, 1982.

ORBACH, SUSIE, *Fat Is a Feminist Issue II: The Anti-Diet Guide to Permanent Weight Loss.* New York: Berkley Books, 1987.

PISCATELLA, JOSEPH, *Controlling Your Fat Tooth*. New York: Workman Publishing Co., 1991.

PISCATELLA, JOSEPH, AND BERNIE PISCATELLA, *Don't Eat Your Heart Out Cookbook*. Boston: G. K. Hall, 1989.

POPE-CORDLE, JAMIE, AND MARTIN KATAHN, *The T-Factor Fat Gram Counter*. New York: W. W. Norton Co., Inc., 1989.

HEALTH-CARE ISSUES

HOGUE, KATHLEEN, CHERYL JENSEN, AND KATHLEEN MCCLURG URBAN, *The Complete Guide to Health Insurance*. New York: Walker and Company, 1988.

INLANDER, CHARLES B., AND ED WEINER, *Take This Book to the Hospital with You: A Consumer Guide to Surviving Your Hospital Stay*. New York: Pantheon Books, 1991.

KLAIDMAN, STEPHEN, *Health in the Headlines: The Stories Behind the Stories*. New York: Oxford University Press, 1991.

STUTZ, DAVID R., M.D., BERNARD FEDER, PH.D., AND THE EDITORS OF CONSUMER REPORTS BOOKS, *The Savvy Patient: How to Be an Active Participant in Your Medical Care*. Mount Vernon, NY: Consumers Union, 1990.

SURGERY AND RECUPERATION (GENERAL)

RYAN, REGINA SARA, *The Fine Art of Recuperation: A Guide to Surviving and Thriving After Illness, Accident or Surgery*. Los Angeles: Jeremy P. Tarcher, Inc., 1989.

PREGNANCY (GENERAL)

RICH, LAURIE A., *When Pregnancy Isn't Perfect: A Layperson's Guide to Complications in Pregnancy*, New York: Dutton, 1991.

SUSSMAN, JOHN R., M.D., AND B. BLAKE LEVITT, *Before You Conceive: The Complete Prepregnancy Guide*. New York: Bantam Books, 1989.

WOMEN'S HEALTH CARE

PISCATELLA, JOSEPH C., *The Fat Tooth Fat Gram Counter* and *The Fat Tooth Restaurant & Fast Food Fat Gram Counter* (2-book set). New York: Workman Publishing Co., 1993.

SHEPHARD, BRUCE D., M.D., F.A.C.O.B., AND CARROLL A. SHEPHARD, R.N., PH.D., *The Complete Guide to Women's Health*, 2nd Ed. New York: Penguin, 1990.

WHITE, EVELYN C., *The Black Women's Health Book: Speaking for Ourselves*. Seattle: Seal Press, 1990.

WOLFE, SIDNEY M., M.D., AND THE PUBLIC CITIZEN HEALTH RESEARCH GROUP WITH RHONDA DONKIN JONES. *Women's Health Alert*. Reading, MA: Addison-Wesley Publishing Group, Inc., 1991.

ORGANIZATIONS (GENERAL)

National Women's Health Network
1325 G Street, N.W.
Washington, D.C. 20005

ORGANIZATIONS (HEART)

Many hospitals have support groups for heart patients which offer activities ranging from educational to social events. Bear in mind that you do not necessarily have to have been treated at that hospital to join. For information, contact your local hospital, or the American Heart Association (consult your telephone book for the local chapter or contact the national organization at 7320 Greenville Avenue, Dallas, TX 75231).
Or contact:
Mended Hearts
7320 Greenville Avenue
Dallas, TX 75231

NEWSLETTERS

Heartline is a monthly newsletter designed for heart patients and others interested in their cardiovascular health. Edited by Dr.

Fredric J. Pashkow, it is published with the active support of the Cleveland Clinic Educational Foundation. $29 per year. For more information, contact the Coronary Club, Inc., 9500 Euclid Ave., E4-15, Cleveland, OH 44195–5058.

Harvard Heart Letter is a monthly newsletter published by the Harvard Medical School Health Publication Group which discusses heart-related topics in depth. $30 per year. Harvard Heart Letter, P.O. Box 420234, Palm Court, FL 32142–0234.

Cardiac Alert is published monthly for the purpose of educating for the prevention of heart disease. It is edited by Dr. Jorge C. Rios, M.D., George Washington University Medical Center. $75 per year. Phillips Publishing, Inc., 7811 Montrose Road, Potomac, MD 20854.

Diet-Heart Newsletter, published quarterly by health-book author Robert Kowalski, offers nutritional information, recipes, and tips. $15 per year. Diet-Heart Newsletter, P.O. Box 2039, Venice, CA 90294.

Index